Psychosocial Interventions for People with Schizophrenia

A Practical Guide for Mental Health Workers

Also by Neil Harris:

Long Term Neuroleptic Treatment and the Role of the Community Mental Health Worker

Psychosocial Interventions for People with Schizophrenia

A Practical Guide for Mental Health Workers

edited by

Neil Harris, Steve Williams
and Tim Bradshaw

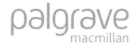

First published 2002 by
PALGRAVE MACMILLAN
Houndmills, Basingstoke, Hampshire RG21 6XS and
175 Fifth Avenue, New York, N.Y. 10010
Companies and representatives throughout the world

PALGRAVE MACMILLAN is the global academic imprint of the Palgrave Macmillan division of St. Martin's Press, LLC and of Palgrave Macmillan Ltd. Macmillan® is a registered trademark in the United States, United Kingdom and other countries. Palgrave is a registered trademark in the European Union and other countries.

ISBN 0–333–77739–5 paperback

This book is printed on paper suitable for recycling and made from fully managed and sustained forest sources.

A catalogue record for this book is available from the British Library.

10   9   8   7   6   5   4   3   2   1
11   10   09   08   07   06   05   04   03   02

Printed and bound in Great Britain by
Creative Print & Design (Ebbw Vale), Wales

Contents

List of Tables   vii

List of Figures   vii

List of Boxes   viii

Notes on Contributors   ix

Foreword   xi

Abbreviations   xiii

Part I
What is Schizophrenia?

1   The Nature of Schizophrenia
    Steve Williams   3

2   Hearing Voices Past and Present – A User's Perspective
    Hywel Davies   18

3   Politics and Policies of Schizophrenia
    Steve Williams   26

Part II
Clinical Skills

4   The Helping Relationship
    Julie Repper   39

5   Case Management
    Ian Wilson   53

6   Neuroleptic Drugs and Their Management
    Neil Harris   68

7   Psychological Treatment for Anxiety and Depression in
    Schizophrenia
    Ian Baguley and Claire Baguley   84

8   Assessment and Therapeutic Interventions With Positive
    Psychotic Symptoms
    Julie Everitt and Ronald Siddle   102

9   Indentifying and Overcoming Negative Symptoms
    Ronald Siddle and Julie Everitt   117

10 Relapse Prevention Intervention in Psychosis
    Alice Knight   130

11 Working With Families
    David Reader   143

Part III
Working and Living in the Community

12 Working and Schizophrenia
    Jenny Droughton and Steve Williams   161

13 Neighbourhood Networking – Working With the
    Community as a Source of Support: A Practical Guide
    Douglas Inchbold   175

Part IV
Special Considerations

14 Dual Diagnosis – Substance Misuse and Schizophrenia
    Mark Holland   189

15 Risk and Serious Mental Health Issues
    Ged McCann and Mick McKeown   205

16 Psychosocial Interventions in Institutional Settings
    Mick McKeown, Ged McCann and Joe Forster   211

Part V
Changing Service – Keeping Going

17 Involving Service Users
    Rachel Perkins   237

18 Training and Clinical Supervision
    Tim Bradshaw   251

Conclusion   267

Index   268

List of Tables

		Page
1.1	Kraepelin, Bleuler and Schneider	7
5.1	Meta-analysis of the outcomes of case management studies	62
12.1	Misconceptions about work and SMI	163
12.2	Models of work, employment or training provision for people with SMI	165
14.1	Helpful interventions at different stages of motivation: A practical crosswalk between the cycle of change and stagewire treatment	196
14.2	Identified needs and intervention with Christine and family	199
16.1	Factors influencing the uptake of PSI in in-patient environments	227
16.2	Practical consequences of organic ward training and development	232
18.1	Learning outcomes and related approaches to teaching and learning used on PSI courses	257

List of Figures

		Page
7.1	Generic cognitive-behavioural formulation for emotional disorder	86
7.2	Cross section of the maintenance cycle of depression	86
7.3	Typical 'thinking errors'	87
7.4	Cross section of the maintenance cycle of anxiety	88
7.5	Example of activity schedule recording sheet	91
7.6	Example of diary sheet	94
7.7	Example of diary for challenging negative automatic thoughts	95
7.8	Example of behavioural experiment diary	96
8.1	Process of therapy	103
8.2	Example of a client's homework for monitoring a symptom	107
8.3	Questions to elicit coping strategies	108
8.4	Range of coping strategies	108

List of Boxes

		Page
4.1	Summary of what service users say they want from services	44
4.2	How to develop effective working relationships with seriously mentally ill people	48
4.3	Adapting standard therapy for work with people with serious mental illness	49
9.1	Interventions	128
17.1	Government policy and service users	237
18.1	Elements of effective PSI training courses	254
18.2	Appropriate course content for comprehensive PSI training courses	255
18.3	Guidelines for developing a clinical supervision contract	260

Notes on Contributors

Claire Baguley is a Cognitive Behavioural Therapist with Tameside and Glossop NHS Trust.

Ian Baguley is Divisional Leader (Mental Health), School of Nursing, Midwifery and Health Visiting, University of Manchester.

Tim Bradshaw is Lecturer, COPE Initiative, School of Nursing, Midwifery and Health. Visiting, University of Manchester and Honorary Nurse Therapist, Merseycare Mental Health Care NHS Trust.

Hywel Davis is Chair of Pembrokeshire Hearing Voices Network, South Wales.

Jenny Droughton is Lecturer, Merseycare Mental Health Care NHS Trust and University of Manchester.

Julie Everitt is a Nurse Consultant for Adult Acute In-patient Care with Merseycare Mental Health Care NHS Trust.

Neil Harris is a Practice Development Nurse for the Community with Manchester Mental Health and Social Care Trust and Honorary Lecturer, School of Nursing, Midwifery and Health Visiting, University of Manchester.

Mark Holland is Lead Nurse with Manchester Mental Health and Social Care Trust.

Doug Inchbold is Development Officer (Health Promotion), Manchester Mental Health Care Partnership.

Ged McCann is Specialist Commissioning (Forensic) Manager, Yorkshire North Yorkshire Health Authority.

Mick McKeown is a Senior Lecturer at the University of Central Lancashire.

Alice Knight is a Trainee Clinical Psychologist, at the University of Manchester.

Rachel Perkins is Consultant Clinical Psychologist, and Clinical Director of Rehabilitation and Continuing Care Service of South West London and St George's Mental Health Trust.

David Reader is a Clinical Nurse Specialist, Psychosocial Interventions for Psychosis, with North West Wales NHS Trust.

Julie Repper is Senior Lecturer at the Sheffield Centre for Health Related Research (SCHARR).

Ron Siddle is Consultant Cognitive Behaviour Therapist for Manchester Mental Health and Social Care Trust.

Steve Williams is Senior Cognitive Behaviour Nurse Therapist, Mental Health Services of Salford, and Honorary Lecturer, School of Nursing, Midwifery and Health Visiting, University of Manchester.

Ian Wilson is Case Manager, Manchester Mental Health Social Care Trust, and Lecturer, COPE Initiative, School of Nursing, Midwifery and Health Visiting, University of Manchester.

Foreword

It is a great pleasure to provide a Foreword for this new volume on psycho-social interventions for people with schizophrenia. The book has been an ambitious enterprise, divided into five sections, and with a total of eighteen chapters. The authors have been well chosen with contributions from managers, user, clinicians, researchers and teachers. Importantly, the user perspective is interwoven throughout, with chapters on hearing voices, the therapeutic relationship and, more specifically, the involvement of users. Unfortunately, (and in common with much National Service Framework-related activity at present), the carer voice is not so well articulated although the chapter by David Reader on family work goes some way to redressing this imbalance. Nonetheless, this is a book that will inspire clinicians to continue the development of skills-based approaches for work with people with a psychosis. Indeed, the section on clinical skills is packed with important and useful information that will be referred to time and again by trainees (and others) from PSI programmes.

The chapter on training in PSI-work points out that the research evidence for the usefulness of such training is only some ten years old but that over the past decade great strides in the area have been made. The number of programmes has proliferated, the number of trainees working in the field has expanded, and much of the post-qualification material taught has now permeated through to pre-qualifying training itself. As might be expected though, this has led to, quite rightly, much debate about the future direction of psychosocial intervention training. Among the many questions that could be posed about PSI training are the following:

(1) Should PSI training aim to improve attitudes towards working with people who have serious mental health problems or should it aim to create highly skilled therapists or both?
(2) Should the central aim of PSI training be to improve users' satisfaction with services? (for example, by helping users' to achieve their personal goals?).
(3) Should PSI be seeking to demonstrate reduction in bed use and improvement in symptoms and social functioning?
(4) Does the recent broadening of PSI training to include policy and organisational issues (e.g. courses at Universities of Birmingham, Sheffield and Manchester) indicate an intention to influence the organisation and philosophy of mental health services as a whole?
(5) Is the evidence base for psychosocial interventions as compelling now as

was once claimed? (see for example the recent Cochrane review of cognitive behaviour therapy for schizophrenia, 2002).

It is in the context above that the conclusion to this book raises the thorny
question of implementation of taught-PSI skills in routine service settings –
an area of the book that might have been developed in greater depth alongside conjecture about the likely service configurations that will arise from the
National Service Framework for Mental Health. For example, the establishment of assertive outreach teams, early intervention services and crisis intervention teams can all be expected to impact significantly on the role and
function of community mental health team workers – traditionally the group
that has been targeted for PSI training to date. Similarly, whilst policy exhor-
tations aim to realise multi-professional training, PSI training has achieved
minimal success in training groups other than mental health nurses. How
should PSI training differ, if at all, for psychologists, mental health nurses, psychiatrists and occupational therapists? – have the boundaries that have defined
professional identity historically now become so blurred that such issues are
no longer important?

But these questions are perhaps better left to the future, and in raising them
in this Foreword, I have no intention to detract from the quality of this excellent volume. What is unquestionable is that PSI training and PSI trainees have
made a major contribution to the lives of people who experience a psychosis.
Trainees instil optimism, work from an overarching theoretical framework,
enable people to develop coping strategies that build on their existing reper-
toires, and attempt to understand the impact of their interventions (Brooker
et al., 2002). This book can do nothing but strengthen PSI practitioners and
trainees' attempts to work with service users to achieve their own goals – the
most significant aim of a high quality mental health service.

Charlie Brooker
Professor of Mental Health, University of Sheffield

Reference

Brooker, C., Saul, C., Robinson, J., King, J. and Dudley, M. (2002) *Is training in
Psychosocial Interventions Worthwhile?* Report of a psychosocial intervention trainee
follow-up study. Submitted for publication.

List of Abbreviations

ACT	Assertive Community Treatment
AIMS	Abnormal Involuntary Movement Scale
BNF	British National Formulary
COPE	Collaboration on Psychosocial Education
CBT	Cognitive Behavioural Therapy
CFI	Camberwell Family Interview
CPN	Community Psychiatric Nurse
CSE	Coping Strategy Enhancement
DAS	Dysfunctional Attitude Scale
DoH	Department of Health
EPC	Epidemiologic Catchment Area
EE	Expressed Emotion
EPSE	Extra Pyramidal Side Effects
ESS	Early Signs Scale
FI	Family Intervention
FQ	Family Questionnaire
GHQ	General Health Questionnaire
HADS	Hospital Anxiety Depression Scale
HoNOS	Health of the Nation Outcome Scales
ICM	Intensive Case Management
IPS	Individual Placement and Support
KASI	Knowledge About Schizophrenia Interview
KGV	Krawiecka, Goldberg and Vaughn Symptom Rating Scale
LUNSERS	Liverpool University Neuroleptic Side Effects Rating Scale
NHS	National Health Service
NIDS	Neuroleptic Induced Deficit Syndrome
NMS	Neuroleptic Malignant Syndrome
PS	Problem Solving
PSI	Psychosocial Intervention
PsyRats	Psychiatric Rating Scales
PVT	Prevocational Training
RAI	Relative Assessment Interview
SANS	Scale for the Assessment of Negative Symptoms
SE	Supported Employment
SFS	Social Functioning Scale
SMI	Serious Mental Illness
TCO	Threat/Control Override

TD	Tardive Dyskinesia
UK	United Kingdom
UKCC	United Kingdom Central Council
WHO	World Health Organization

Part I

What is Schizophrenia?

CHAPTER 1

The Nature of Schizophrenia

STEVE WILLIAMS

Introduction

Why the Nature of Schizophrenia Matters to Grass Roots Workers

The existence of schizophrenic illness has been asserted by the psychiatric system for only one hundred years or so (Kraepelin, 1896), although it is even more recently, that is, since Bleuler's work at the early part of the last century (Bleuler, 1911) that the term with which we are now so familiar became favoured over Kraepelin's original term of 'dementia praecox'. It may be regarded as a fairly arcane matter to discuss in a practical text book issues such as the nature of schizophrenia, and yet the failure to be clear about the status of this term in a scientific and clinical sense, with the associated controversy and polarisation of opinion among mental health professionals concerning what such a term actually means have been unhelpful to people with 'schizophrenic' disorders (Patmore and Weaver, 1990; Wooff *et al.*, 1988).

Why Rejecting the Label of Schizophrenia Can be Unhelpful

Completely rejecting the 'label' of schizophrenia has contributed to the neglect of people whose symptoms or experiences gave them a greatly increased risk of serious problems including suicide, for example (DoH, 1992), by some mental health professionals (and services) who regard such psychiatric labelling as harmful, but too often seemed unable to respond positively to the very real needs of people diagnosed as having schizophrenic illness. At its worst, such rejectionist positions meant that many people diagnosed as having schizophrenic illness, that is, people whose problems in very many cases should give them priority status for access to mental health services, received little or no help or support from professionals in some areas (White, 1985, 1990), or at best the minimum level of intervention possible, often from the most inexperienced and junior member of the team. This neglect of a priority population extended to the carers of people with schizophrenic illness, with some family members of people with a schizophrenic illness even reporting the police as the most helpful agency with which they interacted (White, 1990) rather than the supposedly dedicated mental health services. Indeed, some

3

80 per cent of people with a schizophrenic diagnosis were not even on the caseload of a community psychiatric nurse during these comprehensive surveys conducted in the 1980s and the 1990s.

Why Thinking of Schizophrenia Simply as a Disease Can Be Unhelpful

The emphasis of the disease model in schizophrenia and the associated and erroneous assumptions about 'inevitable' deterioration have also been unhelpful in developing programmes of care that hope to realistically improve the lot of people diagnosed as having schizophrenia. Reliance on notions of disease, with the associated deterministic assumptions about course and outcome have induced a pessimism in mental health workers and services that is unhelpful and unwarranted. It is evident that course and outcome in schizophrenic illness is immensely variable (WHO, 1979a) and that a large part of the variation in outcome can be explained by psycho-social rather than merely biological variables (Warner, 1994; Mari and Streiner, 1994). The assumptions that Kraepelin made about the inevitably deteriorating course of this disorder, assumptions that influenced his very naming of the disorder as *dementia praecox*, are wrong. That we do not need to be so pessimistic about outcome in schizophrenic illness has been demonstrated by studies with very well designed methodologies (WHO, 1979a; Bleuler, 1972; Ciompi and Muller, 1976) but this pessimism too often persists. Contemporary psychiatrists such as Turkington have called for mental health workers to abandon such pessimistic views and catch up with the actual evidence. Of course, other problems with having a disease concept exist, in that it becomes increasingly difficult to square such a concept with the gathering evidence of seemingly schizophrenic symptoms in the normal population (Tien, 1991; Romme and Escher, 1989).

The Aims of This Chapter

This chapter aims to equip readers with an understanding of some of the problems associated with the schizophrenia concept, in particular the criticisms that the concept just does not hang together in any scientific sense (Boyle, 1990). It also aims to help readers understand how the psychiatric establishment have tried to respond to such criticisms by increasing the reliability of psychiatric diagnosis, especially in schizophrenic illness (Wing *et al.*, 1974; APA, 1987, 1994; WHO, 1990). I also aim to review some of the evidence about the existence of apparently schizophrenic symptoms in the 'normal' population (Tien, 1991) mapping this onto contemporary understandings of schizophrenic illness utilising breakthrough (although no longer recent) stress-vulnerability models (Zubin and Spring, 1977; Nuechterlein and Dawson, 1984) which can help mental health professionals respond positively (and with some optimism) to the needs of people with a diagnosis of schizophrenic illness. Ultimately, the aim of this chapter is to enable readers to have an evidence-based and contemporary understanding of the term schizophrenia, which enables them to engage individuals with such a diagnosis in efforts at collaborative health improvement.

The History of the 'Schizophrenia' Concept

At the end of the nineteenth century, German Psychiatrist Emil Kraepelin (Kraepelin, 1896) proposed that his observations and the observations of his contemporaries regarding the condition of large groups of the inmates of the institutions in which they worked could in many instances be explained by a single construct, that of dementia praecox. He argued that the presentation of this disorder could be quite different in affected individuals but that it was still acceptable to infer the same disorder due to similarities in onset, course and outcome. Similarities in onset, course and outcome are actually criteria toward the bottom of any scientific league table for inferring or proving the existence of a supposed disorder for a number of reasons. One reason why such criteria are towards the bottom of acceptability for proving the existence of a disorder in any scientific sense is that while the terms may sound quite scientific, they are actually very difficult to define operationally, that is, it is difficult to be confident that an observation grouped under 'course' by one researcher will be grouped under 'course' by another researcher, or even the same researcher at a different point in time (Boyle, 1990). A further reason why such similarities are way down the league table of establishing a disease process is that such similarities, even where properly observed, enjoy only the status of a syndrome, in a medical sense. A syndrome refers to a *hypothetical* construct, a clustering of symptoms and signs, but significantly without independent medical evidence supporting the hypothesised construct such as the existence of bacteria or organic changes that can be proven to account for the observations made. It enjoys only a lowly status in the league table of scientific certainty because it is often considered to be a *temporarily* useful way of thinking, helpful until such time that scientific advances can help us to identify what is really going on and demonstrate with a degree of scientific certainty the disease entity responsible for the signs and symptoms that have been noted. It is usually acknowledged that such scientific advances will, in all probability, rule out as well as in some of the observations we have currently grouped together given our rather inadequate scientific tools. Scientists usually infer a concept after having made many observations of related phenomena, providing evidence of observations in the field, which suggest a pattern has been observed which may itself be a genuine indication of a real 'cleavage in nature'. Such observations can then be replicated or not as the case may be, and the existence of the hypothesised syndrome further supported or chal- lenged. The problem with Kraepelin's approach was that not only did he try to prove the existence of dementia praecox by use of observations suggesting a syndromal pattern, he actually did this in a back to front manner, that is, he assumed that the existence of the syndrome had been adequately established before providing observations of the putative condition that he then used to further support the existence of the syndrome in the first instance! This back to front and tautological method for establishing the syndrome of schizo- phrenia was further compounded by Kraepelin when he later repeatedly changed his definitions of what was meant by the hypothesised disorder on several occasions, risking giving the impression that this was a very elastic concept capable of expansion or retraction apparently at will:

> Between the 6th and 8th editions of his text Kraepelin further increased the number of behaviours said to be symptoms of dementia praecox. The scale of the increase can be gauged from the fact that in 1896 a discussion of the constructs of demen- tia praecox took up about thirty seven pages . . . in the 6th edition dementia praecox took up seventy seven pages . . . by the 8th edition the discussion had grown to 356 pages. (Boyle, 1990, p. 44)

Leaving aside the scientific status of the syndrome Kraepelin central obser- vation was that dementia praecox (as the name implies) was a condition characterised by an inevitable progressive deteriorating course, intellectual deterioration, poor judgement and destruction of the personality (Kraepelin, 1896). However, this was later challenged by the Swiss psychiatrist Eugene Bleuler (Bleuler, 1911). Working in the relatively benign economic circum- stances that have pertained in Switzerland for most of this century, Bleuler was obtaining social recovery rates (allowing patients with the disorder to work and live independently of the institution) of around 60 per cent compared with Kraepelin's reported 12 per cent. Bleuler also challenged Kraepelin on what were the key features of the disorder, suggesting that thought disruption or derailment, and flat or limited affect/expression of emotion were the char- acteristic features that could be noted in affected individuals. These features, he argued, led to the 'characteristic split between thinking and feeling' that he named 'schizophrenia'. According to Bleuler, symptoms such as delusions and hallucinations were merely by-products of this process. Bleuler sought then to change the core characteristics of the syndrome Kraepelin had observed, after accepting as fact that Kraepelin had indeed observed and described such a syndrome. Once again the procedure is scientifically unsound: if Kraepelin had not observed any common pattern or regularity worthy of the status of syndrome, or indeed had drawn the wrong conclusions about typical features from such observations, surely Bleuler's job was to demonstrate that the (new schizophrenia) syndrome actually existed before commenting on its typical features. Instead, Bleuler accepted Kraepelin's work insofar as it helped to establish that a syndrome of any kind existed, but then challenged his key observations about what signs and symptoms constituted the syndrome. In effect, he suggested that while Kraepelin had established that a syndrome characterised by an inevitable deteriorating course existed, that the syndrome did exist, but without the inevitably deteriorating course! Such a suggestion really required that Bleuler start afresh from the level of observation and establish from the beginning whether a syndrome of schizophrenia did exist, and that its key features were those he had described, but he failed to follow this course of action, relying on Kraepelin's work which he was now calling into question to have already done this for him.

Nearly fifty years after Bleuler, Schneider (1959) tried to establish criteria for the diagnosis of schizophrenia according to two ranks, that is in the first rank the cardinal diagnostic signs for the diagnosis which he stated as being audible thoughts, delusional perceptions and the experiencing of outside influences on the body, and in the second rank all the other symptoms of schizophrenia. The methods he used for divining which phenomena belonged to which rank are unclear and have been criticised by Boyle (1990) as having no obvious scientific merit, and yet this system has remained the basis for the diagnosis of schizophrenia. According to Boyle his concepts also failed to independently 'cluster' in the way expected of a syndrome, and he compounded the early mistakes in this field by assuming, as had Kraepelin himself and Bleuler that the concept of schizophrenia already enjoyed scientific status and

Table 1.1 Kraepelin, Bleuler and Schneider

	Kraepelin 1896	*Bleuler 1911*	*Schneider 1956*
Name of disorder	Dementia praecox	Schizophrenia	Schizophrenia
Key features	Inevitable progressive deteriorating course, intellectual deterioration poor judgement	Thought disruption/ derailment, flat or limited affect/ expression of emotion	Audible thoughts, delusional perception, experiencing outside influences on body
Outcome	Very poor – 12 per cent social recovery	Fair – 60 per cent social recovery	Not specified?
Scientific status of concept	Not established	Not established	Not established
'Independent' medical evidence of concept (micro-organism/ bacteria etc.)	None	None	None

it was his job simply to describe it more precisely, in order to enable other clinicians to recognise it when they observed it.

In summary we can see that Kraepelin, Bleuler and Schneider did not establish that a syndrome known as dementia praecox or schizophrenia existed. What they did instead was to describe what they considered to be key features of a syndrome that they assumed had been established to exist, and that explained many of the bizarre behaviours encountered in the institutions of the(ir) time. Kraepelin had hoped that the biological causes and brain pathology that accounted for the behaviours he had described (so he believed) would eventually be established. This has not been the case, and despite a century of research to establish the causes and explain the pathology of schizophrenia, none of Kraeplin's followers have been able to do so.

Increasing the Reliability of the Diagnosis

The problems of the validity of the schizophrenia concept will not just go away and continue to trouble the psychiatric establishment. On top of this difficulty, another criticism has been advanced, namely that the diagnosis of schizophrenia is applied in a very inconsistent and unreliable way. This criticism is certainly a justified one given the variability in applying the diagnosis historically in the UK, USA and Scandinavian countries for example (Warner, 1994). Sensitive to the charge that the problems with the lack of independent validity of the construct combined with inconsistent diagnostic practices has rendered the term meaningless, the psychiatric profession has attempted to at least establish agreed criteria for the diagnosis of schizophrenia. However, such attempts have had a troubled history. Until after the Second World War no real attempts were made by psychiatrists to ensure their ability to consistently name the same set of behaviours as schizophrenia (indeed this problem was not confined to schizophrenia; other mental disorders were also idiosyncratically and inconsistently described but we will not concern ourselves with that here). Previous to this a crude attempt at establishing a classification system had been attempted under the auspices of the Congress of Mental Medicine in 1885. It did report accordingly, and the report was officially adopted by the renamed International Congress of Mental Science in 1889. It is clear, however, that the classification systems recommended basically represented a consensus view adopted by the committee members with little or no empirical validation in the case of most of the 'diseases' named (Kendell, 1975). The individuals charged with the diagnosis and treatment of mental disorder in the various asylums and madhouses that existed across Europe at this time showed little inclination to be corralled into using this system and relied, as previously, on their own systems such as they were. Some of these individuals undoubtedly used Kraepelin's system and later perhaps Bleuler's but no standard system was used in any consistent, reliable way. Behaviours that led to one diagnosis by one psychiatrist in one asylum did not reliably lead to the same diagnosis elsewhere; indeed different diagnostic labels altogether may have been in use, meaning that not only could they end up with a different diagnosis, but that it might not even be possible to get the same diagnosis as a second psychiatrist never applied that diagnosis, whatever the presenting picture! This unsatisfactory state of affairs has of course been addressed several times since in an attempt to arrive at a degree of professional uniformity in terms of what constitutes schizophrenia, and to apply this criteria consistently (APA, 1952, 1968, 1980, 1987, 1994; WHO, 1948, 1965, 1967, 1973, 1974, 1977, 1978, 1979b, 1985, 1990). While high levels of reliability in applying a diagnosis of schizophrenia have been reported in studies where clinicians have used the same diagnostic tools (e.g. when using the PSE developed by Wing *et al.*, 1974), we should be clear about the limitations of what this means. Such 'evidence' is not empirical as has sometimes been claimed; it merely suggests that when clinicians have been trained to use a particular tool that they can do so reliably. It does not compensate for the lack of validity of the schizophrenia concept in the first instance, and there are no independent criteria that can be applied by way of biochemical or histological tests to validate what is in effect an agreed observation by a group of medical men. In any case, what certainly cannot be substantiated is that the various classification systems in use actually measure the same disorder, and that while they emphasise different cardinal features they are essentially concerned with the same validated illness or disease. In a study by Brockington *et al.* (1978), ten sets of diagnostic criteria were applied to 322 inpatients; reported concordance rates were very low (Kappa 0.29) and would not meet scientific criteria. Without addressing the core concept of the meaningfulness or otherwise of the schizophrenia concept, reliability of diagnosis amounts to nothing more than the systematic application of the current schizophrenia zeitgeist. As Mary Boyle (1990, p. 85) says:

> When members of a particular discipline agree on some aspect of their belief system, one explanation is that they have, for whatever reasons, been convinced by the same authorities. Without independent evidence that the agreement is based on more than shared idiosyncratic beliefs, then nothing else may be assumed.

Schizophrenic Symptoms in the 'Normal' Population

A further problem with the schizophrenia concept is that 'schizophrenic' symptoms appear to exist in the 'normal' population without in any sense being a marker of a descent into psychotic illness (Romme and Escher, 1989; Tien, 1991; Kingdon and Turkington, 1994; Bentall, 1993). Moreover, the symptoms that can be demonstrated to exist in normal populations at levels far beyond that which psychiatry would expect or predict appear to be the symptoms regarded as key or cardinal diagnostic features in some of the major schedules agreed on to increase reliability of diagnosis. Indeed, some authorities (Kingdon and Turkington, 1991) have suggested that an important step in treating people with psychosis is the 'normalisation' of their experiences, that is the attribution of psychotic experiences such as voices and hallucinations to events such as extreme stress, sleep deprivation or biochemical disturbance perhaps due to taking street drugs (see Chapter 8). This process of normalisation is meant to decatastrophise the experience for the sufferer in an attempt to break the vicious cycle of symptoms/anxiety/ arousal/symptoms. These findings further undermine the notion of schizophrenia as a discrete, tightly defined pathology and begin to cast the experiencing of psychotic or schizophrenic symptoms in a new light. In their work with voice hearers, Marius Romme and Sandra Escher note that this experience (voice hearing) is not in fact confined to people with schizophrenia at all:

> We concluded that hearing voices is present in people with very different kinds of diagnoses, and that qualitative characteristics of hallucinations are not specific to a particular psychiatric diagnoses. (Romme and Escher, 1996, p. 140)

Other writers have suggested that hallucinatory experiences are not at all confined to people with any kind of psychiatric diagnoses (Bentall, 1996; Tien, 1991), while there is ample evidence in the grief literature that hallucinatory experiences are a normal part of a grief reaction (Worden, 1994). Psychiatric authorities may argue that hallucinatory experiences, while very common among people with a diagnosis of schizophrenia, are not actually key diagnostic features of the disorder according to Schneiderian premises (i.e. they are second, not first rank, symptoms), but given the lack of validity of the concept in the first instance and the fact that agreed diagnostic systems simply imply shared understandings between leading psychiatrists without independent medical corroboration, such objections are a little obtuse. Different criteria have been applied historically to the experience of voice hearing and for long periods of human history such 'psychotic' experiences have been valued or at least regarded in a neutral way as Hywel Davies, chapter in this book shows (Chapter 2). Beliefs in 'unscientific' phenomena such as the ability of people to transfer thoughts to another person are suprisingly common also in our culture (Cox and Cowling, 1989) and the notion that it is only delusional beliefs that can be shown to be held onto despite contrary evidence cannot be supported; Kingdon and Turkington (1994) suggest that it is only a small proportion of the population that form their beliefs on the basis of scientific rules of reasoning, with the rest of us (perhaps all of us from time to time) forming and maintaining our beliefs perhaps even on important matters on the basis of scant evidence or even despite contrary evidence.

A Contemporary View of Schizophrenia

Given what we have said about the problems with the validity and reliability of the schizophrenia concept, and the growing evidence that psychotic symptoms appear to exist in 'normal' people, is there any point in holding onto the concept at all? Despite the problems that abound in being clear about what we mean by the term schizophrenia, what cannot be denied is that large numbers of people experience a great deal of distress and unhappiness as a result of experiences such as hearing voices and holding delusional beliefs (DoH, 1992). Such individuals do appear to have qualitatively different (worse) experiences as a result of their symptoms than some members of the non-clinical population (Romme and Escher, 1993). People with a diagnosis of schizophrenia have a 10–15 per cent chance of dying as a result of suicide (DoH, 1992) and the early years of the illness may present particular risk (McGorry and Jackson, 1999). Major physical health problems such as heart disease frequently go undetected and untreated in this population and are a significant source of mortality. The social and occupational functioning of most people with such a diagnosis is profoundly affected (Warner, 1994), their social networks are severely reduced (Cresswell *et al.*, 1992) and opportunities for work or meaningful daytime activity are extremely limited. Poverty and social exclusion are routine consequences of the diagnosis for many people (Pilgrim, 1990). For individuals who are compelled to receive treatment (as a result of the failure of the psychiatric system to actively engage them with services in many instances), psychological complications of such compulsory treatment may occur including post-traumatic stress disorder. Side effects of the medication given to help alleviate some of the psychotic symptoms frequently include weight gain and sexual dysfunction (Day and Bentall, 1996). These are not inconsequential side effects for anyone, but considering that schizophrenia is most often first diagnosed in young adults and even adolescents, they are potentially major problems. For most people, medication is still administered by mental health nurses who are inadequately trained to spot side effects or even to properly monitor the effect of the medication on key symptoms or the persons quality of life and therefore aid in the goal of parsimonious treatment, that is, maximum benefit from minimum dosage. Although anti-psychotic medications are all recommended to be prescribed in the absence of other anti-psychotic agents, multiple prescription is commonplace, effectively doubling the side effect profile to which the affected person is exposed, without increasing the anti-psychotic benefits available. Despite internationally replicated studies with tightly controlled methodologies spanning forty years or so demonstrating the immense importance in helping family members and other carers respond positively to the affected person's attempts to constructively deal with their problems (Mari and Streiner, 1994), family members and other carers of people with schizophrenia routinely receive no information or support in helping the person with schizophrenia to cope with distressing symptoms from mainstream services. Not infrequently, such services had no formal obligations of any kind to develop services for this population (CSAG, 1996) (this may be now changing with the recently published National Service Framework for mental health services (DoH, 1999)), and the services that were provided or not were completely dependent on the vagaries, priorities, prejudices and personalities of local mental health services without reference to firm guidelines of any kind. Despite recent growing evidence of the effectiveness of cognitive-behavioural methods of treatment for people with diagnoses of schizophrenia and other psychoses (Wykes *et al.*, 1998), the absence of such treatment tools from the armomatorium available in routine services (if such a term can actually be applied to the extremely narrow treatment options actually available) remains almost complete (CSAG, 1996). What is absolutely evident is that despite the problems with the concept of schizophrenia from any scientific standpoint and the often poor levels of reliability with which the diagnosis is applied, allied to the evidence of psychotic symptoms in the non-clinical population, people who are currently diagnosed as having schizophrenia must remain a high priority for care and treatment by the dedicated mental health services.

But how are mental health professionals to conceptualise schizophrenia and orientate themselves to helping people with this diagnosis given what has been said in this chapter about the concept? A breakthrough in understanding (and treating) the problems of people diagnosed with schizophrenia occurred with the articulation of stress-vulnerability models of schizophrenia (Zubin and Spring, 1977). This early and perhaps crude model suggested that the occurrence of psychotic symptoms in an individual was a result of predisposition to the illness (including a persons genetic make up) combined with exposure to enough stress to trigger the symptoms. While accepting that the schizophrenia concept held water and that genetic predisposition probably determined vulnerability to the development of the disorder, this model also articulated the mediating role of stress in the development of psychotic symptoms. It suggested that even with only average levels of genetic predisposition that psychotic symptoms could occur in affected individuals if they were subject to extreme levels of stress. In addition this model appeared to suggest that it may be possible to prevent the appearance of psychotic symptoms by reducing or modifying the stress that a vulnerable person may be experiencing at any one time. This model has often been regarded as a heuristic or practical one, in that it allowed us to further build onto it as our knowledge about schizophrenia increased, but also to build into the model some concepts that were perhaps generally accepted without being conclusively proven, for example the concepts of the importance of biological vulnerability and stress to the development and outcome of the illness. Of course, these concepts were expressed in very general terms at the time the model was developed given our state of knowledge of how these factors operated in schizophrenia. This model was further refined and elaborated (Nuechterlein and Dawson, 1984) when attempts were made to list some of the *possible* psychological, biological and environmental stressors and protectors that may contribute to the development or non-development of psychotic symptoms in a person at any point in time. Attention is drawn to the possible effect of these factors, all of which have supporting evidence for their importance in schizophrenia, but the exact weighting that they enjoy in terms of their influence is less certain.

Personal Vulnerability Factors

Several factors could increase a persons vulnerability to developing psychotic symptoms and receiving a diagnosis of schizophrenia, including:

- Dopaminergic dysfunction;
- Reduced available processing resources (i.e. being unable to process all the stimulus presented in a particular environment or situation, perhaps leading to confusion or too quick and probably erronous judgements about other people/circumstances);
- Autonomic hyperreactivity (being in a state of heightened arousal with subsequent effects on judgement and decision-making, and anomolous perceptions such as hallucinatory experiences);
- Schizotypal personality traits (a tendency to be aloof/socially isolated, associated with the tendency to misjudge the motives of others without appropriate opportunities for social referencing/comparisons).

Environmental Stressors

The following factors can also increase the likelihood of symptoms occurring:

- Critical or emotionally over-involved attitudes towards the person (being subject for sustained periods of time to high levels of criticism, hostility or emotional over-involvement can lead to a highly stressed state in vulnerable people in which prodromal or frankly psychotic symptoms may emerge or be exacerbated);
- Overstimulating social environment (given the vulnerability to psychotic experiences/frank psychosis a person may have as a result of personal vulnerability factors, including reduced ability to process social stimulus, an environment which is overly stimulating may trigger or exacerbate psychotic symptoms);
- Stressful life events (such events may overload a persons ability to cope).

Personal Protectors

A range of personal factors can protect a person from developing psychotic symptoms, even in the presence of personal vulnerability factors and environmental stressors, and these factors are subsumed under the following headings in this model:

- Coping and self-efficacy (pre-existing coping strategies and a concept of self as an effective person may help minimise the risks of the emergence or exacerbation of psychotic symptoms in a vulnerable person).
- Anti-psychotic medication (have the effect of blocking receptor sites, lowering the overstimulation and therefore reducing the occurrence of psychotic symptoms/prodromal states).

Environmental Protectors

Even with high levels of vulnerability and relatively low levels of personal protection available, individuals may still be protected from psychotic illness by measures aimed at environmental manipulation, such as:

- Effective family problem-solving (reducing aversive home environments by increasing understanding and improving problem-solving skills and the frequency with which they are used may help provide a more manageable environment for a vulnerable person);
- Supportive psychosocial interventions (a range of interventions utilising psychological principles and socially focused treatment strategies such as enabling a person to have meaningful and manageable daytime activity can protect against the re-emergence or exacerbation of psychotic symptoms).

Nuechterlein's model goes on to suggest that these factors or their absence combine and interact, and may produce intermediate states of arousal, which unchecked lead on to prodromal symptoms such as profound sleep disturbance and high levels of arousal, which again lead on, if unchecked to frank psychotic symptoms. Such symptoms affect an individuals social and occupational functioning, and problems in these domains together with the actual experiencing of the symptoms feedback into the outcome of the disorder itself.

Conclusion

Of course, such models do not represent the end point in understanding schizophrenia despite their importance in underlining the role of psychosocial interventions in delaying ameliorating or even preventing the occurrence of psychotic symptoms in vulnerable people. Stress-vulnerability models in schizophrenia can perhaps better be understood as a staging post in our developing knowledge of schizophrenia, convenient stopping places that attempt to summarise the evidence thus far and help to guide our way of thinking and responding to people with a diagnoses of schizophrenia. It may be that rather than summarising all the evidence for 'schizophrenia' in one model that we would be better served by seeking to build explanatory models of particular symptoms such as paranoid delusions, understanding how they work and trying to reverse the maintaining factors as has been advocated by Bentall (1996) and others. This approach is of course predicated on the assumption that schizophrenia is an umbrella term covering disorders that have distinct aetiology, and maintaining psychological factors, and that retention of the term is unhelpful, lumping together as it does disorders with distinct and heterogeneous profiles, thus serving to prevent advancement in our understanding and treatment. While this position has much to recommend it, the stress-vulnerability model is at least a convenient if temporary starting off point in ensuring that people with diagnoses of schizophrenia receive appropriate and helpful psychosocial interventions as advocated and explained in this book. In time, such a unifying concept may prove innapropriate or even unhelpful in the understanding and treatment of psychosis; at the current juncture it appears a helpful concept, and one which this book will utilise.

Suggested Reading

American Psychiatric Association (1994) *Diagnostic and Statistical Manual of Mental Disorders*, 4th edn, Washington, DC, APA.

Boyle, M. (1990) *Schizophrenia; A scientific Delusion?*, London, Routledge.

Pilgrim, D. (1990) 'Competing Histories of Madness', in R.P. Bentall (ed.), *Reconstructing Schizophrenia*, London, Routledge.

Tien, A. (1991) 'Distributions of hallucinations in the normal population', *Social Psychiatry and Psychiatric Epidemiology*, 26, 287–92

Zubin, J. and Spring, B. (1977) 'A new view of Schizophrenia', *J. Abnorm. Psychol.*, 86, 103–26.

References

American Psychiatric Association (1952) *Diagnostic and Statistical Manual of Mental Disorders*, Washington, DC, APA.

American Psychiatric Association (1968) *Diagnostic and Statistical Manual of Mental Disorders*, 2nd edn, Washington, DC, APA.

American Psychiatric Association (1980) *Diagnostic and Statistical Manual of Mental Disorders*, 3rd edn, Washington, DC, APA.

American Psychiatric Association (1987) *Diagnostic and Statistical Manual of Mental Disorders*, revised 3rd edn, Washington, DC, APA.

American Psychiatric Association (1994) *Diagnostic and Statistical Manual of Mental Disorders*, 4th edn, Washington, DC, APA.

Bentall, R.P. (1993) 'Cognitive Models of Voice Hearing', in M. Romme and S. Escher (eds), *Accepting Voices*, London, Mind Publications.

Bentall, R.P. (1996) 'From Cognitive Studies of Psychosis to Cognitive-Behaviour Therapy for Psychotic Symptoms', in G. Haddock and P.D Slade (eds), *Cognitive-Behavioural Interventions with Psychotic Disorders*, London, Routledge.

Bleuler, E. (1911; translated from German into English 1950); *Dementia Praecox or the Group of Schizophrenias*, New York, International Universities Press.

Bleuler, M. (1972; translated into English 1978) *The Schizophrenic Disorders: Long term patient and family studies*, New Haven, CT, Yale University Press.

Boyle, M. (1990) *Schizophrenia; A scientific Delusion?*, London, Routledge.

Brockington, I.F., Kendell, R.E. and Leff, J.P. (1978) 'Definitions of schizophrenia: concordance and prediction of outcome', *Psychological Medicine*, 10, 665–75.

Ciompi, L. and Muller, C. (1976) Lebensweg und Alter der Schizophrenen, Berlin, Springer.

Clinical Standards Advisory Group (1996) *Schizophrenia*, London, HMSO.

Cox, D. and Cowling, P. (1989) *Are you normal?*, London, Tower Press.

Cresswell, C.M., Kuipers, L. and Power, M.J. (1992) 'Social networks and support in long-term psychiatric patients', *Psychological Medicine*, 22, 1019–26.

Day, J.C. and Bentall, R.P. (1996) 'Neuroleptic Medication and The Psycho-Social Treatment of Psychotic Symptoms: Some Neglected Issues', in G. Haddock and P.D. Slade (eds), *Cognitive-Behavioural Interventions with Psychotic Disorders*, London, Routledge.

Department of Health (1992) *The Health of the Nation White Paper*, London, HMSO.

Department of Health (1999) National Service Framework for Mental Health, London, The Stationary Office.

Kendell, R.E. (1975) *The Role of Diagnosis in Psychiatry*, Oxford, Blackwell.

Kingdon, D.G. and Turkington, D. (1994) *Cognitive-Behavioural Therapy of Schizophrenia*, Hove, Psychology Press, Lawrence Erlbaum.

Kraepelin, E. (1896) *Psychiatrie*, 5th edn, Leipzig, Barth.

Mari, J.D.J. and Streiner, D.L. (1994) 'An overview of family interventions and relapse on schizophrenia: meta analysis of research findings', *Psychological Medicine*, 24, 565–78.

McGorry, P.D. and Jackson, H.J. (1999) *The Recognition and Management of Early Psychosis*, Cambridge, Cambridge University Press.

Nuechterlein, K.H. and Dawson, M.E. (1984) 'A heuristic vulnerability-stress model of schizophrenic episodes', *Schizophrenia Bulletin*, 10, 300–12.

Patmore, C. and Weaver, J. (1990) *A survey of community mental health centres*, London, Good Practices in Mental Health.

Pilgrim, D. (1990) 'Competing Histories of Madness', in R.P. Bentall (ed.), *Reconstructing Schizophrenia*, London, Routledge.

Romme, M.A.J. and Escher, S. (1989) 'Hearing Voices', *Schizophrenia Bulletin*, 15(2), 209–16.

Romme, M. and Escher, S. (1993) *Accepting Voices*, London, Mind Publications.

Romme, M. and Escher, S. (1996) 'Empowering People Who Hear Voices', in G. Haddock and P.D. Slade (eds), *Cognitive-Behavioural Interventions with Psychotic Disorders*, London, Routledge.

Schneider, K. (1959) *Clinical Psychopathology*, 5th edn, New York, Grune & Stratton.

Tarrier, N., Beckett, R., Harwood, S., Baker, A., Yusupoff, L. and Ugarteburu, I. (1993) 'A trial of two cognitive-behavioural methods of treating drug resistant residual psychotic symptoms in schizophrenic patients: I. Outcome', *British Journal of Psychiatry*, 162, 524–32.

Tien, A. (1991) 'Distributions of hallucinations in the normal population', *Social Psychiatry and Psychiatric Epidemiology*, 26, 287–92

Warner, R. (1994) *Recovery from Schizophrenia; Psychiatry and Political Economy*, New York, Routledge.

White, E. (1985) *The Second Quinquennial Survey of Community Psychiatric Nurses*, Manchester, University of Manchester Press.

White, E. (1990) *The Third Quinquennial Survey of Community Psychiatric Nurses*, Manchester, University of Manchester Press.

Wing, J.K., Cooper, J.E. and Sartorius, N. (1974) *The Measurement and Classification of Psychiatric Symptoms*, Cambridge, Cambridge University Press.

Wooff, K., Goldberg, D.P. and Fryers, T. (1988) 'The practice of community psychiatric nursing and mental health social work in Salford. Some implications for community care', *British Journal of Psychiatry*, 152, 783–792.

Worden, W. (1994) *Grief Counselling and Grief Therapy*, London, Routledge.

World Health Organization (1948) *International Classification of Diseases*, Geneva, WHO.

World Health Organization (1965) *International Classification of Diseases*, 2nd edn, Geneva, WHO.

World Health Organization (1967) *International Classification of Diseases*, 3rd edn, Geneva, WHO.

World Health Organization (1973) *International Classification of Diseases*, 4th edn, Geneva, WHO.

World Health Organization (1974) *International Classification of Diseases*, 5th edn, Geneva, WHO.

World Health Organization (1977) *International Classification of Diseases*, 6th edn, Geneva, WHO.

World Health Organization (1978) *International Classification of Diseases*, 7th edn, Geneva, WHO.

World Health Organization (1979a) *International Classification of Diseases*, 8th edn, Geneva, WHO.

World Health Organization (1979b) Schizophrenia: *An International Follow-Up Study*, New York, Wiley.

World Health Organization (1985) *International Classification of Diseases*, 9th edn, Geneva, WHO.

World Health Organization (1990) *International Classification of Diseases*, 10th edn, Geneva, WHO.

Wykes, T., Tarrier, N. and Lewis, S. (1998) *Outcome and Innovation in Psychological Treatment of Schizophrenia*, Chichester, Wiley.

Zubin, J. and Spring, B. (1977) 'A new view of Schizophrenia', *J. Abnorm. Psychol.*, 86, 103–26.

CHAPTER 2

Hearing Voices Past and Present: A User's Perspective

HYWEL DAVIES

If an idea at first is not absurd, then there is no hope for it (Albert Einstein)

Introduction

In this chapter historical perspectives on voice hearing are reviewed (the hearing of a voice or voices inaudible to others) and a critical examination of whether voice hearing is an abnormal experience, as currently suggested by most psychiatric practice, is conducted. Some of the popular myths about voice hearers and dangerousness are challenged, and perspectives on voice hearing held by voice hearers themselves are considered. It is suggested that mental health services in the United Kingdom adopt holistic, progressive and intellectually creative approaches towards the voice hearing experience.

Voice Hearing Through the Ages

Voice hearing is a phenomena of human experience and is recorded as far back as 10,000 BC (Jaynes, 1976). In early civilisations, voice hearers were often seen as individuals of a religious and/or spiritual significance. Consequently, voice hearers used to hold significant positions in early societies. These voice hearers were seen by their subjects as being in direct communion with the gods or with God by way of their voice hearing experiences. Temples, monuments, murals, statues, figurines and pyramids in Egypt and, for example, in Central America and South America were built in tribute to voice hearers' 'divine perceptions'. In an age when the mind was considered to have two chambers, that is to be *bi-cameral*, voice hearers ruled the kingdoms of the Egyptians, of the Hittites, of the Maya people and of the Incas. These kingdoms were grand and impressive tributes to the world of the supernatural and to the world of the divine. From Turkey to Peru, from Egypt to Mexico, from Cyprus to Central Asia, the leaders of these early civilisations were 'hallucinatory god-kings' (Jaynes, 1976). In early societies dating to approximately 10,000 BC, voice hearing was consistently seen as a valued and even divine

18

phenomenon. The thesis of Jaynes (1976) includes the fact that 'some of the fundamental, most characteristic, and most commonly observed symptoms of florid, un-medicated schizophrenia are uniquely consistent with . . . the bicameral mind' (p. 408).

In a similar context to the bicameral kingdoms of Egypt, Mesopotamia, of the Maya people and of the Inca people, the heroes of the *Iliad* and prophets of the Old Testament heard from time to time the voices of gods or the voice of God. Paul Baker quotes the example of the *Iliad* (Baker, 1995) with reference to the historic link between voice hearing and spirituality. The *Iliad*, written by Homer, was essentially the story of the Trojan wars. Visions ('visual hallucinations') and voices ('auditory hallucinations') are both present in the *Iliad*. Homer frequently describes a Greek god or goddess appearing to a warrior at an extreme moment in the midst of battle, the apparition then tells the warrior what to do. According to Baker, this type of spiritual phenomenon was not simply a literary device but a reflection of the normality and cultural acceptability of hallucinatory phenomena at this period in history. Similarly, the experiences of the Old Testament prophets were not literary indulgences but reflected apparently 'real' experiences (Joyce, 1920). The abnormal aural and visual experiences of, for example, Ezekiel, Isaiah, Job and Amos were not literary devices or metaphorical, but rather reflected 'real' experiences. If Ezekiel, Isaiah, Job or Amos had been alive in Britain in the twentieth century, they may have been defined by psychiatry as 'schizophrenic'.

While voice hearing phenomena was apparently culturally acceptable, it was still regarded as unusual. Many of the prophets of the Old Testament of the Bible were regarded by the majority of their contemporaries as 'aliens'. Their 'auditory hallucinations' and their 'visual hallucinations' rendered the prophets of the Old Testament 'abnormal'. Joyce summarises the changing attitudes towards voice hearing in the following passage;

> . . . In all early societies, the abnormal mental states of vision and ecstasy were as profoundly impressive to the onlookers as they are to the man who experiences them. Both he and they are convinced that these mysteries are conclusive evidence of intercourse with the spiritual world . . . But now the general attitude towards the attendant circumstances of early inspiration has been completely reversed. The unstable, psychic temperament, with its tendency to fall into trances, instead of arousing respect as of old, is the subject of suspicion. The fact that any claimant to inspiration was subject to trances and other mental disturbances would, in many quarters today, raise doubts as to his sanity, and would certainly weaken the force of his testimony. (Joyce, 1920, p. 430)

Voice hearers, since the time of the prophets of the Old Testament, include Jesus Christ, Mohammed, many saints of the early Celtic church, Joan of Arc, Teresa of Avila and Saint John of the Cross. John Milton's *Paradise Lost* was, according to John Carey (1999), the product of a series of voice hearing experiences. The artistic work of William Blake as a poet, writer, engraver and artist appeared to have been inspired by 'hallucinatory' experiences (Wordsworth Poetry Library, 1994). As a child, William Blake saw a cloud of angels swarming a tree in his native London and, at one stage of his adult life, he believed that the Archangel Gabriel was speaking to him in the garden of his home. Blake received virtually no formal education and his written and visual work appears to have been inspired by voices and/or visions. In 1825 Blake met the diarist Crabb Robinson, who wrote the following about him: 'Shall I call him an Artist or Genius – or Mystic or Madman? Probably he is all' (ibid.). Blake's perceptions as a creative force appear to have been inspired by 'auditory and visual hallucinations'. There have been other voice hearers in the twentieth century of creative note. They include Carl Gustav Jung, Mahatma Gandhi, Sir Winston Churchill, Sir Anthony Hopkins and Zoë Wannamaker (Baker, 1995). Certain twentieth-century voice hearers who have been labelled by psychiatry as 'schizophrenic' include Louis Wain ('the man who drew cats'), John Ogden (the English classical pianist), Peter Green (the founder member of Fleetwood Mac), Syd Barrett (a founder member of Pink Floyd) and Brian Wilson (a founder member of the Beach Boys). Voice hearing is not necessarily an interminable imprisonment for the individual labelled by psychiatry as 'schizophrenic'. Certain twentieth-century 'schizophrenics' have achieved something positive out of something negative in their lives. David Helfgott, the Australian classical pianist was a primary inspiration of the award-winning 1997 film 'Shine'. Labelled by psychiatry as having a 'schizo-affective' disorder, Helfgott subsequently conducted a world tour of his music as a concert pianist. Janet Frame, the award-winning New Zealand writer, transformed her experience of 'schizophrenia' through writing (Frame, 1990). John Nash Jr, game theorist and mathematical thinker, was once labelled by psychiatry as 'schizophrenic' yet, in 1994, he was awarded the Nobel Prize for Economics. The book *A Beautiful Mind* (Nasar, 1998) chronicles Nash's life. There are other 'schizophrenics' who have achieved despite, rather than because of, their circumstances.

Psychiatry has had a troubled and controversial history in terms of describing certain human behaviours as pathological. The nature and definition of mental illness has varied according to the prevailing values of the day. Black slaves who ran away from their duties were deemed by psychiatry at the time to be mentally ill. This psychiatric 'illness' was known by psychiatry as drapetomania (Thomas and Sillen, 1972). Irascibility or impertinence on the part of a black slave was also deemed by psychiatry to be mental illness. This particular psychiatric 'condition' was known as Dysaesthesia Aethiopica. Similarly, vagrancy in Victorian Britain was seen by psychiatry as a mental illness. Epilepsy was once regarded by psychiatric orthodoxy as a mental illness. In the Soviet Union of the twentieth century, certain political dissidents were deemed by Soviet psychiatry to be mentally ill. Similarly throughout the world, homosexuals, lesbians and bisexuals were once regarded by traditional western psychiatry as mentally ill.

Voice Hearing as a Normal Phenomena

Voice hearing can be described as the hearing of a voice or voices inaudible to others. For most of the twentieth century, voice hearing was usually regarded by psychiatric orthodoxy as a symptom of 'schizophrenia'. However, most voice hearers in contemporary society have no contact whatsoever with psychiatric services (Tien, 1991). As stated by Baker (1995), hearing voices is not even a particularly uncommon experience. According to recent research (Tien, 1991) 10–15 per cent of the general population hear a voice or voices over a long period, with 2.3 per cent of individuals (Tien, 1991) hearing a voice or voices at any one particular time. The impact of these voices fall into two types, helpful and unhelpful. Most voice hearers, 66 per cent in Tien's study, perceived the voice or voices as positive or helpful (Eaton *et al.*, 1991), describing the voices as familiar and recognisable. This category of respondent appeared to believe that the purpose of the voices is strengthening and raising their self-esteem. The voices are experienced as life-enhancing and as an understandable aspect of their internal selves. A minority of voice hearers, 33 per cent in Tien's study reported distress or impairment of functioning as a result of voice hearing experiences (Eaton *et al.*, 1991). A minority of voice hearers experienced the voices as aggressive and negative from the onset. For these people the voices are hostile and they are not accepted as part of themselves. They suffer from negative voices that can cause chaos in their minds, demanding so much attention that communication with the outside world is extremely difficult. However, in most circumstances, voice hearing is manageable. Tien's research (1991) illustrated a voice hearing prevalence of 2.3 per cent among the general (non-clinical) population. If this figure is generalised across the entire UK population, about 1.3 million people would hear voices at any one time. It is evident that many/most of these individuals do not consult mental health professionals about their experiences as presumably they experience no distress or manageable distress as a result of voice hearing.

Interesting holistic and progressive work has been carried out in Europe with voice hearers in recent years. The pioneering and emancipatory work of Romme and Escher (1993) is to be applauded by anyone who wishes for psychiatry to approach mental health in a humane, sensitive and historically valid fashion. In the key words of this ground-breaking book, '*Accepting Voices . . .* is "a new analysis of hearing voices outside the illness model. This original research is a powerful challenge to popular stereo-types and psychiatric orthodoxy which inhibits rather than stimulates personal growth"' (Romme and Escher, 1993). For Romme and Escher, psychiatry has to move on from its biochemical obsessions and become a more life-enhancing and more empowering profession.

Marius Romme's decision to approach the issue of 'schizophrenia' and voice hearing in general in a new, yet old?, light was triggered by Patsy Hage, a Dutch psychiatric patient, who emphasised to Romme the reality of her voices. It was Hage, influenced by the writings of Julian Jaynes, who understood the historical context of hearing voices. Moreover, Hage had the controlled intelligence to, in effect, ask Romme, her psychiatrist, 'If you believe in the reality of God, someone whom you have not seen or heard, then why don't you believe in the reality of my voices?' In due course, Romme and Hage appeared on a popular television programme in Holland to talk and to encourage discussion about voice hearing. They got a huge and overwhelming response with 450 Dutch television viewers contacting the television programme stating that they were voice hearers. Most voice hearers, Romme was astonished to learn, had no contact whatsoever with psychiatry.

The Hearing Voices movement in Europe grew partly as a result of Romme's pioneering work with voice hearers in the second half of the 1980s. Today there are more than seventy-five Hearing Voices groups in the UK. Romme's person-orientated work with voice hearers in Holland paved the way for the published work of Paul Baker (1995, 1996) and Ron Coleman and Mike Smith (1997) in the United Kingdom. Similarly John Watkins (1996, 1998) in Australia takes the ramifications of Romme and Escher's work in Holland to a new audience in the Southern Hemisphere. Philip Thomas (1997) rightly calls for a more balanced dialogue between voice hearers and psychiatrists.

In the late twentieth century it could be argued that voice hearers are making a modest 'come-back'. Aidan Schingler, a voice hearer, held an exhibition of his three-dimensional 'schizophrenic' work at Durham Cathedral in August 1997. Ron Coleman, a voice hearer, has lectured extensively in Europe and North America on the issue of voice hearing. Neale Donald Walsch (1995), a voice hearer, produced international best sellers out of his early morning 'conversations with God'.

The struggle to 'normalise' voice hearing can be compared to the collective struggle of earlier decades to combat sexism, racism and homophobia in Britain. Barriers to understanding voice hearing include differences in perception, differences in concepts, different ideas about treatment, unawareness of personal history and lack of an awareness of the relationship between voices and everyday life (Romme and Escher, 1993, pp. 251–2). 'Resignation and fatalism are not the only available responses to hearing voices' (p. 255).

Myths and Facts About Voice Hearers

Many mental health professionals may have unhelpful stereotypes of voice hearers as a result of the media-induced panic concerning voice hearers and violence. This may prevent them challenging such unhelpful stereotypes among the general public, carers and even voice hearers themselves, so it may be useful to try and put the record straight:

(1) Approximately 95 per cent of homicides committed in Britain are committed by people who do not have mental health problems (Audit Commission, 1994).

(2)   The vast majority of people who use mental health services are not violent (ibid.).

(3)   Between 1974 and 1994 the rate of homicide doubled, yet there was no increase in homicides in the same period by people with mental health problems (ibid.).

(4)   In terms of homicide the general public is far more at risk from young men under the influence of alcohol than from people with a mental health problem (ibid.).

(5)   The random killing of a stranger by a psychotic individual is a rare occurrence (Royal College of Psychiatrists, 1996).

(6)   A person without a mental health problem is 400 per cent more likely to commit an act of homicide that a person with a mental health problem (ibid.).

(7)   15 per cent of people with a depressive illness commit suicide (ibid.).

(8)   10 per cent of 'schizophrenics' commit suicide (ibid.).

(9)   A person with 'schizophrenia' is 100 times more likely to commit suicide than to commit an act of homicide (ibid.).

(10) One is thirteen times more likely to be killed by a stranger without mental health problems than by a stranger with mental health problems (Department of Health, 1997).

How the Mental Health System Should Respond to Voice Hearers

Hearing voices is an historical phenomenon that dates to at least 10,000 BC (Jaynes, 1976). In early societies, voice hearers used to be significant individuals. Then after about 1300 BC, according to Jaynes, the view of voice hearing as evidence of spiritual phenomena began to change, and with it the status of voice hearers in society. People who hear voices have, of course, continued to influence society. Most voice hearers are not even in contact with psychiatric services (Tien, 1991). Reported presence of verbal hallucination is clearly not always indicative of mental disorder. Along with other providers of mental health service provision, psychiatry needs to adopt an approach of empowerment rather than control with regard to voice hearers. As many voice hearers have been significant writers, artists and musicians from history, I contend that it may be appropriate for mental health service provision in the United Kingdom to encourage musical, literary and artistic creativity in the mentally marginalised. The organisations Core Arts, Survivor's Poetry and Sound Minds of London undertake this kind of creative work with the mentally marginalised (Core Arts, 1999; Survivor's Poetry, 1999; Sound Minds, 1999).

It is now necessary for mental health service provision in Britain to adopt a more holistic and life-enhancing approach to voice hearing. This new approach should ideally involve historical, economic, personal, social, cultural, sexual and spiritual perspectives. If appropriate, it should involve a literary, artistic or even musical dimension as part of personal growth. Recent publications from the Mental Health Foundation, in the field of holistic consumer wishes (Mental Health Foundation, 1997) and complementary therapies in the alleviation of mental distress (Mental Health Foundation, 1998) are promising contributions to the amelioration of the position of the mentally ostracised, voice hearers included, in contemporary British society. There has been an enormous increase in the popularity of complementary therapies in recent years across society, and it could be that complementary therapies may be able to help those in severe mental distress (Wallcraft, 1999). Historically, voice hearers have sometimes been regarded as saints, prophets, geniuses, mystics, gurus and/or shamen within their societies. United Kingdom mental health service provision should approach the care and treatment of these individuals with an appropriate level of respect.

Suggested Reading

Coleman, R. and Smith, M. (1997) *Working With Voices*, Gloucester, Handsell Publications.

Jaynes, J. (1976) *The Origin of Consciousness in the Breakdown of the Bicameral Mind*, Harmondsworth, Penguin.

Romme, M. and Escher, S. (eds) (1993) *Accepting Voices*, London, Mind.

Thomas, P. (1997) *The Dialectics of Schizophrenia*, London, Free Association Books.

Tien, A.Y. (1991) 'Distribution Of Hallucinations in the Population', *Social Psychiatry and Psychiatric Epidemiology*, 26, 287–92.

References

Audit Commission (1994) *Finding a Place: A Review of Mental Health Services for Adults*, London, HMSO.

Baker, P. (1995) *The Voice Inside: A Practical Guide To Coping With Hearing Voices*, Gloucester, Handsell.

Baker, P. (1996) *Can You Hear Me?*, Manchester, Hearing Voices Network.

Carey, J. (1999) 'Paradise Lost' (Millennium Masterworks), *Sunday Times Culture Magazine*, 8 May, p. 10.

Coleman, R. and Smith, M. (1997) *Working With Voices*, Gloucester, Handsell Publications.

Core Arts (1999) Information Brochure, London, Core Arts.

Department of Health (1997) *Progress Report of the Confidential Inquiry Into Homicides and Suicides by Mentally Ill People*, London, HMSO.

Eaton, W.W., Romanski, A., Anthony, J.C. and Nestads, G. (1991) 'Screening For Psychosis in the General Population With a Self-Report Interview', *Journal of Nervous And Mental Disease*, 179, 689–93.

Frame, J. (1990) *An Autobiography*, London, Women's Press.

Jaynes, J. (1976) *The Origin of Consciousness in the Breakdown of the Bicameral Mind*, Harmondsworth, Penguin.

Joyce, G.C. (1920) *Old Testament Prophecy. Peake's Commentary on the Bible*, T. C. & E. C. Jack.

Mental Health Foundation (1997) *Knowing Our Own Minds*, London, MHF.

Mental Health Foundation (1998) *Healing Minds*, London, MHF.

Nasar, S. (1998) *A Beautiful Mind*, London, Faber & Faber.

Romme, M. and Escher, S. (eds) (1993) *Accepting Voices*, London, MIND.

Royal College of Psychiatrists (1996) Report of the Confidential Inquiry Into Homicides and Suicides by Mentally Ill People.

Sound Minds (1999) Information brochure London, Sound Minds.

Survivor's Poetry (undated) Information Brochure London, Survivor's Poetry.

Thomas, A. and Sillen, S. (1972) *Racism and Psychiatry*, New York, Brunner Manzel.

Thomas, P. (1997) *The Dialectics of Schizophrenia*, London, Free Association Books.

Tien, A.Y. (1991) 'Distribution of Hallucinations in the Population', *Social Psychiatry and Psychiatric Epidemiology*, 26, 287–92.

Wallcraft, J. (1999) 'Complementary Therapies' *Mental Health & Learning Disabilities Care*, 2(10), pp. 351–4.

Walsch, N.D. (1995) *Conversations With God: An Uncommon Dialogue*, Book 1, London, Hodder & Stoughton.

Watkins, J. (1996) *Living With Schizophrenia*, Melbourne, Hill of Content.

Watkins, J. (1998) *Hearing Voices: A Common Human Experience*, Melbourne, Hill of Content.

Wordsworth Poetry Library (1994) *The Works of William Blake*, London, Wordsworth Editions.

CHAPTER 3

Politics and Policies of Schizophrenia

STEVE WILLIAMS

Introduction

Government policy relating to the care and treatment of people with schizo-phrenia profoundly affects the services that are delivered to such people, and the space and creativity that grass-roots workers can occupy and utilise in the goal of collaborative health improvement. Historically, the policy framework concerning the care and treatment of people with schizophrenia has been influenced by a very narrow range of usually medical opinion (Scull, 1979). Indeed, the very acceptance of the concept of schizophrenia itself, as presently under-stood, is the result of the influence of such heavyweight, if particular opinion (and ambition) in this area of human activity. Whether such policy is the historic segregation of the mentally ill along with the incapacitated poor and vagabonds from the rest of the population and then the further separation from the employable poor into the vast 'specialist' state asylums, whose influ-ence in the mental health system is still experienced (in common with many mid-career mental health nurses, I was trained in a large asylum) or modern day attempts at social re-inclusion (DoH, 1999), failure to understand the policy emanating from the centre would be ill advised for those who must face its consequence as user of services, carer or worker. As well as understanding the policies and their implications, individuals who wish to see developments and improvements for people with schizophrenia must be prepared to try to influence such policy or leave the arena as the sole preserve of a narrow, self-interested, establishment perspective. A massive democratic deficit exists, whereby the people who actually use services, or have important carer's roles with people affected by schizophrenia and in many cases those charged with service delivery on the ground have struggled to get their viewpoint heard. Being informed about official policy and its general direction can help users, carers and grass-roots workers present cases about services that need to be developed for people with schizophrenia, take opportunities as they arise to improve services and challenge too often ill-informed middle management (and sometimes senior management) interpretations of government policy that may be unhelpful to people with schizophrenia and their carers.

Aims of This Chapter

Understanding the historic development of policy and practice and the current zeitgeist will not in itself democratise the mental health system, but without it such political progress will be impossible, and it is for this reason this chapter is included in this book and its consideration is recommended to those who work in, use or are affected by the mental health services. This short chapter aims to review the history of policy development towards the mentally ill, and spend some time considering contemporary policy and its implications. Near the end of this chapter is a checklist of developments that grass-roots workers can lobby for confident that such developments are policy congruent is provided.

The Development of Policy Towards the Mentally Ill

Perhaps the mentally ill, like the poor, have always been with us, but official policy towards them and attempts at their control or treatment are actually quite recent developments in terms of human history (Scull, 1979). Before the 1600s, people who were regarded as being mad, and quite possibly including people who would now be diagnosed as having schizophrenia or other psychotic conditions, lived among other people in their communities. From time to time they may have received attention from those communities, some of which may have been motivated by a desire to be supportive. The support that mentally ill people may have received would of course have been highly variable, and one perspective on the history of the development of policy towards the mentally ill from a mainstream psychiatric opinion cites a parish record stating '. . . a payment to the wardens for purchase of cord to bind a woman who was furiously mad . . .' (Freeman, 1993).

It was from the middle of the seventeenth century throughout Europe that the mentally ill began to be systematically segregated from the rest of society, along with the poor and criminal elements within the various 'houses of correction' established in the major centres of population. While historians differ in their interpretations of the motives in doing so across France, Germany and England during the same period, it appears clear from historical records that such institutions were concerned with the newly swollen numbers of people without work or other means of support to be found in degraded circumstances in most of the major cities. Before this period, it appears evident that the mentally ill (or 'the mad' to use the lexicon of the time) were not segregated from the rest of society in any official or systematic way.

> Confinement was an institutional creation peculiar to the seventeenth century . . . in the history of unreason it marked a decisive event: the moment when madness was perceived on the social horizon of poverty, of incapacity for work, of inability to

integrate with the group; the moment when madness began to rank amongst the problems of the city. (Foucault, 1967, pp. 63–4)

Treatment of the varied inmates of these new institutions generally involved work, which was meant to re-impose the sort of self-discipline evidently lacking in the poor, vagabonds and the mad. Of course, such work was also meant to help with the costs of maintaining such institutions, as well as being thera-peutic in itself. A further aim in establishing such institutions may have been to act as a deterrent to those who would not (or could not) work but per-sisted in begging. Marxist historians such as Scull (1979) have suggested that these institutions tried to generate within the inmates the qualities most suited to the new working methods and relations that were beginning to replace the age old agrarian traditions at least in the centres of population, that is, self dis-cipline and the work ethic.

Whatever the motives for the confinement of the poor and the mentally ill within institutions across Europe, there can be no doubt as to the huge growth in such institutions during the second half of the seventeenth century and the eighteenth century; on the eve of the French Revolution such institutions were to be found in 32 provincial cities, while in the UK there were 126 work-houses by the end of the eighteenth century, only one hundred years after the first was founded in Bristol in 1697.

Once the mentally ill had been identified as a problem and confined in this way, the social context in which approaches to their care and treatment would be framed had been established and continues to persist today.

Specialist Asylums and Moral Management

The British County Asylum Act of 1808 recommended the establishment of public speciality asylums for the mentally ill or insane. This was partly to offset the rising costs of caring for pauper lunatics who could not be managed within standard workhouses and were often transferred to private madhouses (Warner, 1994). Despite the encouragement, cajolement and frank punish-ment used by the workhouses to get their inmates economically active, many of the mentally ill inmates of these institutions could not gear themselves to the rhythms of the labouring day, whatever the rewards or punishments subsequent to such activity. They were of no value in the workhouse, unable to contribute to work to offset the costs of their 'care' and creating the wrong impression on important visitors and other inmates alike.

Conventional histories of psychiatry often begin at about this point, where enlightened medical men try and treat the mentally ill or insane in a humane and effective manner. Pinel's removal of restraints in Bicetre in Paris only one year after it had become an establishment purely for the insane and Tuke's establishment of moral management at the retreat in York are seen as such moments of enlightenment, even liberation. Foucault (1967) in his powerful critique of what Sedgewick (1982) has labelled 'public relations' versions of psychiatry reminds us that Pinel, Tuke and their contemporaries actually left the mentally ill still confined in the asylums, that demanding self-restraint on behalf of the mentally deranged person was meant to replace physical restraint (which was still available and even referred to as a last resort) and that moral management was much more available to the middle classes than the pauper lunatic.

Warner's (1994) political economy of schizophrenia refers to the fact that moral treatments appeared in different industrialised countries at about the same time, including Britain and France but also Italy and the United States, and suggests that the economic picture is most helpful for understanding this apparent coincidence. After the revolution in France, for example, the mentally ill were separated from criminals and other elements with whom they had been confined and were expected to be located in the areas where the labour force was lacking. His analysis basically suggests that whenever unemployment rates fall in advanced industrial economies, there is much more political interest in rehabilitating people otherwise fairly marginal to the productive process such as the chronically mentally ill. The relative costs of such rehabilitative ventures are offset against the benefits of returning the person to a productive economic life. The philosophies of the age reflect and are shaped by this economic imperative according to Warner, although advocates of moral or enlightened treatment may very well not be aware of this hidden process. A comparison is drawn by Warner of the values and ethos of the moral management epoch of the early 1800s with the social psychiatry movement after the Second World War, and these movements separated by one hundred years and more do appear to have several common values and features.

While moral management in the publicly financed institutions never matched the ideal as practised at the retreat and other privately financed institutions for middle-class patients, it did have a brief flowering. During the 1850s in England most of the county asylums had officially ended using physical restraints and staffing ratios seemed to be marginally improving. It has been suggested that such improvements were also motivated by the desire to legitimise the reduction of outdoor relief as part of the new Poor Law Commission policy, and that once legitimised the specialist asylums were expanded beyond their true utility in terms of size, and resources per inmate gradually cut back. Whatever the reason, by the mid 1860s moral treatment approaches were no longer available at most publicly financed institutions for the mentally ill.

Medical Power and the Mentally Ill

William Tuke who established the retreat in York was a retired tea merchant, and perhaps more importantly a Quaker, not a 'mad doctor' of any kind. Medical dominance in the realm of the care and treatment of the mentally ill was not established and little practised at this time. Medical ambition however, there clearly was, and in 1856 the General Medical Bill was finally passed by Parliament after several failed attempts. Counties had been required to provide asylums for the mentally ill since 1845 and most of Britain's asylums were built in the next 25 years, so the mentally ill and their care, treatment and control was an increasingly important area of concern, and potential professional status. This Bill can be seen to have established medical authority over deviant behaviour, and it is important to note that this was done in the complete absence of any evidence concerning medicines efficacy at treating such deviancy. Attempts were made at about this time and later, to describe and categorise the most extreme kinds of behaviour that the mentally ill exhibited, and these extreme kinds of behaviour became known eventually as schizophrenia. Such descriptions, including the very earliest work by luminaries such as Kraepelin, failed to meet normal scientific standards for claiming to have discovered or observed a medical disorder (see Chapter 1).

From this time until the present, medicine has had a huge influence over the care and treatment of mentally ill people, through the asylum years and on to the current era of community care. In its early days of dominion over the mentally ill, physical methods of treatment were preferred, consistent with the hypothesised aetiology of schizophrenia and the medical nature of psychiatry. Methods of treatment favoured by mainstream psychiatry over the decades have included ECT and more recently neuroleptic medication. The medical domination of the mentally ill has led to treatment and research paradigms which have understated the influence on the cause and outcome of psychosis of a wide range of psychosocial stressors including family environment (see Chapter 11) and social stressors such as the availability and structure of paid work, especially for working-class people (see Chapter 12) for example. This has even been the case when other treatment approaches have demonstrated high levels of effectiveness, such as with family intervention (see Chapter 11). Over-medicalising psychosis has contributed to a total lack of focus on the actual experiences of people with psychosis and their priorities;

> Another implication of the discourse on madness being left today in the expert hands of psychiatrists is the tendency to individualise what are social processes. Thus, for instance, in the never ending debate about more precise descriptions of schizophrenia and the endless search for the cause of this disease, the most important dimensions of the lives of mad people are underscrutinised. Most psychiatric patients in the community are poor, unemployed or unemployable, homeless or living in poor accommodation, exploited by government-funded landlords, and often sad, lonely and frightened. (Pilgrim, 1990, pp. 223–4)

Of course, other consequences of the over-reliance on medical paradigms to understand and treat psychosis have included the toxic effects of asylum living on the self-efficacy of people with psychosis, and the powerful and unwanted side effects of drug treatment including irreversible effects such as tardive dyskinesia (Day and Bentall, 1996). Mainstream accounts of the history of medical involvement with the mentally ill often make relatively light of iatrogenic disorders such as institutionalisation and tardive dyskinesia, and not infrequently make rather grandiose claims about neuroleptics emptying the asylums, discounting or downplaying the likely effect of changing social policy and full employment patterns (pre-dating the widespread prescription of neuroleptics) on discharge rates (Warner, 1994).

Psychiatrists are not alone in being implicated in the over-medicalisation of psychosis. Clinical psychologists (with some notable exceptions) have appeared content for most of their history to leave the field of psychosis to the psychiatrists, while they themselves concentrated on less intractable disorders such as depression and anxiety. This has recently changed, as several chapters in this book illustrate. Lay people too and society in general are also implicated, being too often unconcerned about what happened to marginalised people such as the mentally ill in the industrial age as long as it happened out of sight.

Contemporary Policy

While contemporary government policy towards mental illness in the United Kingdom has officially favoured community care over hospital treatment for over forty years, significant shifts in the policy emanating from the centre are still clearly detectable and significant for all involved in mental health services. The direction of change in mental health services has been clear since the 1950s and certainly since the 1959 Mental Health Act, which allowed for most mental illness treatment to be on a voluntary basis. The direction of change to community-based, local services and away from institutional care was finally enshrined in legislation in the 1975 White Paper *Better Services for the Mentally Ill* (DHSS, 1975). During the 1970s and the 1980s, there was a big growth in community orientated mental health resources, in particular of community psychiatric nurses. At the same time the closure programme of the large county asylums accelerated, and by the mid to late 1980s concern was being expressed that the needs of people with severe psychiatric problems and even disabilities were not being prioritised (Audit Commission, 1986).

Government reports and policies (Griffiths, 1988; DoH, 1991) attempted to address the needs of the most psychiatrically disabled people living in the community by improving the co-ordination and management of the diverse agencies and professional groups involved in mental health provision, sometimes by free-market inspired notions of competition for contracts, sometimes by concepts borrowed from the experience of mental health services in the United States. A return to the asylum was not on offer: mental health services had better learn how to care for vulnerable people living in the community, one way or another. *The Health of the Nation White Paper* was published in 1992 (DoH, 1992), and this document identified mental illness as one of the five key areas for action. Three primary targets were set for mental illness:

- To improve significantly the health and social functioning of mentally ill people;
- To reduce the overall suicide rate by at least 15 per cent by the year 2000;
- To reduce the suicide rate of severely mentally ill people by at least 33 per cent by the year 2000.

Guidelines were provided by the government to help health and other bodies meet these targets in the form of key area handbooks. The second edition of the handbook for mental illness (DoH, 1994) suggests that these targets can be met through using up-to-date treatment approaches including psychotherapies as well as 'improved physical treatments', changes in treatment settings (i.e. more community care and less asylums) and changes in working patterns (i.e. more multidisciplinary and cross-agency working and less fragmentation of services). There is no real emphasis in this document on social intervention in terms of the alleviation of social exclusion, poverty and unemployment playing any part in reaching these targets. The zeitgeist clearly perceived improvements in public health as being achieved by better uptake and utilisation of health technologies and clearer control and management (by way of market models) of mental health professionals/agencies. Mental illness is perceived as an individual problem requiring individual treatment approaches (including family intervention). Although the targets appear to be *public* health targets/ improvements, and although the link between social disadvantage/exclusion and poorer morbidity/mortality (including suicide) has been repeatedly and incontrovertibly established (Townsend, 1979; DHSS, 1980; Health Education Council, 1987), interventions in the social realm find no place in this policy. The influence of politics on policies and therefore on the lives of mentally ill people is evident.

In September 1999, the government published its National Service Framework for Mental Health (NSF) (DoH, 1999). Much more comprehensive in its aims than the three targets identified in the key area handbook referred to above, the NSF sets seven standards across the field of mental health. The standards are associated with mental health promotion, primary care/access to services, appropriate care and treatment for severely mentally ill people, the needs of carers and the prevention of suicide. Guiding values and principles are identified across these standards including:

- involving service users and their carers;
- delivering high quality and effective treatment in a non-discriminatory and accessible way;
- community safety (including staff and carers);
- promoting independence;
- well co-ordinated, publicly accountable and continuous services that empower and support staff.

Compared to the documents published in the 1990s, there is reference to 'social exclusion' both causing and being an avoidable consequence of mental health problems. Health and Social Services are expected to actively promote mental health, by working at the level of the individual *and* the community. The language of the market has gone, but services will be actively and closely monitored, according to this document, to ensure that they are delivering on this agenda. While 'quick fix' solutions are not part of what this document recommends (there is reference to a ten-year 'modernisation agenda'), progress is expected to be made against milestones to ensure that there is a truly national health service, and unacceptable variations in standards of service must be eradicated. While space precludes a full review of this important document, it is perhaps worth considering the milestones associated with the standards most *directly* relevant to the client group under discussion.

Standards four and five of the NSF are concerned with effective services for people with severe mental illness. The aim of these standards is to ensure that people with severe mental illness are adequately supported in the community and have access to a hospital bed (or equivalent) locally and without undue restriction. A series of milestones are identified which should indicate good progress towards the achievement of these standards, which include:

- protocols between primary care/specialist services concerning the management of people with severe mental illness (SMI);
- assessment and access arrangements in place for people with SMI in contact with criminal justice system;
- good and timely access to psychological therapies;
- access to and appropriate use of new anti-psychotics;
- full range of rehabilitation services (education, training, occupation, social support, supported housing) in place and accessible where indicated;
- early intervention, assertive outreach and crisis services available where indicated locally;
- assessment of full range of bed needs and investment planned to meet shortfall;
- reduction of bed occupancy rates (below 95 per cent) and out of area admissions.

Standard six is concerned with 'caring about carers'. Its aim is to ensure that those people who play important carers' roles for people with SMI have their needs assessed and where appropriate met by health and social services. Associated milestones for this standard include:

- identification of carers and assessment of their needs;
- development of a carers care plan;
- carers should have had the care plan for the person they provide care to explained to them, understand the nature of the illness and know how to contact services;
- carers should express satisfaction with services;
- carers should be involved in service review and development.

The NSF is clearly an important document for people who use mental health services, care for those that use them or work in them. Indeed, it is probably an important document for the public at large given the emphasis on common mental health problems and mental health promotion. While this document continues to describe approaches to the care and treatment of the historically marginalised (severely) mentally ill, it also describes approaches to mental health for the community at large. In that sense, it is a *public health* approach to mental health, and while it remains very concerned about the appropriate care, treatment and supervision of severely mentally ill people (not least from a public safety perspective), this is regarded as the bottom line. Once such services have been properly organised and provided, attention can be focused on people with less severe but distressing (and sometimes disabling) mental health problems. This document also makes reference to the imminent need for a root and branch review of the mental health legislation, suggests new arrangements for the management of mental health services (emphasising strong links with primary care and the value of specialist mental health trusts) and highlights the investment available in light of the changes required.

Policy Congruent Checklist of Potential Service Developments

- Social inclusion schemes and action (supported housing/vocational schemes).
- Comprehensive and coherent mental health services (assertive outreach/crisis teams/easy access to hospital beds).
- Access to hospital beds or respite (in area admissions/functional bed use).
- Staff empowerment (appropriate training and supervision).
- Partnerships with users and carers (shared care plans fully explained/involvement in service planning and development).
- Access to psychological therapies for users of services (without unacceptable delays).
- Education for carers (structured psycho-education).
- Identifying carers needs (by way of assessment and CPA).
- Access to new neuroleptics (where indicated by non-response/high side-effect profile).
- Standardised prescription regimes (minimising prescription regimes above those recommended).
- Early intervention services (utilising psycho-social interventions to minimise hypothesised 'secondary' disability).
- Developing competence of primary care team with people with psychosis.

Conclusion

An understanding of the history of policy development towards the mentally ill, and the motivations of such policy can help provide a context for the current zeitgeist. Understanding the current zeitgeist is a step toward empowering people who use mental health services, care for people with mental health problems or work in such services. Current official policy appears to offer real opportunity for comprehensive psychosocial treatment paradigms for the severely mentally ill. Historic analysis suggests that such opportunities for paradigm shifts in the understanding and treatment of mental illness occur for relatively short periods of time as a result of a particular set of economic and political circumstances. It is important that users, carers and workers who wish to endorse and support such paradigm shifts take advantage of such benign conditions while they exist. Courage will be required to overcome the tendency of human beings to assume that the current way of understanding and treating mental illness (or other social/political issues) is the natural or correct way (Wilkinson, 1996). Such assumptions may make policy and political progress much more difficult and should be resisted in the interests of open-mindedness and objectivity.

Suggested Reading

Department of Health (1999) *National Service Framework for Mental Health*, London, The Stationery Office.\

Foucault, M. (1967) *Madness and Civilization*, London, Tavistock.

Pilgrim, D. (1990) 'Competing Histories of Madness', in R.P. Bentall (ed.), *Reconstructing Schizophrenia*, London, Routledge.

Scull, A. (1979) *Museums of Madness*, London, Allen Lane.

Warner, R. (1994) *Recovery from Schizophrenia*, London, Routledge.

References

Audit Commission (1986) *Making a Reality of Community Care*, London, HMSO.

Day, J.C. and Bentall, R.P. (1996) 'Neuroleptic medication and the psycho-social treatment of psychotic symptoms: some neglected issues', in G. Haddock and P.D. Slade, *Cognitive-Behavioural Interventions with Psychotic Disorders*, London, Routledge.

Department of Health (1991) *The Health of the Nation*, London, HMSO.

Department of Health (1992) *The Health of the Nation White Paper*, London, HMSO.

Department of Health (1994) *The Health of the Nation: Key Area Handbook, Mental Illness*, London, HMSO.

Department of Health (1999) *National Service Framework for Mental Health*, London, The Stationery Office.

Department of Health and Social Security (1975) *Better Services for the Mentally Ill*, London, HMSO.

Department of Health and Social Security (1980) *Inequalities in Health; Report of a Research Working Group (The Black Report)*, London, HMSO.

Foucault, M. (1967) *Madness and Civilization*, London, Tavistock.

Freeman, H. (1993) 'The history of British community psychiatry', in C. Dean and H. Freeman (eds), *Community Mental Health Care*, Trowbridge, Gaskell.

Griffiths, R. (1988) *Community Care: Agenda for Action*, London, HMSO.

Health Education Council (1987) *The Health Divide*, London, HMSO.

Pilgrim, D. (1990) 'Competing Histories of Madness', in R.P. Bentall (ed.), *Reconstructing Schizophrenia*, London, Routledge.

Scull, A. (1979) *Museums of Madness*, London, Allen Lane.

Sedgewick, P. (1982) *Psychopolitics*, London, Pluto Press.

Townsend, P. (1979) *Poverty in the United Kingdom: A Survey of Household Resources and Standards of Living*, Harmondsworth, Penguin.

Warner, R. (1994) *Recovery from Schizophrenia*, London, Routledge.

Wilkinson, R.G. (1996) *Unhealthy Societies: The Afflictions of Inequality*, London, Routledge.

Part II
Clinical Skills

CHAPTER 4

The Helping Relationship

JULIE REPPER

Introduction

Although the literature on 'effective' interventions for people with schizo-phrenia is slowly increasing, there is a dearth of guidance for practitioners struggling with the day-to-day implementation of these specific approaches. In the current move towards evidence-based practice, emphasis on the *outcome* of different interventions has led to the neglect of accounts describing the *process* of their delivery. Central to this process is the relationship between mental health worker and service user. Indeed, the successful delivery of any intervention depends upon this relationship, yet little has been written about the development of helpful relationships with people who have serious mental health problems, or the effect of the relationship on service user defined outcome.

This chapter begins with some of the reasons why relationships with people who have serious mental health problems have been ignored; it goes on to explore the importance of the 'helping relationship' in the delivery of effec-tive support for people with serious mental health problems; it then draws on first person accounts to consider aspects of the relationship that are valued by services users; and finally, it discusses ways of making 'therapeutic' relation-ships accessible for people who have cognitive and emotional impairments.

Background

Until relatively recently, counselling and psychotherapeutic approaches had not been pursued with people who have serious cognitive and emotional difficul-ties. Traditionally, mental health professionals have been taught that it is at best pointless and at worst damaging to discuss symptoms with a schizophrenic client (Scharfetter, 1980). Yet, when the very phenomena causing the most distress is ignored, the potential for a trusting relationship is severely limited. As Campbell (1998) writes, from his experience as a service user, this is closely linked to the subordination of madness and disability within society as a whole:

> Is it possible to restore these people to full humanity when we actually fear their dif-ference so much and when they themselves secretly feel less than human? How can

you validate the mad when you are ignorant of their experience and ignore what they tell you about it?. . . If you do not recognise a central part of an individual except in terms of disease, it will be difficult for that person to be anything but of a different order to you, and of a lower order to you. (p. 246)

It has also generally been believed that because of their impaired mental state people with schizophrenia are unable to collaborate in a working relationship (Wolpe, 1958). If what they say is not worth taking seriously, then talking therapies are not worthwhile. If their views are seen as inconsistent, invalid and unrealistic, they need to be told what they want and how to achieve it. Deegan (1988) writes of the experience of being told repeatedly that recovery was not an option for her:

We were told that we had an incurable malady and that we would be 'sick' or 'disabled' for the rest of our lives. We were told that if we continued with recommended treatments and therapies we could learn to 'adjust' and 'cope' from day to day. (p. 13)

She goes on to describe her response to this: denial, despair and eventually largely self-inspired hope, culminating in her present recovery, and active campaigning for recognition of the capacity of all people with mental health problems to recover. But service users who do not go along with the diagnoses and prescriptions of their doctors can become locked into a 'catch-22' situation: they are deemed to have no insight if they disagree with their psychiatrist, yet in order to earn the 'gift' of insight, they have to submit to others' opinions, labels and treatments. Campbell (1998) writes:

The concept of insight – perhaps lack of insight would be more appropriate from the psychiatric perspective – is one of the most powerful and insidious forces eroding our position as competent creative individuals.

A further reason for the reliance on drugs, asylum and practical help rather than psychotherapy, lies in the way in which mental health problems have been understood. For many years, schizophrenia was conceptualised as a biological disorder which could only be treated by drugs, and which, by definition, would not be amenable to psychotherapy. During the late 1960s and the 1970s there was some interest in the effect of psychodynamic psychotherapy for schizophrenia, but since this approach achieved very little success (for reviews, see Gunderson, 1979; Gomes-Schwartz, 1984) it was rapidly discarded. A range of less intensive supportive psychotherapies, all of which rely on a therapeutic alliance between therapist and client achieved similarly unimpressive results – in terms of *professionally* defined outcomes – but confirmed the value that clients placed upon their relationship with the therapist. For example, Rogers *et al.* (1976) compared the process of client centred therapy with 'schizophrenic' and 'depressed' clients. They reported that whereas 'depressed' clients focused on self-exploration, the 'schizophrenic' client:

> seems to be seeking a relationship he can trust, and it is the therapist's potential as a trustworthy, caring person which appears important to him. (p. 76)

In a review of the literature on the helping relationship and the 'schizo-phrenic client', Goering and Stylianos (1988) suggest that the success of newer rehabilitative strategies with people who have schizophrenia is due to a com-bination of both 'technical' (behaviourally defined) and 'interpersonal' (relationship-based) variables. Client-centred/insight-orientated approaches alone are not successful (probably because they are too ambiguous and complex on a cognitive level), but psychosocial approaches that focus on the acquisition of skills and social competency are successful, not merely because they remedy psychological and social deficits, but because they provide a context in which a strong helping relationship can develop. In a structured, task/behaviour-orientated, 'here and now', reinforcement-based intervention (typical of those now termed 'psychosocial interventions') the client is not overwhelmed by the confusing type of therapy offered, and the therapist has a clear structure to work in. Thus, Goering and Stylianos (1988) conclude, the process of recovery may be due to the experience of the relationship pro-moted by the technique, as much as by the mastery of the new skills promoted by psychosocial interventions.

While this may be the case, it is also true to say that accounts of rehabilita-tive psychosocial interventions, while paying lip service to the need for a 'working collaboration', or the identification of 'mutually defined goals', rarely describe in any detail the relationship underlying the intervention. Through-out healthcare, the growth of 'evidence-based practice' has led to an empha-sis upon interventions that can be clearly defined, with measurable outcomes. Highly structured, behavioural interventions are far more amenable to defini-tion and measurement than such vague aspects of relationships as 'develop-ing a therapeutic alliance', 'inspiring hope', or 'exploring social opportunities'. Therefore fundamental components of valued and effective relationships have been ignored in favour of detailed descriptions of 'technical' aspects of care, and it is generally assumed that change is achieved through the acquisition of knowledge or skills, or modification of the environment rather than as a result of the relationship: the relationship is of secondary importance, and assumed to be relatively easy to develop. But it is possible that the nature and strength of the relationship that develops between the therapist and the client may be one of the most potent therapeutic ingredients of effective rehabilitative interventions. Certainly, the success of any work with a person who has mental health problems, whether it be assistance with the basics of day-to-day life, formal therapy, treatment or emotional support, depends upon the relation-ship we have with the person we are helping. And establishing a relationship, based upon a degree of trust and mutual understanding, with a person who has serious emotional and cognitive difficulties, is neither simple nor easy.

The Delivery of Effective Support for People with a Diagnosis of Schizophrenia

The importance of the relationship between worker and service user is clearly illustrated by research into psychosocial interventions for people with serious mental health problems. The high drop-out rates encountered in family work (Fadden, 1998) and the early CBT trials (Tarrier *et al.*, 1993) contrast markedly with the high levels of engagement reported in case management research (Ford *et al.*, 1995). Clearly engagement – relationship building – is an essential aspect of working with people who have serious mental health problems. Interventions can only be considered successful if they can be rendered acceptable to those who are deemed to require them. Chadwick *et al.* (1996) discuss in detail the problem of engaging clients with psychosis in cognitive behavioural therapy, and they propose a number of practical solutions and suggestions for overcoming the problems. Fowler *et al.* (1998) suggest that the key to providing successful CBT lies in establishing a psychotherapeutic relationship in which the client feels understood and involved, but concede that this may be problematic when there is an initial mismatch between client and therapist views:

> The solution involves a flexible approach to therapy which is sensitive to the client's beliefs and emotions and starts from the client's perspective. . . . The formation of a trusting relationship is the foundation stone for later work. (p. 126)

Birchwood *et al.* (1992) similarly examine the reasons for families' reluctance to engage in therapy and make recommendations for practice. As Fadden (1998) summarises:

> Much attention is paid at the start to establishing a collaborative, working relationship with all family members, including the person with schizophrenia. A positive, non-blaming attitude on the part of the therapist helps to establish a working alliance where the family and therapist together attempt to find new ways of coping and effective solutions to problems faced. (p. 116)

Despite the relatively high early drop-out rates, for clients who remain in treatment, CBT and family intervention are much more likely than case management to lead to improved symptoms and social functioning (to compare 'success' of different interventions, see Cochrane Collaboration reviews: Marshall *et al.*, 1997; Marshall and Lockwood, 1998; Mari *et al.*, 1996; Jones *et al.*, 1998). Evidently the most effective support comprises appropriate specific/'technical' interventions within the context of an engaging, support-ive and ongoing relationship.

This suggestion receives further support from the results of CBT research trials. Tarrier *et al.* (1998) compared clients receiving non-specific counselling with those receiving CBT. Both groups improved over the intervention period. Differences between the two groups only emerged at follow up, when clients who had received CBT maintained improvements and those who had received non-specific counselling deteriorated. It appears that the development of a warm trusting relationship between worker and service user is a *necessary* part of delivering effective support, but on its own, it is not *sufficient* to effect optimum and sustainable changes.

What Service Users Want From Their Relationship With Mental Health Workers

Service users are clear about what they want from services and what they find helpful and unhelpful in services. However, their accounts bear little resem-blance to the lists of interventions that professionals seek to provide in order to relieve symptoms and 'improve social functioning'. Rather, people who use services want: choice; accessibility; advocacy; equal opportunities; income and employment; self-help and self-organisation (Read, 1996). In a study of users' perceptions of their *unmet* needs, Estroff (1993) found the most common to be: an adequate income, intimacy and privacy, a satisfying sex life, meaningful work, a satisfying social life, happiness, adequate resources and warmth. The same themes were echoed in a study of what users wanted from mental health staff: better information and choice, more accessible help, and practical help with: income and benefits, finding employment; housing; daily living skills; childcare; and help in accessing appropriate specialist services (Duggan *et al.*, 1997). Shepherd *et al.* (1995) also found that service users and service providers had different priorities: users valued help to come to terms with their problems and assistance with housing, finance, social networks and physical health, while professionals placed greater emphasis on professional support, treatment and monitoring.

Clearly, if we are to provide helpful and meaningful support for people with mental health problems, we have to work *collaboratively*, towards *common* goals. The service user has to see some point in engaging in the relationship, and his or her self-defined needs and wishes need to be the starting point. It is unlikely that these will become apparent in a formal assessment meet-ing. Informal, frequent, contact with the service user in different settings, dis-cussions rather than interrogations, are likely to reveal a rich picture of them as a person – not merely a breakdown of their problems: their views, experi-ences, social networks and social life, self-concept, understanding of their problems, and aspirations. As Strauss (1994) describes, people's subjective experience of schizophrenia cannot be accessed by formal interviewing tools

---

Box 4.1   Summary of what service users say they want from services

- Information
- Choice
- Accessible services
- To be valued and treated as an equal
- Advocacy
- Practical help
- Equal opportunities
- Income
- Employment
- Housing
- Help with benefits
- Skills for self help
- Opportunity to develop an informed plan about the treatment and support that they would like to receive if they reach a crisis
- Close relationships
- Satisfying social life
- Childcare
- Physical health care

---

and rating scales; far more is revealed by open, flexible and informal contact.

This would appear to be confirmed by the results of a series of focus groups conducted to elicit users' and carers' views of the core competencies of mental health workers (IHCD for NHSE NW Office, 1998). They prioritised the values and attitudes of workers over 'technical' skills. Values that they listed included respect, optimism, ability to manage the power imbalance between users and professionals, belief in the value of a trusting relationship, ability to 'let go' of the service user, flexibility, openness, and the ability to work across traditional boundaries. It is these interpersonal skills that have been recognised in surveys of users' views about mental health nurses. Users of a rehabilitation service identified mental health nurses as providing practical help (cooking, cleaning, budgeting, dressing, bathing) caring (and continuing to care whatever they did), counselling (talking, chatting, social chit-chat), medication and liaison with other professionals (Meddings and Perkins, 1999).

Although these users did not consider their 'talk' with nurses to be particularly specialised, they did find it beneficial. This 'ordinary' talking was also valued in a survey of 516 people who had all been admitted to psychiatric hospital on at least one occasion (and 120, more than six times). Rogers and Pilgrim (1994) reported that nurses were viewed more favourably than other mental health professionals (32.4 per cent respondents said nurses had helped the most, and 59.4 per cent were either satisfied or very satisfied with nursing care). The quality of nursing care regarded most highly was talking, listening and ordinary relating; physical care and practical help; and, non-intervention or flexibility – tolerating some rule breaking. Interestingly, student nurses were preferred as they engaged in seemingly genuine empathic relationships.

While the manner in which the most effective help can be provided differs from relationship to relationship, Repper *et al.* (1994) identified four main principles of effective working relationships with people disabled by long-term mental health problems. In an in-depth study of clients and case managers working on four sites they identified four consistent themes in the development of relationships that service users valued: realism, taking a long-term perspective, a positive, empathic understanding of the client, and client-centred flexibility (see also Perkins and Repper, 1996). These principles provide a useful framework for exploring the development of effective helping relationships with people who have serious mental health problems.

Creating Effective Relationships

While it is essential to maintain hope, optimism and long-term aspirations, it is also important for workers to be *realistic* about the pace and nature of the change that can be expected. For some people maintenance of functioning may be a worthy goal, for others it may be possible to work slowly towards independent employment, for yet others, help to enhance their quality of life may represent a big change. People who have serious mental health problems may not make a steady improvement that continues to full recovery. Their ability to cope may fluctuate over time. They may experience periodic relapses, or they may deteriorate whenever they try to cope with a certain level of independence, or if they stop taking medication, but they need support throughout: an ally to recognise their achievements when they are succeeding and to provide a safe and positive response when things do not go so well. At times of crisis, it is often tempting for us to blame the client for failing, or to withdraw from the client in disappointment, or through a sense of having, ourselves, failed. But if we can be realistic about what might be expected, and if we can try to understand events by knowing the clients' beliefs and aspirations, then we may be better able to provide the continuity of relationship and confidence in them that they need. In addition, realism can help to stop demoralisation – on the part of service users and workers: if goals are realistic, targets are achievable, and reinforcement is built into steps that are meaningful and rewarding to the client, then failure is less likely to occur.

While the 'cure' based culture may not be as pervasive as a decade ago, the constant search for solutions and therapies that lead to discharge and independence can make service users and providers feel demoralised when they fail to realise this. In finding ways of remaining realistic, users' accounts of recovery can be helpful. Recovery does not mean that all suffering has disappeared, or that all symptoms have been removed, or that functioning has been completely restored. It is marked by:

> . . . an ever-deepening acceptance of our limitations. But now, rather than being an occasion for despair, we find our personal limitations are the ground from which spring our own unique possibilities. This is the paradox of recovery . . . that in accepting what we cannot do or be we begin to discover what we can be and what we can do . . . recovery is a process. It is a way of life. It is an attitude and a way of approaching the day's challenges. (Deegan, 1992, p. 8)

Linked to the need to be realistic about what might be expected, is the importance of *taking a long-term perspective* with people who frequently only develop trusting relationships slowly, over long periods. People with serious mental health problems frequently find it difficult to build relationships. They may experience voices and delusions which make them 'paranoid'; many have experienced neglect and abuse as children and young adults; and most people with long-term difficulties have suffered rejections and discrimination as a consequence of their mental health problems. Relationships with families, friends and employers have become distorted or lost, and they have often experienced a sense of failure within mental health services they have been referred to (and often rejected by) different supports when they 'failed to respond' in the expected manner (see Repper and Perkins, 1996; Repper *et al.*, 1998). They require a trusting relationship on a long-term basis, to have time to:

> break goals down into smaller steps, not to rush, to understand setbacks as just part of the 'journey', and to realise that 'what does not work today might work tomorrow. (Repper *et al.*, 1994)

Change can be very slow, and workers need to retain a confident and positive perspective when the client becomes demoralised and weighed down with multiple difficulties of seemingly insurmountable proportions. One of the difficulties for workers trying to maintain a long-term perspective is that clients have often been in the service longer than they have, and it is only if they are prepared to commit themselves to working in a service for several years that they can see the full extent of changes in the people using that service. Yet again, it is users who provide the most helpful accounts of learning to live for the day, valuing themselves as they are rather than striving to achieve impossible heights, accepting that there is time to try different strategies for coping (see Koehler and Spaniol, 1994).

In order to build a collaborative relationship with people who often have very different experiences of life, mental health workers have to be willing to explore the way they see their situation in a *positive and empathic* manner. This involves a genuine curiosity, a preparedness to listen non-judgementally, a belief in their rights and in the need to acknowledge their strength and address their aspirations. If we can understand their experiences and their views, it helps us to understand what sort of help they want – or why they might not want help at all. Campbell (1998) speaks of service users' need for 'reciprocity' and this is echoed in surveys of users' views. Rogers and Pilgrim (1994) found service users particularly valued being 'treated as an equal', people 'taking time to listen', demonstrating empathy and understanding. Similarly, Johnson (1995) reported that people seriously disabled by longstanding mental health problems clearly articulated the qualities that they valued most in staff: demonstrating 'genuine interest', talking to them 'as a person rather than merely about their mental state', 'sharing a sense of humour'.

Finally, Repper *et al.* (1994) found that *flexibility* was essential. People's needs change over time, they change their minds about what they want to do, they may want to try several different strategies at one time, and none at all at another.

> The worker therefore has to continually evaluate what the person needs on this particular occasion and how this can best be provided, treading the thin line between under-provision (or neglect) and over-provision (or deskilling the person), whilst allowing the client to guide the process by prioritising their needs and wishes. (Perkins and Repper, 1996, p. 49)

This is particularly pertinent in the implementation of CBT or family psychosocial intervention skills. In a recent evaluation of PSI training, Repper (2000) found that formal strategies were often difficult to implement with clients who were most disabled by cognitive and emotional impairments. When people were distracted by their voices or delusions, or when they were extremely anxious, trainees found it difficult to implement taught skills in a planned way. Rather, they had to tailor their support to the clients' needs on that particular occasion. This required adapting their skills sensitively: on some occasions it was possible to work on coping strategies for voices or delusions, on others it was necessary to sort out a practical – financial relationship or housing problem, on others it was necessary to provide a short supportive visit and arrange to visit again shortly. One of the most useful ways of demonstrating that a person's wishes and views are taken seriously is to undertake practical tasks that they consider important. Clients interviewed in the study of case management (Repper *et al.*, 1994) spoke of their ability to trust those workers who 'proved' their usefulness in simple practical ways: getting bills sorted out, helping them to write letters, getting the washing machine fixed.

It is essential that clients have some control over the support that they receive. They may not always be able to decide on the frequency or duration of visits, but given full information they can be helped to makes choices about the nature of support that can be provided. Service users are often most anxious about the decisions that others make for them if they deteriorate. Developing – and adhering to – an informed plan, an 'advance directive', about the treatment and support they would like if they reach a crisis, is a further way of enabling them to have control of their lives, particularly if this is coupled with active discussion of ways in which they can recognise and avert crises (Harris, 1999).

**Box 4.2   How to develop effective working
relationships with seriously mentally ill people**

- Start from the clients perspective
- Adopt a positive non-blaming attitude
- Maintain hope and optimism
- Be realistic about the pace of change that can be expected
- Be sensitive to the clients beliefs and emotions
- Adopt a flexible and collaborative approach
- Be prepared to offer simple practical interventions, for example getting bills sorted out
- Show warmth and understanding
- Accept that trust may only develop slowly
- Offer long term support
- Achieve a balance between support and offering specific skilled interventions

---

Making 'Therapy' Accessible

People who are seriously disabled by their mental health problems may find it difficult to cope with the expectations of specific therapy sessions. Getting there at the arranged time and date; concentrating for the required length of time; remembering what happened in the previous session; practising home-work as required and reporting on progress may present difficulties. Rather than deny therapy on the basis that they are not 'up to it', the therapy needs to be rendered accessible.

First, it may be unrealistic to expect a person with serious mental health problems to benefit from a time-limited, sessional therapy that is symptom-focused without establishing a trusting relationship and ensuring that other key aspects of their lives are stable. Hogarty *et al.* (1995) have developed 'personal therapy' in an attempt to overcome the limitations of specific intervention approaches. This is a staged treatment that aims to give individuals the awareness and coping strategies to control their symptoms, but the first phase is designed to develop a supportive relationship and stabilise external factors such as housing, benefits, medication and expectations of the family. This 'joining' phase lasts between three and six months and represents:

> the establishment of a therapeutic alliance that communicates an empathic under-standing of the patient's difficulties as well as hopefulness about the patient's recovery. (p. 383)

Second, if a person finds it difficult to organise themselves in relation to the world, it may be necessary to provide therapy in the person's home rather than

> ## Box 4.3 Adapting standard therapy for work with people with serious mental illness
>
> - Stabilise external factors that may be causing the person stress (e.g. housing, benefits, medication etc.)
> - Allow time for rapport and trust to develop
> - Consider offering therapy in the patients home
> - Adapt the length and frequency of sessions according the persons ability to maintain concentration
> - Be creative in developing approaches to help the person remember what has been taught in sessions and to apply self help strategies between sessions

expecting them to arrive at an office at a prearranged time. Alternatively, reminders, telephone calls, and/or help with transport might make it possible for them to get there – but it cannot be assumed that all people have a telephone in their house, or that they keep a diary of appointments.

Third, for some people the demands of a standard, hour-long, therapy session are too great. They may find the intensity of interaction distressing, they may become agitated and their symptoms may be exacerbated (Perkins and Dilks, 1992). Their ability to handle sessions may vary from week to week as their problems fluctuate. The therapist needs to be sensitive to signs that the individual is finding it difficult to cope, and be willing to take a break, stop the session, or change the nature of the demands placed upon the client.

Fourth, for those who find it difficult to remember previous sessions, or have problems practising skills discussed between sessions, it may be useful to write down or audio-tape record key points. Reminders stuck on the fridge, the door, or even upon particular objects that are causing disturbance may be helpful. With the client's approval, it can be helpful to involve a friend or family member to help practice coping strategies, or problem-solving skills. Interventions are more likely to be successful if others who spend time with the client are aware of what they are being taught, or the structure of sessions. While a weekly therapy session cannot ensure that a person eats, gets to work or has a bath, therapeutic interventions can be reinforced on an opportunistic basis by the people who are helping the individual get on with the necessities of life.

Conclusion

Services, approaches and interventions can only be successful, helpful or 'effective' if they are contributing to recovery. Service users describe recovery as a process of making sense of what has happened to them, reconstructing a positive identity, accepting, living with and growing beyond the limits of their mental health problems (e.g. Leete, 1989; Young and Ensing, 1999). This is not something that can be 'done to' a person, it is something that users must do for themselves: a deeply personal process that is unique to every individual; '. . . a matter of rising on lopped limbs to a new life' (Deegan, 1988).

Clearly being on the receiving end of mental health services is very different from administering them. Anyone seeking to define service users' experiences, categorise their symptoms, prescribe and evaluate their treatment might be seen as detracting from the proactive role of each individual in their own recovery. Yet, service users accounts do not discount help, rather, they illuminate the nature of support that best facilitates their own journeys. They do not define the role of mental health workers, rather, they characterise the values, attitudes, supports, facilities, and resources that they require – within and outside mental health services. Of paramount importance in the helping relationship is the mental health worker's belief in their capacity to recover – whatever the manifestation and seriousness of their problems; a willingness to be clear, honest and informative; a desire to learn from each individual what they feel, think and want; and, an ability to use this information in the manner most helpful to that person.

Further Reading

Egan, G. (1990) *The Skilled Helper: A Systematic Approach to Effective Helping.* Monterey, CA, Brookes Cole

Goering, P.N. and Stylianos, S.K. (1988) 'Exploring the helping relationship between the schizophrenic client and the rehabilitation therapist', *American Journal of Orthopsychiatry*, 58(2), 271–80.

Perkins, R.E. and Repper, J.M. (1996) *Working Alongside people with Long-Term Mental Health Problems*, Cheltenham, Stanley Thornes.

Young, S.L. and Ensing, D.S. (1999) 'Exploring recovery from the perspective of people with psychiatric disabilities', *Psychosocial Rehabilitation Journal*, 22, 219–31.

References

Birchwood, M., Cochrane, R., Macmillan, J.F., Copestake, S. and Kucharska, J. (1992) 'The influence of ethnicity and family structure on relapse in first episode schizophrenia', *British Journal of Psychiatry*, 161, 783–90.

Campbell, P. (1998) 'Listening to clients', in P.J. Barker and B. Davidson (eds), *Ethical Strife*, London, Arnold.

Chadwick, P., Birchwood, M. and Trower, P. (1996) *Cognitive Therapy for Delusions, Voices and Paranoia*, Chichester, Wiley.

Deegan, P. (1988) 'Recovery: The lived experience of rehabilitation', *Psychosocial Rehabilitation Journal*, 11, 11–19.

Deegan, P. (1992) 'The independent living movement and people with psychiatric disabilities: Taking back control over our own lives', *Psychosocial Rehabilitation Journal*, 15, 5–19.

Duggan, M., Ford, R., Hill, R., Holmshaw, J., McCulloch, A., Warner, L., Muijen, M., Raftery, J., Strong, S. and Wood, H. (1997) *Pulling Together: The Future Roles and Training of Mental Health Staff*, London, Sainsbury Centre for Mental Health.

Estroff, S. (1993) *Community Mental Health Services: Extinct, Endangered or Evolving?* Paper presented at the conference 'Mental Health Practices in the Nineties – Changes and Challenges', Silver Springs, MD, USA.

Fadden, G. (1998) 'Family Intervention in Psychosis', *Journal of Mental Health*, 7(2), 115–22.

Ford, R., Beadsmoore, A., Ryan, P., Repper, J., Craig, T. and Muijen, M. (1995) 'Providing the safety net: Case management for people with a serious mental illness', *Journal of Mental Health*, 1, 91–9.

Fowler, D., Garety, P. and Kuipers, L. (1998) 'Cognitive therapy for psychosis: formulation, treatment effects and service implications', *Journal of Mental Health*, 7, 123–33.

Goering, P.N. and Stylianos, S.K. (1988) 'Exploring the helping relationship between the schizophrenic client and the rehabilitation therapist', *American Journal of Orthopsychiatry*, 58(2), 271–80.

Gomes-Schwartz, B. (1984) 'Effective ingredients in psychotherapy: Prediction of outcome from process variables', *Journal of Consulting and Clinical Psychology*, 46, 1023–35.

Gunderson, J.G. (1979) 'Individual Psychotherapy of schizophrenia', in A.S. Bellack (ed.), *Schizophrenia: Treatment, management and rehabiliation*, Orlando, FL, Grune & Stratton.

Harris, A. (1999) 'Crisis avoidance', *OpenMind*, March/April, 12.

Hogarty, G., Kornblith, S., Greenwald, D., DiBarry, A., Cooley, S., Flesher, S., Reiss, D., Carter, M. and Ulrich, R. (1995) 'Personal therapy: A disorder relevant psychotherapy for schizophrenia', *Schizophrenia Bulletin*, 21(3), 379–93.

Institute for Health Care Development (IHCD) (1998) *Core competencies for Mental Health Workers*, NHS Executive Office North West.

Johnson, B. (1995) *Therapeutic attitudes: The client's perception*, unpublished research diploma dissertation, University of Nottingham.

Jones, C., Cormac, I., Mota, J. and Campbell, C. (1998) 'Cognitive behaviour therapy for schizophrenia', *The Cochrane Library*, 4 (26 August).

Koehler, M. and Spaniol, L. (1994) *Personal Experiences of Recovery*, Boston, Center for Psychiatric Rehabilitation.

Leete, E. (1989) 'How I perceive and manage my illness', *Schizophrenia Bulletin*, 15, 197–200.

Mari, J.J., Adams, C.E. and Streiner, D. (1996) 'Family intervention for those with Schizophrenia', in C. Adams, J. Mari and P. White (eds), *Schizophrenia Module of the Cochrane Database of Systematic Reviews*, Oxford, The Cochrane Collaboration.

Marshall, M. and Lockwood, A. (1998) 'Assertive community treatment for people with severe mental disorders', *The Cochrane Library*, London, BMJ Publications.

Marshall, M., Gray, A., Lockwood, A. and Green, R. (1997) 'Case management for people with severe mental disorders', *The Cochrane Library*, Issue number 3, London, BMJ Publications.

Meddings, S. and Perkins, R. (1999) 'Service user perspectives on the "rehabilitation team" and roles of professionals within it', *Journal of Mental Health*, 8, 87–94.

Perkins, R. and Dilks, S. (1992) 'Worlds Apart: Working with severely socially disabled people', *Journal of Mental Health*, 1, 3–17.

Perkins, R.E. and Repper, J.M. (1996) *Working Alongside People with Long-Term Mental Health Problems*, Cheltenham, Stanley Thornes.

Read, J. (1996) 'What do we want from mental health services', in J. Read and J. Reynolds (eds), *Speaking Our Minds*, Milton Keynes, Open University Press.

Repper, J. (2000) *Translating Policy into Practice: Evaluating a multidisciplinary training in psychosocial interventions for working with people who have serious mental health problems*, unpublished PhD thesis, University of Manchester.

Repper, J., Cooke, A. and Ford, R. (1994) 'How can nurses build trusting relationships with people who have severe and long-term mental health problems? Experiences of case managers and their clients', *Journal of Advanced Nursing*, 19, 1096–104.

Repper, J., Perkins, R., Owen, S. and Robinson, J. (1998) ' "I wanted to be a nurse . . . but I didn't get that far": Women with serious ongoing mental health problems talk about their lives', *Journal of Psychiatric and Mental Health Nursing*, 5(6), 505–9.

Rogers, A. and Pilgrim, D. (1994) 'Service users' views of psychiatric nurses', *British Journal of Nursing*, 3, 16–18.

Rogers, C., Gendlin, E., Kiesler, D. and Truax, C. (1976) *The Therapeutic Relationship and its Impact*, Westport, CT, Greenwood Press.

Scharfetter, C. (1980) *General Psychopathology*, Cambridge, Cambridge University Press.

Shepherd, G., Murray, A. and Muijen, M. (1995) 'Perspectives on schizophrenia: A survey of user, family care and professional views regarding effective care', *Journal of Mental Health*, 4, 403–22.

Strauss, J.S. (1994) 'The person with schizophrenia as a person II: Approaches to the subjective and complex', *British Journal of Psychiatry*, 164, (Suppl. 23), 103–7.

Tarrier, N., Beckett, R., Harwood, S., Baker, A., Yusopoff, L. and Ugarteburu, I. (1993) 'A trial of two cognitive behavioural methods of treating drug resistant residual symptoms in schizophrenia. I: outcome', *British Journal of Psychiatry*, 162, 524–32.

Tarrier, N., Yusupoff, L., Kinney, C., McCarthy, E., Gledhill, A., Haddock, G. and Morris, J. (1998) 'Randomised controlled trial of intensive cognitive behaviour therapy for patients with chronic schizophrenia', *British Medical Journal*, 317, 303–7.

Wolpe, J. (1958) *Psychotherapy by reciprocal inhibition*, Stanford, Stanford University Press.

Young, S.L. and Ensing, D.S. (1999) 'Exploring recovery from the perspective of people with psychiatric disabilities', *Psychosocial Rehabilitation Journal*, 22, 219–31.

CHAPTER 5

Case Management

IAN WILSON

Introduction

Case management has been defined as a process where a single person takes responsibility for maintaining a long-term supportive relationship with a patient, regardless of where the patient is and regardless of the number of agencies involved (Intagliata, 1982). Its function is to assist patients to identify, secure and sustain the range of internal and external resources they need to live as independent a life as possible in the community (Rapp and Kisthardt, 1991). There are similarities with the concept of a 'key worker' as described in *Building Bridges* (Department of Health (DoH), 1995) and at times the two terms appear interchangeable. This method of service delivery has proved to be particularly important in the configuration of services for those patients with severe and enduring mental health problems such as schizophrenia.

This chapter

- outlines the historical origins of case management;
- describes six models of case management, which incorporate the theoretical principles of this method of service delivery;
- presents a brief summary concerning the efficacy of case management;
- describes the role and function of a case manager;
- discusses how case management integrates into the day-to-day working of a team;
- examines future trends for case-managed services.

Historical Context

The origins of case management as a means of engaging and delivering care to people with severe and enduring mental ill health (SMI) can be found in the USA in the 1960s and the 1970s. The closure of the large state asylums and the subsequent de-institutionalisation of service provision for 'long stay' patients caused concerned clinicians to look for models of delivering continuous, comprehensive and flexible community care (Burns and Santos, 1995). The Community Mental Health Centre (CMHC) Construction Act (1963; USA) allowed for the development of local mental health centres (Bloom,

1984). Work in these centres led to a growing recognition among clinicians of the range of services required to meet the diverse needs of the mentally ill population. At the same time it became clear that patients with SMI were finding it increasingly difficult to access the services they required (Mechanic, 1991). Those patients with SMI, who had been largely cared for in the former institutions, were unable to advocate for their own needs, were reluctant to seek out psychiatric help and were difficult to engage and to keep track of when they did (Mueser *et al.*, 1998). In response to these factors, a new service function developed, that of case management which in turn evolved a new type of professional – the 'case manager'. Since its inception comprehensive and sophisticated models of case management have been developed which allow for the provision of clinical, social and rehabilitative services within the role.

Case Management in the United Kingdom

In the UK context, case management was advocated as a means of solving the problems of a fragmented and poorly co-ordinated service for patients with SMI living in the community (Audit Commission, 1986). By the end of the 1980s this approach became framed in the legislation *Caring for People* (DoH, 1990).

In order to minimise conflicts of interest, the guidelines emphasised that case managers should not be involved in the delivery of care, leading the way to the development of 'brokerage' models of service delivery. However, further legislation focused on the need for patients with SMI to receive more 'active' methods of case management (DoH, 1994), while the introduction of the Care Programme Approach further emphasised the need for adequately co-ordinated services. In *Building Bridges* (DoH, 1995) recommendations were made regarding the role of key worker for patients with SMI. This document acknowledged that this role is likely to be time consuming and intensive; the development of a therapeutic relationship, especially through the use of assertive outreach, is seen as essential and case loads are encouraged to be kept at 'manageable' levels, though what these should be in practice has been the source of much debate among both researchers and clinicians.

What is 'Case Management'?

The role and functions of case management have been discussed in depth by authors such as Onyett (1992) and Morgan (1993). Several authors have tried to summarise the concept of case management; here are two examples:

> Case management services are activities aimed at linking the service system to a con-
> sumer and at co-ordinating the various system components to achieve a successful

outcome . . . case management is essentially a problem solving function designed to ensure continuity of services and to overcome systems rigidity, fragmented services, mis-utilisation of certain facilities and inaccessibility. (Onyett, 1992)

A client level strategy for promoting the co-ordination of services, opportunities and benefits. The major outcomes of case management are; the integration of services and achieving the continuity of care. (Moxley, 1989)

The goals of case management include the enhancement of physical survival, personal growth and community participation; and recovery from, or adaptation to, mental illness. Case managers should ideally be involved in all aspects of their patient's physical and social environments, including housing, psychiatric treatment, healthcare, benefits entitlement, transport, families and carers and social networks (Kanter, 1989).

Models of Case Management

Although there is no universally agreed typology of case management (Marshall *et al.*, 1996), as this method of service delivery has developed in clinical practice so different models have developed. At least six separate models have been described (Mueser *et al.*, 1998) which will be briefly described below. Although all these models appear to share a common purpose, 'to help patients to survive and optimise their adjustment to the community' (Mueser *et al.*, 1998), they differ significantly in their clinical practice.

The Brokerage Model

The original case management model was the brokerage model. Here the primary functions are assessment of need, to refer the client to agencies in order to fulfil these needs, and co-ordinate, monitor and evaluate the input of these services. (Intagliata, 1982). This was in direct response to the perceived needs of patients who had to negotiate the complicated system of fragmented care which existed in the USA following the closure of mental hospitals. With this model there is an implicit expectation that groups of clinicians and services exist 'out there' (somewhere!) who are able to actually work with patients. This model is typically employed by case managers with large case loads who tend to have very little contact with their clients.

The Clinical Case Management Model

In response to the drawbacks of the purely brokerage model, the clinical case management model was developed to allow case managers to become actively involved as clinicians providing direct services (Harris and Bergman, 1988).

Their involvement has been described as offering services in the following areas:

- Engagement, assessment and planning;
- Environmental interventions; linking into community resources, consultation with family members and other carers;
- Maintaining and increasing social networks;
- Advocacy and communication with other professionals;
- Direct work with the patient, including:
  - individual 'talking' therapies;
  - training in independent living skills;
  - psycho-education.
- Monitoring of mental health and crisis intervention (Kanter, 1989).

The main departure from the brokerage model is the acknowledgement that the case manager has the skills to become a clinician in their own right (Mueser *et al.*, 1998).

Assertive Community Treatment (ACT)

This comprehensive, multidisciplinary team approach, with the teams themselves typically including nurses, occupational therapists, social workers and psychiatrists, aimed to provide all services *in vivo* (in the patients' own homes, or in 'community facilities' instead of in offices or hospital bases). The basic tenets of this approach include

- low patient to staff ratios (often put at 10:1 rather than the more usual 30:1 or even higher);
- team working of groups of patients rather than individual case loads;
- services delivered by the ACT team themselves instead of being routinely brokered out;
- time unlimited services – a commitment to work with patients over many years if necessary.

This model invariably employs assertive outreach and routinely offers a range of skills training in activities of daily living, management of medication and symptoms, support and education for families, along with 24-hour crisis support. The community team typically assumes full service responsibility for each patient.

There is a great deal of variation within services that call themselves 'ACT' teams, with some teams formally deciding to develop modifications to address the particular needs of their community or patient profiles. Other services find that local factors guide the development process which results in a dilution of ACT principles. This can happen by default due to financial restrictions in setting up the service and maintaining it, or by the reluctance of clinicians to change their roles in ways that reflect the needs of a community support system rather than more institutionalised models of care. There can also be wider political and societal barriers to implementation (Hoult, 1990). The variation in individual ACT teams creates difficulties when attempting to analyse the results of experiments into the efficacy of this kind of service delivery (Mueser *et al.*, 1998).

Intensive Case Management

The wish to address the perceived needs of patients who have ongoing complex needs and who consume large amounts of time and resources has led to the development of the intensive case management model (ICM) (Surles *et al.*, 1992). This model is designed to address the needs of patients who are hard to engage in community support but have frequent contact with emergency services. The ICM model employs low patient/staff ratios, utilises assertive outreach and offers practical assistance in daily living skills.

A major difference between the ICM and ACT models is that the former focuses on individual case loads rather than team management. ICM thereby can enhance engagement and continuity of care as well as limiting the amount of 'redundant' communication between team members, which can be anticipated in an ACT model, where clinicians often employ twice daily meetings to hand over patient information (Onyett, 1992). The drawback of ICM is the heavy responsibility borne by the individual clinician, with the resultant risk of 'burn-out' and feelings of lack of support resulting from isolation from other team members.

The Personal Strengths Model

The personal strengths (also known as the 'development-acquisition' model) identifies patients' strengths and focuses on their interests, abilities and competencies rather than their deficits, weaknesses and problems, as has often been the case with services in the past. The patient is viewed as the primary director of the helping process and all patients are believed to be able to change and grow. The relationship between the case manager and the patient is considered essential to the delivery of successful outcomes. An assertive outreach approach is invariably used to help promote effective engagement. Finally, the entire community is viewed as a valuable resource rather than an obstacle to success (Rapp, 1988).

The benefits of a strengths model approach include the establishment of goals agreed by the patient rather than imposed by the professional, leading to fewer traumatic and negative contacts with services and increased satisfaction with services (Rapp and Wintersteen, 1989).

The Rehabilitation Model

There is one final model of case management, the rehabilitation model (Anthony *et al.*, 1993). As with the personal strengths model, there is a strong emphasis on the wishes of the patient rather than those of the professional; however, by drawing up a comprehensive rehabilitation plan, based on a thorough assessment of the patient's goals and needs, there is a clear focus on addressing deficits in functioning, in turn improving the chances of the patient achieving successful community tenure. The case manager is expected to contribute the least possible input to achieve successful outcomes, thus promoting independence and autonomy.

Important Issues in the Process of Case Management

Engagement

The initial stage in the relationship between the client and case manager is, like any other relationship, a period of tentative and guarded interactions and responses. In these early contacts the aim of the case manager is to 'engage' the client in a collaborative therapeutic relationship, to demonstrate the benefit that the client can derive from continued involvement with the case manager.
    Elements of the engagement process include

- information regarding the service being offered; the service's account-ability to the person, the collaborative nature of the working alliance, the range of interventions available;
- an explanation of how the service may help the person create opportunities;
- a demonstration of the practical usefulness and reliability of the case manager (the achievement of a practical success at this stage cannot be overestimated);
- to make a genuine human contact with the patient on a personal level and show a degree of empathy with their situation.

When patients were asked to list elements they appreciated when engaging with a worker they said that a display of humour, a willingness to self-disclose, being able to show warmth, honesty, empathy and a genuine interest in the patient, helping with immediate tangible needs, being willing to meet out of the worker's office and trying to do 'fun' things together were what they were looking for (Sainsbury, 1995). Providing practical support *in vivo* can foster engagement while maintaining housing tenure. For instance, a patient whose house is unhygienic may be threatening his physical health, upsetting his neigh-bours and jeopardising his tenancy, all at the same time. Working alongside the patient to address this problem can often be extremely beneficial and has been cited as the type of intervention most appreciated by patients.

Case Vignette

Martin's first five years of contact with mental health services was charac- terised with violent, chaotic and self-destructive behaviour, frequent hospi- tal admissions following non-adherence to treatment and poor engagement with healthcare professionals. He had a reputation as a difficult and unpre- dictable person who had a poor prognosis.

He was transferred from a generic CPN's case load and assigned a case manager working within an intensive case management service. His guarded and sometimes hostile manner resulted in a lengthy engagement period. A breakthrough was achieved when he was introduced to the LUNSERS side-effect rating scale. Martin had been suffering from erectile dysfunction for some months and his case manager advocated on his behalf for a change in medication, which eliminated the problem. This initial tangible benefit had a positive effect on the therapeutic relationship. A warmer, more trust- ing relationship developed where informal and social activities became more frequent. Gradually, Martin began to discuss his residual psychotic symp- toms and standardised assessments were introduced, accepted and com- pleted. Further psycho-education sessions incorporating information about the stress-vulnerability model resulted in improved adherence to medication and agreement to participate in symptom monitoring and the implementa- tion of strategies to address auditory hallucinations.

This case vignette highlights the importance of taking a patient considered approach and working at a pace the client dictates. Martin only felt comfort- able to discuss auditory hallucinations nine months after the initial meeting, although this had been a continual problem, and after he had experienced tangible benefits of the relationship, for example, the elimination of his disturbing and embarrassing side effect.

Assertive Outreach

An important function of most intensive case management models is that of assertive outreach. It will often be necessary to consider some degree of assertive outreach when the potential consequences of loss of contact or non- engagement with the service are likely to be negative. Attempting to run a service where patients are not systematically contacted and followed up is likely to prove ineffective with patients who disengage rapidly from care. Clinicians have little or no scope to enforce adherence with treatment in the community. They must therefore develop strategies to win over users by engaging them on their own terms. This usually involves overcoming scepticism and mistrust. Many service users with high levels of need experience difficult contacts with professional mental health workers. It is often necessary to allow for periods of resistance and testing by reluctant users. Perseverance at this time can lead to an enhancement of relationships in the long term. Occasionally clinicians find themselves offering a service to a patient who consistently rejects that service. A judgement is made at this point regarding whether the person finds it hard to survive without the service and also whether they are able to make rational and realistic decisions. There are obvious implications about users' rights and the motivations of case managers who decide to override those rights. Issues of informed consent are a key feature in this context. Patients do have the right to make 'poor' decisions, but can real autonomy for patients be fostered in a climate of paternalistic or authoritarian service provision? If a case manager fails to continue assertively to engage a patient who is clearly in distress and confusion, could they be viewed as being negligent of their duty? Many assertive case management teams have strict protocols about assertive outreach. The refusal to engage with the service does not necessarily mean that the service is withdrawn. Rather, creative new approaches to foster engagement are consistently offered. However, there will always be individual patients who consistently refuse to engage with services no matter what. In practice, these patients sometimes end up undergoing compulsory admissions, often to secure accommodation. Alternatively, they end up in the prison system or move to other districts with no planned transfer of care and are effectively lost to services unless and until crisis occurs.

Functions of the Case Manager

There is broad agreement on the core components of the case managers role which Challis and Davies (1986), suggested were as follows.

Assessment

Assessment is a continual process that works on an informal level, for example, in unstructured discussions, or more formally using standardised assessment schedules. Working from the general, developing a 'life picture' of the person, to the particular, focusing on one discrete aspect of the person's life, like symptoms, social functioning or medication side effects, the case manager collects information which is used to direct the prioritisation of work or monitor progress. This process is not only concerned with identifying the patient's needs; the wishes and strengths of the patient, from both a psychological and environmental perspective, are essential pieces of information to be included in the package of care negotiated with the patient. Assessment information is only worthwhile if it is used in a collaborative process that empowers the patient as well as the case manager.

The types of standardised assessments used are numerous. They include global assessment of needs; assessment of symptoms (e.g. the KGV; Krawiecka *et al.*, 1977, modified by Lancashire, 1998); assessment of social functioning (e.g. The Social Functioning Scale; Birchwood *et al.*, 1990); medication issues (e.g. LUNSERS; Day *et al.*, 1995; Drug Attitude Inventory; Hogan *et al.*, 1983).

Planning

The information gained by assessment is used to prioritise work and select interventions. Working with the expressed needs of the client, work should be focused on problems which are clearly defined and amenable to measurement, for the purposes of evaluation. When goals are set they must be realistic and achievable. An important consideration in the planning process is the need to convey an appreciation of the long-term perspective; that some goals will take time to achieve, 'that setbacks are part of the journey . . . and what doesn't work today might work tomorrow' (Repper *et al.*, 1994). An over ambitious intervention programme increases the expectation to achieve targets. This in turn can result in feelings of stress, reduce the motivation to work towards a goal and expose the person to feelings of failure and personal helplessness in achieving change.

The 'Care Programme Approach' has placed the importance of co-ordinated services at the forefront of most services' planning requirements. However it is organised, it is only truly useful when it is developed collaboratively.

Direct Work With the Client

Undertaking work with the client naturally follows the assessment and planning process. Much has been written about interventions performed by case managers. The quality of interventions offered by individual workers is vital to the effectiveness of the service being offered. There has been a steady development of interest in the delivery of a range of psychosocial interventions for patients with SMI based on the stress-vulnerability model and incorporating cognitive behavioural family interventions, cognitive therapy for residual symptoms of psychosis and early warning signs packages. Training in these interventions through initiatives such as Thorn (Lancashire *et al.*, 1997), although essentially multidisciplinary in approach, has tended to focus on improving the skills of community staff and the majority of those trained have been community psychiatric nurses (Brooker *et al.*, 1994). There has been an emphasis on the development of case management as a vehicle to deliver these interventions and to configure services based on this approach. Case management appears the ideal framework to promote a psychosocial service. Its focus on working with patients in the long term, its explicit commitment to the engagement process and to the importance of the therapeutic relationship to enhance the delivery of care, and the clinical flexibility which allows time-consuming interventions such as family intervention to take place, are all easier to achieve within a case-managed service.

Other areas for direct interventions to be employed by case managers include medication management, housing needs, specialist benefit advice and strategies to work with patients who habitually use street drugs. Each of these interventions requires some degree of specialist knowledge and has training implications.

Review and Evaluation

The former is the method by which the case manager's role maintains continuity of service by tracking the work undertaken with the client and their support network. The latter measures the impact of services on the client's life.

Ongoing assessment of strengths and needs can indicate discrepancies between assessed needs and provision and missed opportunities by not utilising a new found strength. Shortfalls in service provision are also highlighted. Explicitly stated goals, personnel, and time-scales in the care plans provide a framework to review and evaluate a person's total service. Service reviews, involving key people and the client, should occur every six months, more often if necessary. The case manager plays a central role in these reviews, both in the presentation of information and in utilising information gained by the process. The case manager plays a vital role in evaluating whether or not an intervention has had positive and beneficial effects on the clients' life.

What Makes Case Management Effective?

Many research studies have investigated the efficacy of case management (for detailed reviews, see Holloway *et al.*, 1995; Mueser *et al.*, 1998; Burns and Santos, 1995).

The findings of Mueser *et al.*'s (1998) meta-analysis of 75 studies into the efficacy of case management are summarised in a Table 5.1.

Table 5.1 Meta-analysis of the outcomes of case management studies

Outcome area	Improved	No change	Worse
Time in hospital	14	8	1
Housing stability	9	2	1
Jail/arrests	2	7	1
Medication adherence	2	2	0
Symptoms	8	8	0
Substance abuse	1	5	0
Social adjustment	3	11	0
Vocational functioning	3	11	0
Quality of life	7	6	0
Patient satisfaction	6	1	0
Relative satisfaction	2	2	0

Source: Mueser *et al.* (1998).

Huxley (1993) identifies the following key features of successful case management services:

- a specific target group of clients;
- clear and specific objectives in relation to the outcomes of care
- a specific evidence based model of case management

For example – the resettlement of long-term residents of a psychiatric hospital (objective), who suffer from SMI (target group), using the rehabilitation model of case management (specific model), or work with clients with a dual diagnosis (specific target group) to maintain contact, and facilitate harm reduction (service objectives) using an ACT (specific model).

How Does Case Management Fit Into Team Working?

In order to implement a service adopting a case management system a number of complex issues need to be addressed. First, although cost effective as a means of service delivery (Nelson *et al.*, 1995) compared to standard care, it is still a costly form of treatment to implement initially. It has proved to be of particular cost effectiveness for those people who suffer from enduring and complex needs and frequently use hospital based services, conditions such as dual diagnosis or those at particular risk of harm to self or others. Therefore, targeting difficult to engage patients has been seen as an effective way of using case management as a service delivery system.

It is always problematic when attempting to adapt new methods of working from one healthcare system to another, and this has been true of case management. The successful examples of case managed services within the NHS have proved to be those that have not become bogged down with trying to implement models such as ACT or personal strengths in a wholesale way. Instead, the successful examples of case management have been eclectic in their design, tailoring their services to fit into existing services and resources, as well as utilising the existing skills of their workers in ways that have empowered and supported them.

The establishment of an intensive case managed service aimed at patients with SMI can cause problems with existing services. There is a natural reaction to any new model of care by existing services and there is the possibility that some clinicians will see it as a criticism of their own care. This negative reaction can be intensified if it is decided to 'graft on' case managers to existing community services, where clinicians tend to have had generic case loads and high numbers of patients. Case managers may find themselves having to constantly justify their protected case load size and their time consuming efforts to engage with clients while 'traditional' style CPNs continue to manage large and often extremely complex case loads of their own.

Further problems arise when questions of admission and discharge occur. In a truly autonomous ACT team it has been required practice for that team to assume complete control over all admissions and discharges. In an ideal situation this has led to these teams assuming full responsibility for staffing their own acute admission beds. In practice within the NHS this has seldom proved possible. Instead, case managers must become sophisticated at developing working relationships with the wider service and often have to prove themselves to medical and in-patient nursing teams before they can expect clinicians to trust their judgements or show a willingness to work flexibly with them.

Conclusion

As Marshall (1996) states, case management in the UK is not just an intervention; rather it is a government policy. He goes on to describe the Care Programme Approach as having developed standard case management for all, regardless of level of need or clinical priorities. This cogent criticism of the way services have been generally structured reflects an under-resourced and heavily bureaucratic community care system. It should not, however, detract from the positive aspects of well-resourced and targeted assertive community services, of which there are a number of fine examples throughout the country. It is clear that there is not one single 'perfect' community care model to suit all service settings. Developing hybrid models to reflect the needs of particular areas and patient groups is a possible way forward to make the most of available resources. However, whatever the structure of the service, it is possibly of secondary importance when compared to the relationship that develops between the patient and the case manager. Research suggests that patients themselves place their relationships with workers above any consideration of service structures (Solomon and Draine, 1994). There is yet to be conclusive proof that the patient case manager alliance can actually contribute to the outcome of interventions in terms of improving social functioning or reducing symptoms. Despite this, case management of patients with SMI allows workers to engage with their patients in long term relationships. This enables the uptake of a range of innovative and creative psychosocial interventions which can give clinicians, patients and their families hope for the future.

Further Reading

Brooker, C. and Repper, J. (eds) (1998) *Serious Mental Health Problems in the Community: Policy, Practice and Research*, London, Bailliere Tindall.

Morgan, S. (1993) *Community Mental Health: Practical Approaches to Long-term Problems*, London, Chapman & Hall.
Onyett, S. (1992) *Case Management in Mental Health*, London, Chapman & Hall.
Stein, L.I. and Santos, A.B. (1998) *Assertive Community Treatment of Persons with Severe Mental Illness*, New York, W.W. Norton.
Burns, T. and Guest, L. (1999) 'Running a Assertive Community Treatment Team', *Advances in Psychiatric Treatment*, 5, 348–55.

References

Anthony, W.A., Forbess, R. and Cohen, M.R. (1993) 'Rehabilitation Oriented Case Management', in M. Harris and H. Bergman (eds), *Case Management for Mentally Ill Patients: Theory and Practice*, Chur, Switzerland, Harwood Academic.
Audit Commision (1986) *Making a Reality of Community Care*, London, HMSO.
Birchwood, M., Smith, J., Cochrane, R., Wetton, S. and Copestake, S. (1990) 'The Social Functioning Scale, The Development and Validation of a New Scale of Social Adjustment for Use in Family Intervention Programmes with Schizophrenic Patients', *British Journal of Psychiatry*, 157, 853–9.
Bloom, B.L. (1984) *Community Mental Health: an Introduction*, Belmont, CA, Brooks Cole.
Brooker, C., Falloon, I., Butterworth, A., Goldberg, D., Graham-Hole, V. and Hillier, V. (1994) 'The Outcome of Training Community Psychiatric Nurses to Deliver Psychosocial Interventions', *British Journal of Psychiatry*, 165, 222–30.
Burns, B.J. and Santos, A.B. (1995) 'Assertive Community Treatment: An Update of Randomised Trials', *Psychiatric Services*, 46, 669–75.
Challis, D.J. and Davis, B.P. (1986) *Case Management in Community Care*, Aldershot, Gower.
Day, J.C., Wood, G., Dewey, M. and Benthall, R.P. (1995) 'A Self Rating Scale for Measuring Neuroleptic Side Effects', *British Journal of Psychiatry*, 166, 650–3.
Department of Health (1990) *Caring for People – Community Care in the Next Decade and Beyond*, London, HMSO.
Department of Health (1994) *Working in Partnership – Collaborative Approach to Care*, London, HMSO.
Department of Health (1995) *Building Bridges*, London, HMSO.
Harris, M. and Bergman, H.C. (1988) 'Misconceptions About The Use of Case Management Services by the Chronically Mentally Ill: A Utilisation Analysis', *Hospital and Community Psychiatry*, 39, 1276–80.
Hogan, T.P., Awad, A.G. and Eastwood, R. (1983) 'A Self Report Scale Predictive of Drug Compliance in Schizophrenics', *Psychological Medicine*, 13, 177–83.
Holloway, F., Oliver, N., Collins, E. and Carson, J. (1995) 'Case Management: A Critical Review of the Outcome Literature', *European Psychiatry*, 10, 113–28.
Hoult, J. (1990) 'Dissemination in New South Wales of the Madison Model', in I.M. Marks and R. Scott (eds), *Mental Health Care Delivery: Innovations, Impediments and Implementation*, Cambridge, Cambridge University Press.
Huxley, P. (1993) 'Case Management and Care Management in Community Care', *British Journal of Social Work*, 23, 365–81.

Intagliata, J. (1982) 'Improving the Quality of Community Care for the Chronically Mentally Disabled: the Role of Case Management', *Schizophrenia Bulletin*, 8, 655–74.

Kanter, J. (1989) 'Clinical Case Management: Definitions, Principles, Components', *Hospital and Community Psychiatry*, 40, 361–8.

Krawiecka, M., Goldberg, D.P. and Vaughan, M. (1977) 'A Standardised Psychiatric Assessment Scale for Rating Chronic Psychiatric Patients', *Acta Psychiatrica Scandanavia*, 55, 299–308. Modified by Lancashire (1998).

Lancashire, S. (1998). *The KGV(M) Symptom Scale Version 6*, unpublished paper, University of Manchester.

Lancashire, S., Haddock, G., Tarrier, N., Baguley, I., Butterworth, C.A. and Brooker, C. (1997) 'The Effects of Training in Psychosocial Interventions for Community Nurses in England', *Psychiatric Services*, 48, 39–41.

Marshall, M. (1996) 'Case Management: a Dubious Practice', *British Medical Journal*, 312, 523–4.

Marshall, M., Gray, A., Lockwwod, A. *et al.* (1996) 'Case Management for People with Severe Mental Disorders', in C. Adams, J. Anderson and M.J. de Jesus (eds), *Schizophrenia Module of the Cochrane Database of Systematic Reviews*, Oxford, Update Software.

Mechanic, D. (1991) 'Strategies for Integrating Public Mental Health Services', *Hospital and Community Psychiatry*, 42, 797–801.

Morgan, S. (1993) *Community Mental Health: Practical Approaches To Long-term Problems*, London, Chapman & Hall.

Moxley, D.P. (1989) *The Practice of Case Management*, London, Sage.

Mueser, K.T., Bond, G.R., Drake, R.E. and Resnick, S.G. (1998) 'Models of Community Care for Severe Mental Illness: a Review of Research on Case Management', *Schizophrenia Bulletin*, 24, 37–74.

Nelson, J., Sadelar, C. and Cragg, S.M. (1995) 'Changes in Rates of Hospitalisation and Cost Savings for Psychiatric Consumers Participating in a case management Program', *Psychosocial Rehabilitation Journal*, 18, 113–23.

Onyett, S. (1992) *Case Management in Mental Health*, London, Chapman & Hall.

Rapp, C.A. (1988) *The Strengths Perspective of Case Management With Persons Suffering from Severe Mental Illness*, NIMH, University of Kansas, cited in S. Morgan (1993), *Community Mental Health Practical Approaches to Long-term Problems*, London, Chapman & Hall.

Rapp, C.A. and Kisthardt, W.E. (1991) 'Bridging the Gap Between Principles and Practice', in S.M. Rose (ed.), *Case Management and Social Work Practice*, New York, Longman.

Rapp, C.A. and Wintersteen, R. (1989) 'The Strengths Model of case management: Results From Twelve Demonstrations', *Psychosocial Rehabilitation Journal*, 13, 23–32.

Repper, J., Cooke, A. and Ford, R. (1994) 'How can nurses build trusting relationships with people who have severe and long-term mental health problems? Experiences of case managers and their clients', *Journal of Advanced Nursing*, 19, 1096–104.

Sainsbury Centre for Mental Health (1995) *Community Support for Mental Health – Module 5: Engagement and Relationships*, London, Sainsbury Centre.

Solomon, P. and Draine, J. (1994) 'Satisfaction with Mental Health treatment in a Randomised Trial of Consumer Case Management', *Journal of Nervous and Mental Disease*, 182, 179–84.

Surles, R.C., Blanch, A.K., Shern, D.L. and Donohue, S.A. (1992) 'Case Management as a Strategy for Systems Change', *Health Affairs*, 11, 151–62.

CHAPTER 6

Neuroleptic Drugs and Their Management

NEIL HARRIS

Introduction

Neuroleptic drugs, also called antipsychotic drugs, are the mainstay treatment for schizophrenia. This type of drug is prescribed in acute episodes to control the distressing positive symptoms, hallucinations, delusions and thought interference and when given long-term for maintenance therapy its role is to prevent relapse. The importance of neuroleptic medication and its role in relapse prevention has been well established (Davis, 1975). However, a significant number, 30–40 per cent of people suffer relapses despite taking neuroleptics (Leff and Wing, 1971).

Within many models of case management the management of this medication is an important role. For mental health professionals to be effective in this role four conditions need to be satisfied:

- acquisition of knowledge about neuroleptics;
- skills of assessment and interventions used in comprehensive medication management;
- the development of a way of working which places the sufferer at the centre of the treatment process;
- the ability to culture a therapeutic relationship with the sufferer.

Historical Perspective

The development and introduction of neuroleptic medication in the 1950s has had an important effect on the treatment and management of people with schizophrenia. Before this people were subjected to bizarre treatments such as insulin-coma therapy, hot and cold baths, and revolving chairs. The introduction of neuroleptics can be seen as a significant factor in enabling a more liberating regimen in the care of the mentally ill. They have been seen as important in facilitating the change of focus from in-patient to community care; reducing the duration of in-patient care and the frequency of relapse.

Types of Neuroleptic Medication

Recent descriptions of neuroleptic medication form two main categories; conventional or classical neuroleptic (the older generation of neuroleptics) and 'atypical' neuroleptics, the newer preparations. Since their development in the 1950s and '60s conventional neuroleptics are the main treatment for schizophrenia. They can be administered orally or by long-acting injection. The major difficulty with these drugs is the wide range of side effects they can produce at the same dose levels that produce positive therapeutic effects. Some clients' experience of side effects can be as distressing and debilitating as the positive symptoms they replace, so compromising the benefit the drugs have in controlling the illness. Atypical neuroleptics are more recently developed medications and can be seen as a breakthrough in the treatment for schizophrenia. Some doctors advocate their direct replacement of conventional neuroleptics (Kerwin, 1994). Relative to conventional neuroleptics, atypicals are more expensive, however, taking a long-term view, these initial costs are offset by the overall cost reduction brought about by improvements in the course of the illness, requiring fewer in-patient days (Thomas and Lewis, 1998, Grey *et al.*, 1997). Compared with conventional neuroleptics they produce side effects at a much reduced level. More specifically, extra-pyramidal side effects are not usually observed at clinically effective doses. However, side effects are not eliminated completely and new problems can be brought about by their prescription.

How These Drugs Work

To understand how these drugs work we need to look at the biochemical theories about the causation of schizophrenia. To understand the biochemical theories we need to know a little about how the nervous system works.

Messages are sent to different parts of the brain by bundles of nerve cells or neurons. There can be a chain of neurons connecting one site of the brain to another. The neurons are not connected physically and the space between them is called the synaptic gap. The message continues its journey across this space by using a chemical link – *neurotransmitter*. Several different neurotransmitters have been found. In the 'receiving' neuron the messages carried by the neurotransmitters, are specialist 'receptors'. A number of these receptors have been identified; they are known as, D_1, D_2, D_3, D_4.

The consensus view is that an overactivity of the 'dopamine' neurotransmitter, caused by either abnormal dopamine production, increased release of dopamine from nerve endings or increased numbers or sensitivity of dopamine receptors, is involved in the development of schizophrenic symptoms – the dopamine hypothesis of schizophrenia. A number of nerve tracts have been found to use the dopamine neurotransmitter. In two of these tracts, the *mesolimbic* and *mesocortical* pathways are thought to be implicated in schizophrenic symptoms. Disturbance in the mesolimbic system can produce a reduction in a person's ability to selectively attend to incoming environmental stimuli. Damage to the *limbic* system, sometimes called 'the seat of emotion', can result in hallucinations, disturbed thoughts and emotions as well as paranoia and self and perceptual distortions (Warner, 1994).

Neuroleptic medication, such as chlorpromazine and haloperidol (conventional neuroleptics), block the transmission of the nerve signal to the dopamine receptors; the drugs are said to be dopamine antagonists. The problem is, that while the neuroleptic blockades D_2 receptors in the mesolimbic system, improving psychotic symptoms, it is also blockading D_2 receptors in other parts of the central nervous system, such as the *striatum* and *substantia nigra*, causing the production of extra-pyramidal side-effects. The drugs are not targeted towards the specific receptors which produce positive therapeutic results but blanket blockade of many receptors.

Another neurotransmitter, serotonin or 5-hydroxytryptamine (5-HT), abundant in the central nervous system, has been implicated in the effectiveness of the newer neuroleptic medications. It has an influence on levels of arousal, the sleep-wake pattern and mood. Again several receptor sites have been identified for serotonin – $5HT_1$, $5HT_2$, $5HT_3$, etc. It is the ability of these newer medications, for example clozapine, olanzapine, and risperidone, to bind with a range of the dopamine and sertonin receptors that results in reduced levels of extra-pyramidal side effects and, unlike the conventional neuroleptic, have been seen to have a positive effect on negative symptoms.

Pharmacokinetics

There can be a wide variation in the effect a drug can have on different individuals. Many factors contribute to this variation – age, weight and constitution, diet and smoking, alcohol and caffeine intake (Hubbard *et al.*, 1993) as well as interactions with other drugs. Following administration of a single dose of medication a tenfold difference in blood level can be measured (Silverstone and Turner, 1991). It can be seen, therefore, that the effect a drug has on a person is not a matter of dosage alone.

The subjective view a person has regarding the action of the drug is of considerable clinical significance. A person's experience of individual preparations and the effects of dose changes become important considerations in making treatment decisions, thus emphasising that treatment must be planned in collaboration with the sufferer.

Side Effects of Neuroleptic Medication

Neuroleptic drugs produce a wide range of adverse effects, which can sometimes be viewed by the sufferer as more troublesome than the symptoms they are prescribed to treat. These side effects affect many bodily systems and people can experience them in a mild form but they can be severe, and physically and socially disabling. All of these drugs cause side effects.

Following is a brief overview of the main neuroleptic side effects.

Extra-pyramidal Side Effects (EPSE)

This group of side effects is divided into four main groups: dystonia, akathisia, psuedo-parkinsonism, and tardive dyskinesia:

Dystonia

A sustained contraction of muscles, usually of the head and/or neck but can occur in any muscle. Abnormal movements that can accompany this reaction are not uncommon. When the condition affects muscles of the eye it is known as *oculogyric crisis*. Acute dystonic reaction can last for several hours if not treated.

Akathisia

Twenty per cent of people receiving neuroleptics experience this symptom (Braude *et al.*, 1983). The symptom is characterised by feelings of inner restlessness and the compulsion to move. Some people have described this feeling as though they want to 'jump out of their skin'. Typical restless movements can accompany these feelings and include rocking from foot to foot, walking on the spot or pacing up and down. When the person is sitting they may shuffle their feet or 'tramp' them up and down. In severe cases the sense of inner restlessness can cause the sufferer to feel extremely disturbed and agitated.

Pseudo-parkinsonism

Stiffening of the limbs, tremor of the hands, and/or head, and a mask-like facial expression represent the core symptoms of this side effect. In addition people can experience an increase in salivation. Akinesia is part of the pseudo-parkinsonism syndrome. It includes reductions in spontaneous movements, speech, and motivation. People with this symptom have been described as apathetic and sufferers themselves have described their feelings as becoming 'dulled'.

Tardive Dyskinesia (TD)

A syndrome characterised by involuntary movements usually restricted to the face and neck but sometimes extends to the trunk and limbs. It has been reported to occur in approximately 20 per cent of people taking conventional neuroleptic medication (Brown and White, 1991). Usually the side effect is mild, non-progressive and reversible, however, for some people the condition progresses to a distressing and irreversible state. At this level of severity the syndrome can affect walking, breathing, eating and talking.

Autonomic Effects

Postural hypotension can occur with associated dizziness. Sedation can be marked.

Anticholinergic Effects

Symptoms of this classification of side effects may be present, and include stomach upset, constipation, dry mouth, blurred vision, and difficulty in passing water.

Sexual Side Effects

Sexual side effects can affect both men and women and it has been reported that up to 60 per cent of people prescribed conventional neuroleptics can experience sexual side-effects (Mitchell and Popkin, 1982).

Weight Gain

A common effect with neuroleptics is weight gain, up to 80 per cent of people treated with chlorpromazine put on weight (Bazire, 2001/02). Atypicals can cause weight gain, with olanzapine between 10–40 per cent of people can put on up to 12 kilograms (Bazire, 2001/02).

Dysphoria

Several reports describe the distressing feelings people experience when taking this type of medication; a dysphoric response. People complain of feeling dull, unable to think, with a permanent hangover. Feelings of being slowed down in body, thought and reduced drive. Clients can distinguish these feelings from depression and anxiety and attribute them to the neuroleptic. The side effect is dose related.

Neuroleptic Malignant Syndrome (NMS)

This is a rare but potentially fatal adverse effect. The condition includes muscular rigidity, raised temperature, fluctuating levels of consciousness and fast pulse. An estimation of 1 per cent of all people who take neuroleptic medication develop NMS (Cohen *et al.*, 1985). The condition must be treated as a medical emergency, treatment stopped, and in-patient care for observation is necessary.

Agranulocytosis

Is a rare and potentially fatal blood disorder, which reports have suggested affect 1 in 300,000 people taking conventional neuroleptics. This risk is increased to 1–2 per cent for people taking Clozapine. This risk is offset by a rigorous blood-monitoring process.

Neuroleptic Induced Deficit Syndrome (NIDS)

NIDS is a recently coined name given to a group of neuroleptic side effects which, as the term suggests, combines effects which reduce the person's social, behavioural and cognitive functioning. These would include the symptoms of akinesia, dysphoria, and the subjective feelings associated with akathisia (Lewander, 1994).

What Works Best?

Clozapine, an atypical neuroleptic, has been shown to be the most effective neuroleptic in treating both positive and negative symptoms (Clozapine Study Group, 1993). It has been demonstrated that between 30–60 per cent of 'treatment-resistant clients' can benefit from clozapine when treated for up to one year (Kane, 1992) with most clients responding within six months (Morrison, 1996).

All of the other neuroleptics are as equally effective as each other, the choice of drug, therefore, is governed by the response of the individual. The client and care team need to be prepared to try alternative drugs until the 'right' one is found – that which achieves the therapeutic goal with the minimum of adverse effects.

Treatment Strategies

There are many factors taken into account in deciding a treatment regimen: route of administration, drug, dose, use of poly-pharmacy, discontinuation, adjunctive medication and reducing dosage. No consensus has been agreed regarding optimum dosage and length of treatment in maintenance therapy shows wide variability.

The practice of poly-pharmacy; the prescription of more than one neuroleptic, is not uncommon in clinical practice. Prescribing more than one neuroleptic can produce a cumulative adverse effect (Pratt, 1998) and is not recommended (BNF, 1999). There are exceptions when this is acceptable, for example, when changing from one drug to another.

Successful drug regimens are a product of discussions and observations. It may be the case that a person has been successfully managed on a regimen of conventional neuroleptics which have not produced any side effects; in this case the person can continue on this prescription (Thomas and Lewis, 1998).

Ten per cent of people diagnosed as suffering from schizophrenia, who are not prescribed neuroleptics, do not relapse in the five years following their last episode (Kissling, 1992), although identifying these people is problematic. In keeping with the principle that sufferers should be prescribed the least medication they need to remain relapse free, two strategies have been investigated; continuous low dosage and intermittent or targeted treatment (Schooler, 1993).

In continuous low dosage people are given lower doses in relapse prevention treatment than during an acute episode. Symptoms are easier to treat if a person is receiving a small dose of medication rather than none at all and the dose can be increased when symptoms or early warning signs appear and then reduced when they subside.

Targeted or intermittent treatment is based on the idea that people only need treatment during periods when they are experiencing symptoms or when early warning signs emerge.

Both these strategies carry more risk of relapse than with more conventional strategies, more so the targeted treatment strategy. There are many circumstances when a client may be seen to be unsuitable for either of these strategies. For example, in the case of targeted strategy, some of the factors which would deem a person unsuitable for this regimen would include those who exhibit dangerous behaviour during relapse or those who are unwilling or unable to play an active part in the treatment process and monitoring of symptoms. The adoption of these strategies requires a high level of service commitment with staff that are skilled in the techniques needed for these strategies.

Many drug regimens are supplemented with additional types of medication, often referred to as adjunctive medication. Most commonly anticholinergic medication, for example benztropine (Cogentin) or procyclidine (Kemadrin) is prescribed to treat side effects. Lithium and Carbamazepine have also been advocated in treatment. Anti-depressants have been used and although their use has been associated with the re-emergence of psychotic symptoms, for clients who are considered 'stable' this is rare (Siris, 1993).

Relapse prevention treatment is a complex and difficult process. Many factors need to be taken into account in finding the correct medication and in identifying the nature of the presenting clinical picture. For example, the following case study illustrates one of the difficult clinical circumstances found during the process of management. This case reflects a perplexing presentation of signs and symptoms and the intricate and overlapping syndromes that can be present. These symptoms could suggest the person is depressed and/or agitated, or may reflect a syndrome of negative schizophrenic symptoms, or they may be a combination of side effects of neuroleptic medication – 'NIDS'.

Case Study

Fred had his first and only acute episode of schizophrenia when he was 48 years-old. His paranoid symptoms were brought under control with Chlorpromazine 400 milligrams (mgs) a day. Over the next four years his medication continued to be adjusted and was stabilised on:

- Faverin 50 mgs twice a day;
- Amitryptyline 50 mgs at night;
- Depixol 60 mgs intramuscularly, fortnightly;
- Procyclidine 10 mgs intramuscularly with the depot injection;
- Procyclidine 5 mgs daily for four days following the injection.

He was adherent to his prescribed medication. His wife 'supervised' its administration.

Initial work with Fred concentrated on completing a comprehensive range of assessments. The results were given to Fred and with his permission, to Jane his wife. Medication was targeted as a priority area.

Education regarding his illness and medication was given to both Fred and Jane. This was undertaken in their home in an interactive, question and answer format and took several weeks to complete. Updates and recaps of information were given at regular intervals and they were encouraged to introduce difficulties, questions and queries as they arose. Fred's mental state enabled him to give consent for the treatment. Discussions including his treatment history and mental state generated a lot of useful information:

- Fred's medication history indicated many instances of sensitivity to neuroleptics; a test dose of 12.5 mgs of Depixol had left him suffering with high levels of extra-pyramidal symptoms, so bad that his wife had thought he had had a stroke. A prescription of sulpiride had resulted in high levels of sedation.
- There had been an absence of positive symptoms since the initial acute episode.
- LUNSERS side effect rating scale revealed a high level experience with side effects.
- The education process resulted in Fred and Jane prioritising medication as the initial target for intervention and their aim was to reduce the number of medications prescribed and achieve a lower dose.

As a result of this information, and supported by effective family intervention, a formulation was agreed:

Fred's high sensitivity to neuroleptic medication leads to high side effect profile and decreased social functioning. A staged reduction in neuroleptic dose with continuing education sessions, goal setting, and work with early warning signs, together with a comprehensive programme of assessment and monitoring, will improve Fred's side-effect profile and increase his level of activity.

Clear about their treatment goal Fred and Jane asked the keyworker to communicate the information to his consultant. At the following out patient appointment the results of assessment and rationale was provided and the wishes of Fred and Jane were explained. Details of the treatment plan were discussed and finalised. The current regimen includes

- Risperidone 4 mg/day;
- Amitriptyline 50 mg at night.

Staged changes and reductions in medication were monitored. Early warning signs (see Chapter 10) were identified and built into a package of standardised assessments including, mental health state, social functioning and side-effects. Goal planning enabled Fred to become involved in the domestic running of the house and he slowly gained interest in an old hobby. Subjective reports from Jane report he has become more alert and the 'twinkle in his eye has come back'. Fred reports that he feels more motivated and his thoughts were again 'flowing freely'. Score on the Social Functioning Scale (Birchwood *et al.*, 1990) shows an improvement, KGV psychopathology assessment (Krawiecka *et al.*, 1977) shows a continued absence of positive symptoms and reductions in the symptoms associated with a negative syndrome; flattened affect, psychomotor retardation. Depression has moved from mild to sub-clinical level. However mild symptoms of orofacial tardive dyskinesia were present. His side effect profile had been reducing, demonstrated by repeated assessment with LUNSERS. Subjective reports from Fred and Jane indicate that previously low levels of activity and social functioning have improved as the medication has reduced.

In this case evidence suggested that side effects were implicated in Fred's problems. By trying different medications and reduction in dosage improvements have been made. If depression had been diagnosed he may have been inappropriately prescribed anti-depressants, alternatively assigning these observations as negative symptoms may have attracted the use of PSIs, or considered as permanent long-term deficits. This complex clinical presentation takes time to tease out.

Adherence

Given the importance of neuroleptics in preventing relapse adherence to medication is an important area in schizophrenia, non-adherence is often cited as a major contributor to relapse and mental health crisis (Kissling, 1992).

Evidence suggests for people suffering from schizophrenia the rate of non-adherence is 50–80 per cent (Kane, 1985; Bebbington, 1995). The reasons why people do not take prescribed medication are various.

Personal factors including, attitude, and understanding of the illness, cultural and personal beliefs, symptoms and level if insight and cognitive impairment. The influence of family and friends have an impact. There are issues regarding the medication itself, such as exposure to side effects, their effectiveness with symptoms and complicated and lengthy regimens. Factors within the care team have an influence on adherence, relationships between client, prescriber and case manager, exclusion from treatment decisions, various aspects concerning treatment setting and a negative attitude to the disorder and its treatment.

Principles for Practice

The principles of good practice in long-term neuroleptic therapy can be brought under two main headings. These principles will be given here along with their implications for intervention.

Principle 1

> For those people who derive a benefit from medication, it should be prescribed at the lowest possible dose needed to achieve the optimal therapeutic effect, that is, relapse prevention

As the role of medication changes in the transition between acute treatment and relapse prevention, adjustments can be made to the medication prescribed or the dose. It may be recognised that clients who have achieved a stable mental state may benefit from a reduction in dose. However, there are difficulties in adjusting drug dosages.

- Decisions regarding dosage are difficult when a client is clinically stable as the dose cannot be titrated against a clinical response (Marder, 1992)
- There is great variability in the pharmacokinetics between individuals prescribed – what dose suits one person may not suit another – a drug regimen is an individually tailored prescription
- There is a great variability in the time between a person discontinuing medication and the onset of acute illness; taking up to six months – therefore, reducing the medication to what is, in effect, a sub-therapeutic dose may not be detected for some time.
- Side effects such as tardive dyskinesia and akathisia can begin to emerge as dosage is reduced, as neuroleptic and anticholinergic medication can 'mask' the symptoms. If the possibility of this is not expected it can cause the person, family and care staff to think that the person's mental state is deteriorating as a result of the dose reduction

There are many areas of work that can provide information that can help to overcome these difficulties and minimise the risk:

Maintain Accurate Records of Medication Prescription

- Include the types of medication, dosage and frequency, and details about the reasons why medication is prescribed, changed or discontinued. The best guide to what medications are effective is previous medication history.

Undertake Appropriate Assessments

- *Continuous informal assessments*, to look at things like, for example, physical and environmental conditions, changes in attitude, lifestyle changes. Information gathered here could be important in the selection of drug and issues related to adherence.
- *Standardised assessments:*
  - ○ Mental Health Assessment – Regularly and accurately assessing a persons mental health state is of vital importance in the process of titrating a dose down to its optimal level or in developing a treatment rationale for dosage reduction. Global psychopathology assessments such as the KGV (Krawiecka *et al.*, 1977) can be used. Case managers need to be trained to use this measure. For assessment or monitoring of specific symptoms other tools can be used, such as the Hospital Anxiety and Depression Scale (HADS) (Zigmond and Snaith, 1983), and Calgery Depression Scale (Addington *et al.*, 1993). This last assessment the Calgery Depression Scale has been specially developed to detect depression in people who have a diagnosis of schizophrenia. It can prove useful in differentiating between depression, negative symptoms and NIDS.
  - ○ Assessment for neuroleptic side-effects – The LUNSERS (Day *et al.*, 1995) provides an overview of a persons experience of side effects. This self-rating scale gives an overall score, reflecting a persons experience of side effects. It can further highlight particular troublesome side-effects or side-effect groups. This might then prompt the assessment of these side effects with a more specific tool such as, the Abnormal Involuntary Movement Scale (AIMS) (NIMH, 1975), a scale for Extrapyramidal symptoms (Simpson and Angus, 1970), or a scale for akathisia (Barnes, 1989).

Attend to Physical Health

Ensure that the person has a physical check-up every twelve months and keep a general check on physical health and attend to complaints of physical illness.

Make the client aware of possible drug interactions with over-the-counter medication.

Use Early Warning Signs

- Work with the person, and their family if appropriate, to identify and utilise their early warning signs of a deteriorating mental health state (see Chapter 10). Monitoring for these signs as a formal intervention can enable reduction in doses or increases in medication should signs of relapse emerge. Successful work in this area can offset the risks associated with low dose drug strategies if this was considered to be the best treatment option available.

Use Interventions that Minimise Non-adherence

Interventions aimed at improving adherence should be undertaken when the client is in receiving an adequate, effective and safe medication regimen.

- Attend to complaints of side effects. Advise and assist the person to min-imise side effects. Many side effects are dose related, dosage can be reduced without a loss in therapeutic effect.
- Counteract the problems of forgetfulness by linking the administration of oral medication to specific times of the day. Seek to administer oral medication at once a day. Utilise buzzing pill boxes and dosette boxes.
- The provision of information regarding the persons condition and treatment.

Principle 2

> Treatment is a collaborative process between the client, the prescriber and the case manager/keyworker, facilitated through a genuine and trusting relationship

The development of a long-term, trusting relationship has been described as 'central' to the process of facilitating client's understanding and involve-ment in their treatment and engagement in strategies that enable successful management.

The call for clients to become active participants in the planning and devel-opment of their treatment and care packages has been detailed in many reports, policy documents and guidelines (DoH and RCN, 1994; DoH, 1994, 1996, 1999). These documents support the position that a genuine, trusting and collaborative therapeutic relationships between members of the multidiscipli-nary team and the client is not only desirable but will improve care and sig-nificantly contribute to the goal of client autonomy. Central to the position of autonomy, the individual's right to self-determinism, the right to choose and make decisions about their lives, is the concept of informed consent.

In the majority of cases consent will be uncontested, but a small number of cases will require a thorough examination of the relevant circumstances. The client's subjective views about medication effects are important in the decision-making process regarding the prescription of drugs, therefore, agreeing to take medication appears to be the essence to successful treatment. The process of consent should be seen as a necessary precursor to the successful development of the therapeutic alliance, may positively affect the client's adherence to treatment, and contributes to the client's increase in self esteem, and feelings of personal control (Brabbins *et al.*, 1996).

Weighing the balance between the risks and benefits of taking medication is sometimes a difficult decision to make. The fundamental questions involved in the decision a person makes regarding taking this form of treatment include;

- What is their illness history – frequency and nature of acute episodes?
- What effect does taking the drug have on the person's life?
- Do they feel they derive a benefit from taking the medication?

Consent

One of the fundamental aspects for the prescription of treatment, and one of the most difficult and controversial, in the context of schizophrenia, is that it is given on the basis of 'informed consent'. The *Guidelines for Mental Health and Learning Disabilities Nursing* (UKCC, 1998) states *the nurse*

. . . has three overriding professional responsibilities with regard to obtaining consent

1. *the nurse* must, acting in the best interest of the client, obtain consent before *s/he* gives treatment or care;
2. ensure that the process of obtaining consent is rigorous, transparent and demonstrates a clear level of professional accountability;
3. all discussions and decisions relating to obtaining consent must be recorded accurately.

These responsibilities can be extended to all disciplines acting as case managers and it would seem that, in adopting this principle the case manager has a substantial role in ensuring that the issue of informed consent is addressed. Discussions regarding who should obtain consent from the client should take place between the prescriber of medication and case manager.

The components of obtaining consent consist of three elements; the provision of information, the absence of duress in the decision-making process, and a judgement regarding an individuals competence to give consent.

Medication and PSI

Neuroleptic medication and PSIs are complementary, interactive, treatments and as such case managers need to give sufficient attention to both areas. To concentrate on PSIs alone may undermine the positive effects these interventions can confer. To embark on a programme of PSIs, without ensuring that sufficient input has been undertaken to establish the client's optimum medication regimen, can have an impact on the effectiveness of the interventions, for example, certain anticholinergic medications can impair memory, affecting a person's capacity to learn. Lower doses of neuroleptic medication may facilitate the client gaining the full benefit of PSIs as a result of reduced levels of secondary negative symptoms and side effects associated with the concept of NIDS (Liberman *et al.*, 1998).

Conclusion

The process of medication management is complex and time consuming. It entails the case manager developing an understanding and knowledge regarding the medication itself, the ability to assimilate this information with respect to individual clients and provide evidence to support the prescription of beneficial medication regimens. In carrying out this role the mental health worker needs to adopt a sensitive approach in dealing with issues relevant to this area of work. For example, although it is considered safe to inform clients about tardive dyskinisia, imparting this information after the person has been taking the medication for a prolonged period can cause alarm or anger in clients or their relatives (Chaplin and Kent, 1998).

The individual variability found in drug treatment and the changes that can occur in the process of consent necessitate that the approach is continuous and long term.

Further Reading

Bazire, S. (2001/02) *The Psychotropic Drug Directory*, Salisbury, Quay Books.
Harris, N. (1998) *Long-term Neuroleptic Treatment and the Role of the Community Mental Health Worker*, Salisbury, Quay Books.
Harris, N., Lovell, K. and Day, J.C. (in press) 'Long-term Neuroleptic Treatment and Informed Consent', *Journal of Psychiatric and Mental Health Nursing*.

References

Addington, D., Addington, J. and Maticka-Tyndale, E. (1993) 'Assessing Depression in Schizophrenia: The Calgery Depression Scale', *British Journal of Psychiatry*, 163 (suppl. 22), 39–44.
Barnes, T.R.E. (1989) 'A Rating Scale for Drug-Induced Akathisia', *British Journal of Psychiatry*, 154, 672–6.
Bazire, S. (2001/02) *Psychotropic Drug Directory*, Salisbury Quay Books.
Bebbington, P.E. (1995) 'The Content and Context of Compliance', *International Clinical Psychopharmacology*, 9 (suppl. 5), 41–50.

Birchwood, M., Smith, J., Cochrane, R., Wetton, S. and Copestake, S. (1990) The social functioning scale: the development and validation of a scale of social adjustment for use in family intervention programmes with schizophrenic patients *British Journal of Psychiatry*, 157, 853–9.

Brabbins, C., Butler, J. and Bentall, R. (1996) 'Consent to Neuroleptic Medication for Schizophrenia: Clinical, Ethical and Legal Issues', *British Journal of Psychiatry*, 168, 540–4.

Braude, W., Barnes, T. and Gore, S. (1983) 'Clinical characteristics of Akathisia: A systematic investigation of acute psychiatric inpatient admissions', *British Journal of Psychiatry*, 143, 139–50.

British National Formulary (BNF) (1999) British Medical Association and Royal Pharmaceutical Society of Great Britain, 38.

Brown, K. and White, T. (1991) 'The Psychological Consequences of Tardive Dyskinesia: The Effect of Drug-Induced Parkinsonism and the Topography of Dyskinesic Movements', *British Journal of Psychiatry*, 159, 399–403.

Chaplin, R. and Kent, A. (1998) 'Informing patients about Tardive Dyskinesia', *British Journal of Psychiatry*, 172, 78–81.

Clozapine Study Group (1993) 'The safety and efficacy of clozapine in severe treatment-resistant schizophrenic patients in the UK', *British Journal of Psychiatry*, 163, 150–4.

Cohen, B., Baldessarini, R. and Pope, H. (1985) 'Neuroleptic Malignant Syndrome', *New England Journal of Medicine*, 313, 163–6.

Davis, J. (1975) 'Overview: maintenance therapy in psychiatry – 1 schizophrenia', *American Journal of Psychiatry*, 132, 1237–45.

Day, J., Wood, G., Dewey, M. and Bentall, R. (1995) 'A self rating scale for measuring neuroleptic side-effects; validation in a group of schizophrenic patients', *British Journal of Psychiatry*, 166, 650–3.

Department of Health and the Royal College of Nursing (1994) *Good Practice in the Administration of Depot Neuroleptics*, London, DoH/RCN.

Department of Health (1994) *Working in Partnership. A Collaborative Approach to Care*, London, HMSO.

Department of Health (1996) *Building Bridges: A guide to arrangements for interagency working for the care and protection of severely mentally ill people*, London, HMSO.

Department of Health (1999) Modern Standards and Service Models – National Service Frameworks, London, The Stationery Office.

Grey, R., Gournay, K. and Taylor, D. (1997) 'New Drug Treatment for Schizophrenia: Implications for Nursing Practice', *Mental Health Practice*, 1, 20–3.

Hubbard, J., Midha, K. and Hawes, E., *et al.* (1993) 'Metabolism of phenothiazine and butyrophenone antipsychotic drugs: A review of some recent research findings and clinical implications', *British Journal of Psychiatry*, 163 (Suppl. 22), 19–24.

Kane, J.M. (1985) 'Compliance Issues in Outpatient Treatment', *Journal of Clinical Psychopharmacology*, 5, 22–7.

Kane, J.M. (1992) 'Clinical efficacy of clozapine in treatment of treatment refractory schizophrenia: an overview', *British Journal of Psychiatry*, 160 (Suppl.), 41–5.

Kerwin, R.W. (1994) 'The new atypical antipsychotics: A lack of extra-pyramidal side-effects and new routes in schizophrenia research', *British Journal of Psychiatry*, 164, 141–8.

Kissling, W. (1992) 'Ideal and Reality of Neuroleptic Relapse Prevention', *British Journal of Psychiatry*, 161 (Suppl. 18), 133–9.

Krawiecka, M., Goldberg, D. and Vaughan, M. (1977) 'A standardised psychiatric assessment scale for rating chronic psychotic patients', *Acta Psychiatrica Scandinavica*, 55, 299–308.

Leff, J.P. and Wing, J.K. (1971) 'Trial of maintenance therapy in schizophrenia', *British Medical Journal*, 3, 599–604.

Lewander, T. (1994) 'Neuroleptics and the Neuroleptic Induced Deficit Syndrome', *Acta Psychiatrica Scandinavica*, 380 (Suppl.), 3–13.

Liberman, R., Marder, S., Marshall, B.D., Mintz, J. and Kuehnel, T. (1998) 'Biobehavioural Therapy: Pharmacotherapy and Behaviour Therapy in Schizophrenia', in T. Wykes, N. Tarrier and S. Lewis (eds), *Outcome and Innovation in Psychological Treatment of Schizophrenia*, Chichester, Wiley.

Marder, S. (1992) 'Pharmacological Treatment of Schizophrenia' in D. Kavanagh (ed.), *Schizophrenia: an Overview and Practical Handbook*, London, Chapman & Hall.

Mitchell, J. and Popkin, M. (1982) 'Antipsychotic drug therapy and sexual dysfunction in men', *American Journal of Psychiatry*, 139, 633–7.

Morrison, D. (1996) 'Management of Treatment Refractory Schizophrenia', *British Journal of Schizophrenia*, 169 (suppl.), 15–20.

National Institute of Mental Health (1975) 'Abnormal Involuntary Movement Scale', *Early Clinical Drug Evaluation Unit Intercom*, 4, 3–6.

Pratt, P. (1998) 'The Administration and Monitoring of Neuroleptic Medication', in Brooker and Repper (eds), *Serious Mental Health Problems in the Community. Policy, Practice and Research*, Baillière Tindall, London.

Schooler, N. (1993) 'Reducing dosage in maintenance treatment of schizophrenia: review and prognosis', *British Journal of Psychiatry*, 163 (Suppl.), 58–65.

Silverstone, T. and Turner, P. (1991) *Drug Treatment in Psychiatry*, London, Routledge.

Simpson, G. and Angus, J. (1970) 'A rating scale for extrapyramidal side effects', *Acta Psychiatrica Scandinavica*, 44, 11–19.

Siris, S. (1993) 'Adjunctive medication in the maintenance treatments for schizophrenia and its conceptual implications', *British Journal of Psychiatry*, 163 (Suppl.), 66–78.

Thomas, C. and Lewis, S. (1998) 'Which Atypical Antipsychotic?', *British Journal of Psychiatry*, 172, 106–9.

UKCC (1998) *Guidelines for Mental Health and Learning Disabilities Nursing*, London, UKCC.

Warner, R. (1994) *Recovery from Schizophrenia*, London, Routledge.

Zigmond, A. and Snaith, R. (1983) 'Hospital Anxiety and Depression Scale' *Acta Psychiatrica Scandinavica*, 67, 361–70.

CHAPTER 7

Psychological Treatment for Anxiety and Depression in Schizophrenia

CLAIRE BAGULEY AND IAN BAGULEY

Introduction

Individuals diagnosed as suffering from schizophrenia can experience high levels of depression and anxiety (Birchwood and Iqbal, 1998). These may be concurrent Axis I disorders, be a consequence of experiencing the trauma of positive symptoms, or relate to issues of loss and social humiliation. The presence of emotional disorder can complicate the presentation of illness, reduce functioning, lower quality of life, and ultimately lead to increased stress levels, which may contribute to the relapse and maintenance of the schizophrenic illness (Wing *et al.*, 1992).

Providing care within a psychosocial model could be the first step in the prevention of secondary depression and anxiety. The model normalises symptoms and experiences, and encourages the client to be active in their own treatment (Baguley and Baguley, 1999). This in turn helps to encourage self-efficacy, maintain self-esteem and hope about the future.

However, there are times when an individual may need active intervention to directly target symptoms of anxiety and depression. A cognitive-behavioural approach provides a simple, evidence-based framework within which the mental health nurse is able to work collaboratively with the client on these problems.

This Chapter aims to introduce mental health workers to the basic principles of the cognitive-behavioural approach for working with symptoms of anxiety and depression. An outline of the stages of assessment, formulation and intervention is given, followed by a case example.

Background to the Cognitive-Behavioural Model of Depression and Anxiety

Ellis (1962) and latterly Beck (1976), Beck *et al.* (1979) and Beck and Emery (1985) are widely considered to be the most influential early clinicians in developing cognitive-behavioural models for depression and anxiety. During the course of his clinical practice Beck observed a fundamental difference between the way depressed people appraised information from their surroundings compared to those who were not depressed. He found clues to this in their thoughts, which he identified as typically, automatic, negative, self-critical and over-generalised in content. Through further analysis he identified links between these negative automatic thoughts and an individual's underlying core beliefs or schema. Beck identified that the themes of core beliefs fall into three areas – beliefs about the self, the world and the future. These are referred to as the 'Cognitive Triad'. Through early experience and ongoing interaction with surroundings these core beliefs are developed and maintained from birth into adult life (Beck, 1976).

From these observations the central theme of the cognitive-behavioural model arose, this being that emotional disorder occurs as a result of chronic or profound misattribution of meaning to events and situations (Beck *et al.*, 1979).

Thus, for example, for one person being surrounded by a large football crowd might trigger thoughts and images of the forthcoming football match and the possibility of their team winning, resulting in feelings of excitement. For another person within the same crowd, their thoughts may be focused on the potential danger of such a large number of people gathered in one place, resulting in feelings of anxiety.

Importantly, this model encourages a view of emotional disorder that also recognises the importance of behaviour and physiology particularly in understanding the maintenance of emotional disorders. Classic maintaining behaviours include avoidance, withdrawal, reassurance seeking and checking. Additionally, individuals can develop their own idiosyncratic safety behaviours, such as carrying favoured objects or wearing particular clothing.

Beck's generic model of emotional disorders (see Figure 7.1) provides a framework for understanding the interaction between all the aspects of the individual, including early experiences and core beliefs. This is clinically useful, as it helps to organise information and form hypotheses about the development and maintenance of a client's problems.

Cognitive-behavioural therapy (CBT) is most potent when the therapist works with the client to discover the links and maintaining factors between thoughts, feelings, physiology and behaviour. For each individual the content of these will vary according to their individual history and experiences. However, there are common patterns that characterise the maintenance of depression and anxiety. These are conceptualised in the simple diagrams below.

Figure 7.2 shows a cross section of the maintenance cycle of depression. The model illustrates how negative thoughts influence and combine with mood, physiology and behaviour to produce a vicious cycle which keeps the depression going. Typical negative automatic thoughts might be 'I'm useless', 'It's all my fault', 'Everything goes wrong for me', 'Life is hopeless'. These thinking errors have been identified as falling into several broad categories (Beck *et al.*, 1979) (see Figure 7.3).

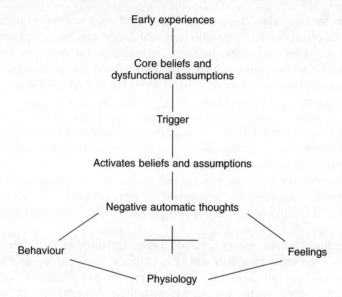

Figure 7.1 Generic cognitive-behavioural formulation for emotional disorder
(Beck, 1979)

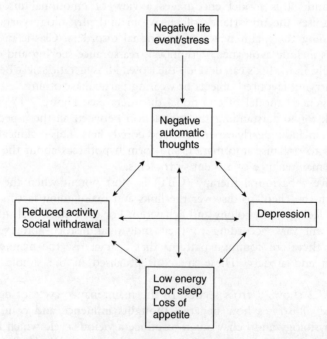

Figure 7.2 Cross section of the maintenance cycle of depression

- *Arbitrary inference*: Coming to a conclusion without complete evidence.

- *Over-generalisation*: Applying a conclusion drawn from a specific event to a range of unrelated situations.

- *Selective Abstraction*: Focusing on a particular piece of evidence rather than viewing the whole.

- *Personalising*: Interpreting events as meaning something about the self.

- *Magnification* and overemphasising the importance of negative information.

- *Minimisation* and under valuing positives.

- *Catastrophizing*: Thinking of the worst possible outcome and overestimating how likely it is to happen.

- *Mind-reading*: Assuming you know the people are thinking negatively about you with no evidence.

Figure 7.3 Typical 'thinking errors'

In the context of a sufficiently difficult or traumatic life event these thoughts will frequently occur in most individuals. However, the duration, intensity and subsequent harmful effects that they have will be influenced by previously held beliefs and coping styles.

Anxiety disorders are similarly maintained by the interaction of these four elements (see Figure 7.4). Individuals suffering from anxiety and panic typically focus inwardly on normally occurring bodily sensations (Clarke, 1986). The individual experiencing anxiety and panic symptoms will classically over estimate the dangerousness of the symptoms and their effects, and underestimate their ability to cope and the availability of rescue factors (Salkovskis, 1996). Typically cognitions relate to bodily or social harm. Often these automatic thoughts are experienced in the form of images (Hackman, 1997). The more imminent the perceived threat the more heightened the anxiety (see Figure 7.4).

Clinical Approaches

Engagement

As with any therapeutic intervention, to be effective it is essential that the worker has good interpersonal skills, and approaches the client from a respectful, empathic and collaborative position. Time must be spent explaining the CBT model and socialising them to a psychological enquiring perspective.

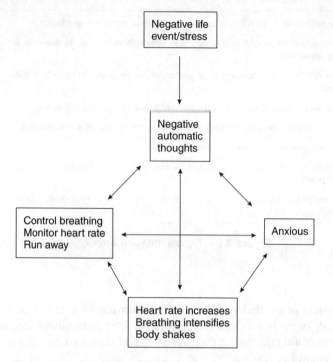

Figure 7.4   Cross section of the maintenance cycle of anxiety

Assessment

Individuals suffering from schizophrenia can suffer from anxiety and depression at any stage of their illness. This could be pre-morbidly, that is, before the onset of their first episode of illness, during the acute phase of the illness, or during the recovery phase. As such it is important to include these areas in routine mental health assessment at first contact, review and discharge planning.

Once anxiety or depression has been identified as a problem area more detailed assessment based on the cognitive behavioural model will be necessary before active intervention can begin.

Hawton *et al.* (1991) give a comprehensive overview of the cognitive behavioural assessment protocol. In addition to the baseline assessment, in order to develop an individualised formulation of emotional disorder, the mental health worker must work with the client to collect detailed information about the thoughts, physiological effects and behaviours that form the maintenance cycle.

Information can be gathered from several useful sources. The client can be asked directly about thoughts, feelings, behaviour and physiological sensations. The mental health worker can also elicit further evidence during their interactions with the client. Things to observe for include bodily reactions such as changes in breathing, posture, flushing or mannerisms. Changes in affect can be good evidence of the occurrence of 'hot' cognitions, for example the client may suddenly become tearful or angry. Enquiring in a direct and supportive manner what is going through their mind at these times will help ellicit these thoughts.

In addition, listening to the language that a client uses and the way they behave within session can provide important clues to underlying cognitive themes and maintaining behaviours.

Diaries can be an extremely useful tool for collecting information, and helping the client to discover the links between thoughts, feelings, physiology and behaviour. The diary should be kept as simple as possible, and the client should be encouraged to record periods of mood change along with possible triggers, associated physical sensations, thoughts and coping behaviours.

These diaries can then be used in session with the client to find examples to focus questioning on. This form of questioning is sometimes referred to as critical incident replay.

Having identified the most recent incident of mood change the therapist asks the client to recall where they were, what they were doing and asks direct questions about thoughts, feelings, physiology and behaviour. This process is described in more detail later in the chapter.

Other useful information can be found by undertaking a historical review of the client's life to include critical incidents, relationships with others and ways of coping. Also, speaking to relatives and carers can provide a further perspective on these issues, and possible contributing environmental and relational factors.

Goal Setting

Having established sufficient assessment of the client's problems it is important to establish shared goals for working together. Often clients will make vague very general statements such as 'To be less depressed' or to 'Go out more'. The mental health worker should work with the client to define goals that are realistic and achievable. Useful questions to ask might be:

- What would you be doing differently if you were less depressed?
- What sorts of things would you be doing if you were going out more?

The aim of goal setting is to have agreement on the areas of importance, and to provide markers for progression through therapy. They should be simple, achievable and as precise as possible, and approached by tackling the easiest first.

Formulation

Formulation is central to CBT intervention. It is the term used to describe the fitting together of the information gathered from assessment and ongoing information gathering to create a shared understanding of the links between thoughts, feelings, behaviour and physiology for the individual client. It is the step which applies the simple generic model to the individual client, and as such provides a 'map' of the problem that helps to decide in which areas interventions should be targeted (Butler, 1998).

It is always useful to begin formulating as soon as possible, if only in a basic way to identify one element of the maintenance cycle. Formulation should be simple, relevant to the problem and based upon the client's experiences. As further information is discovered about the client it should be put into the formulation. Apparent contradictions should be used as an opportunity to review the formulation and revise it as necessary. As such the formulation should be flexible, dynamic, and continually shared with the client for discussion and debate.

Cognitive Behavioural Interventions

Once a shared formulation is in place there are some simple CBT interventions that can be usefully employed to intervene in the maintenance cycles of depression and anxiety.

Activity Scheduling

One of the most common consequences of depression is lack of motivation resulting in social withdrawal, lethargy and reduced exposure to activities that energise and provide pleasure. Additionally depression may inhibit recall of positive events making it difficult for the client to remember positive experiences from memory in order to enhance their mood. All of these factors combine to maintain low mood. This problem is particularly prominent with severe depression, and can contribute to high levels of withdrawal and hopelessness.

Activity scheduling aims to intervene directly in this maintenance cycle. In the first instance it can be most useful to intervene at a behavioural level. However, the technique also works at a cognitive level by encouraging the client to learn about the effects of their behaviour on their levels of depression, and by energising the client makes cognition more accessible. Because of this it is a useful intervention to use prior to trying to use interventions that focus more directly on cognition.

There are four important steps in activity scheduling; collecting data about current functioning; rating of levels of mastery and pleasure for each activity; examination of data in order to identify helpful and unhelpful activities; and scheduling activity to maximise helpful activities and reduce unhelpful activities. Each of these components will be explained in detail.

The first step of data collection is best achieved by providing the client with a diary sheet dividing the day into hourly chunks (see Figure 7.5).

	Mon.	Tue.	Wed.	Thurs.	Fri.	Sat.	Sun.
6–8							
8–10							
10–12							
12–2							
2–4							
4–6							
6–8							
8–10							
10–12							

Figure 7.5 Example of activity schedule recording sheet

The client is asked to briefly record over the week what they were doing at each point in the day.

Second, the client is asked to make two ratings about the activity on a scale of 1–10. First, how much pleasure they gained from the activity, and second, how well they felt that they mastered it. By making these ratings the client starts to focus their thinking onto the different effects of activity, and highlighting pleasurable and rewarding activity, which they may not be able to remember because of biased memory recall.

An extra blank section may be left at the end of the diary to record important things noticed by the client that they might want to discuss further in the next session.

To the depressed client this task can seem daunting and because of this, time must be spent explaining the reasons for collection of the information, and showing by demonstration what is intended. This should be followed by discussion of any problems they can foresee with the task. Solutions to potential problems should be agreed with the client before they leave the session.

The third step involves examination of the diary with the client. First, they should be asked about their reactions to the task, and whether they have learned anything about their depression from the process of recording their activity. The discussion should then widen to look at types of activity the client has been engaged in and accompanying ratings of mastery and pleasure. From this it should be possible to begin to identify activities which produce little reward, long periods of inactivity and activities which have positive benefit. This information should be discussed in terms of how it links with the maintenance cycle of their depression.

This then leads to the fourth step of scheduling activity. This involves using data from the diary to collaboratively pre-plan weekly activity to include more helpful and less unhelpful activities. The plan should sensibly include a balance between activity and rest at appropriate times of the day. This plan should be written onto the diary sheet and homework set between sessions to try out this plan and record resulting mastery and pleasure. This should be reviewed at the following session and revised according to the client's observations about the effect that it is having on their mood.

Identifying and Examining Negative Automatic Thoughts

People suffering from anxiety and depression commonly experience thoughts that are negatively biased. These thoughts affect mood, behaviour, and physiology. As such, working with the client on the content of their thoughts, and how they respond to them can be an extremely useful way to make helpful changes in the whole system of feelings, behaviour and physiology.

The aim of identifying and challenging negative thoughts is to help the client become more aware of the effect of their thinking on the maintenance of their problem, and through this to become better equipped to challenge them as they occur. This may sound like a simple task, however thinking about one's thoughts is in fact very difficult for most people. The majority of thoughts are automatic, occur rapidly and are outside of our immediate consciousness. As such it is a skill which needs to be learnt.

In order to work with negative automatic thoughts clients must be helped to recognise them as they happen. They could be occurring rapidly at any time, in any situation, even during a session, so the clinician should work with the client to find a simple way of 'capturing' them. Initially, time must be spent discussing with the client the nature of the relationship between thoughts and feelings, and explaining that everyone has their own way of thinking about things that can be helpful and not so helpful. In order to illustrate and normalise the link it can be helpful to give some everyday examples at this stage. An example might be presented like this:

> *Everyone has negative automatic thoughts at certain times. For example, a very common one is triggered by a policeman knocking on the door. Most people will say that when this has happened to them they will automatically start to think the worst like 'I've done something wrong', or 'something bad has happened'. These thoughts will then make them begin to feel frightened, they might start to feel their heart racing, hands shaking or breathing getting rapid. This will then influence their behaviour by perhaps avoiding answering the door and pretending not to be at home. However, nine times out of ten, none of these things are true, and in fact the policeman has just called to tell them that they've left their car unlocked. Can you see how the way we think about things can directly affect how we feel, how our body reacts and what we do to cope with it?*

It is helpful to follow this by using the client's own experiences to illustrate how this phenomena applies to their own situation. The first step should be to try to identify with the client a recent example of a distressing event – it might even be something that has occurred during your session!

Cognitive behavioural work is underpinned by a questioning style of interaction often referred to as Socratic dialogue or guided discovery (see Chapter 8).

Start by getting a clear description of where the client was and what they were doing. This then leads to breaking the example down into the four areas of thoughts, feelings, physiology and behaviour. Often it can be useful to start by looking at feelings and moving through physiology, followed by thoughts and behaviour, as generally people are more likely to notice emotion and bodily experiences before the underlying thoughts.

Useful questions to ask might be:

- Can you think of a time recently when you felt particularly anxious or depressed?
- Where were you?
- What were you doing?
- Can you remember how you felt? For example anxious, depressed, angry?
- What sensations did you notice in your body?
- What was running through your mind at the time?
- What were you saying to yourself about what was happening?
- What would be the worst that could happen?
- What did you do to cope with how you felt?
- What was the outcome of this and how did you feel after?

As you are doing this exercise the information should be recorded on a diary sheet (see Figure 7.6). As you can see there is a column for each area that you have asked about. This will form the basis of a thought log, which can be used to help the client continue to try to capture thoughts as homework. It is also helpful to ask for ratings on a scale of 1–10 of level of mood and belief in the thought. Sometimes change occurs in small amounts and these ratings can highlight gradual changes rather than looking for all or nothing results.

When you have collected information about the content of your client's negative thoughts and their style of thinking you can then move onto the second stage of examining the information. This stage involves looking at the diaries with the client to identify particular themes and recurring patterns in trigger situations, thought content and ways of responding to these thoughts. The aim being to develop with the client an understanding of their problems that shows the link between their negative thoughts, emotional and physical state and behaviour.

Once you have a shared agreement on the nature of the links, you are in a position to introduce the third stage of challenging negative thoughts and trying to find more accurate and helpful perspectives.

There are several ways to approach challenging negative automatic thoughts. A basic principle to bear in mind is that it is always more helpful if the client is able to generate their own challenges with the help of Socratic questions.

Date/time	Situation	Bodily	Feelings	Thoughts and images	Coping strategies
	What, Where When?	Sensations	What were your emotions? (1–10)	What was running through your mind? Belief rating 1–10	What did you do?

Figure 7.6 Example of diary sheet

It can be useful to provide the client with a list of common thinking errors (Chapter 8) in order to help them identify those which apply to them. This may be followed by looking in detail at an example from the diary records, and discussing alternative ways of thinking about the trigger situation.

Useful questions to ask might be:

• What thinking error are you using there?
• What might be a more helpful way to think about the situation?
• Is there other information about the situation which you are ignoring?
• What would you say to a friend who was thinking these thoughts?

The client should be encouraged to identify their own alternative thoughts, using their own language. Once a suitable alternative has been found, the client should then be asked how being able to think this might change their feelings about the situation. Ask the client to re-rate their feelings and their belief in the alternative thought. Their response should show that there would be some mood change, even if at this stage it is not sustained. If their mood does not change discuss why, perhaps you have not used their words or it is too glib, work with the client to find something that fits better.

To reinforce this learning, this exercise can be followed by a homework assignment. Using the diary format the client should be asked to add a further two columns in which they can record alternative thoughts and re-rate their feelings (see Figure 7.7). These diaries can then be reviewed during subsequent sessions.

Date and time	Situation What, Who, Where?	Bodily feelings	Thoughts/ images What was running through your mind? Belief rating 1–10	Feelings What were your emotions? (1–10)	Alternative thoughts belief rating 1–10	Re-rated feelings How does thinking this way alter your feelings? (1–10) What do need to do about this now?

Figure 7.7 Example of diary for challenging negative automatic thoughts

Challenging automatic thoughts is a skill. The client should be helped to find ways of remembering the new challenges to their negative thinking, and be encouraged to practise it. A useful technique can be to write down the new perspectives on a small card they can carry with them or stick on their wall.

Behavioural Experiments

Behavioural experiments are a method by which the client is encouraged to experience feared situations, with the aim of gathering more information and to test out inaccurate or catastrophic predictions.

Using the information gathered from the assessment of negative automatic thoughts, key predictions and beliefs will become evident. For example, an anxious person might commonly be thinking that being dizzy is a sign of impending collapse. Alternatively, a depressed person might avoid confrontation because they will be ridiculed.

These beliefs must be stated as explicitly as possible, along with ratings of belief. It is then necessary to discuss with the client how they might find out

Date and time	Prediction What are you expecting to happen?	Experiment What did you do?	Outcome What actually happened? What have you learned?

Figure 7.8 Example of behavioural experiment diary

more about the subject in order to reach a more informed opinion. It is here that the experimental approach is important. Clients are not challenged directly, but are encouraged to become their own scientist, looking for new evidence and comparing it with their predictions about frightening situations.

The procedure follows an experimental model of investigation. It starts by eliciting the client's prediction or hypothesis of what will happen, along with a belief rating in the degree of certainty. The designated experiment is then carried out, followed by discussion of how the actual outcome compared with the predicted outcome and what the client has learned.

This is then followed by a re-rating of degree of conviction in the original prediction. A useful format for recording this procedure is shown in Figure 7.8.

When constructing a behavioural experiment, two factors must be taken into account. First, careful consideration should be given to how long the client will have to stay in the situation to be sure nothing will happen. Second, the client will have to be assisted in dropping all overt or covert safety behaviours. If not addressed these will serve as 'get-out' clauses for dismissing the evidence. For example, the client anxious about dizziness might complete the experiment, but only after taking an anti-depressant tablet. Typically, he might acknowledge that he did not collapse, but believe that things would have been different if he had not taken the tablet, or if he had stayed there longer. Consequently, the belief remains intact.

Where there are several feared situations the clinician should work with the client to order them in degrees of difficulty. Arranging them in this hierarchy allows the client to gain some confidence in the approach by working on the least difficult tasks first.

Imaginal exposure and role-play can also be used to prepare the client for in-vivo tasks. Additionally, rehearsal experiments could be conducted within the consulting room, and the therapist should be prepared to model experiments wherever necessary.

Consolidating Progress and Building on Cognitive Behavioural Interventions

It is important to stress to the client that learning to deal with negative automatic thoughts and unhelpful coping behaviours is a long-term process that they need to continue to practise. At times of stress old ways of thinking and behaving will automatically re-emerge.

In anticipation of this it can be helpful to encourage the client to think about what they have learned and keep a written record, sometimes this is referred to as a 'blueprint'. This should continue to be done in a Socratic manner, by asking a series of questions to focus the client on what they have learned so far. Useful questions to ask are:

- From our work together what have you learned about your problems and how they keep going?
- What are the early warning signs of you becoming anxious/depressed?
- What sorts of unhelpful thoughts and behaviours tend to occur when you are anxious/depressed?
- What sorts of questions are useful to ask your-self to help you think differently about situations?
- How can you continue to build up your self-help skills? What might lead you to become anxious/depressed in the future?
- If this occurs what will you do about it, what help might you need and who can give you this?

Case Example

John was a 19-year-old student who had been discharged from hospital where he had been detained on Section Two of the mental health act for four weeks. During this time he was treated with neuroleptic medication for auditory hallucinations and paranoid delusions. Both of these symptoms were alleviated with medication. John was discharged home with follow-up by a mental health nurse. The first signs of further difficulties were highlighted by John's parents. They expressed concern to the nurse that John had not left the house since leaving hospital. They had tried to encourage him but this just seemed to make him more irritable and withdrawn. They were very worried he might be suffering a relapse of his psychotic illness.

The mental health nurse spoke at length with John and conducted an assessment. This revealed that John was experiencing panic attacks, he referred to them as 'nerve attacks'. She asked John when had he last experienced one of these 'nerve attacks' and he explained one had occurred earlier that day after his father had asked him to go the shop.

The nurse questioned John in a step-wise manner about his physical sensations, thoughts, feelings and coping behaviours. He described a feeling of fear accompanied by a quickening heart rate, breathlessness and tightness across his chest. He found it difficult to be clear about his thoughts. The nurse asked him 'what would be the worst that could happen?' John replied that he might collapse in the street. When asked about images he described a mental picture of being laid in the street surrounded by people laughing.

In order to cope John stayed in his room and pretended that he had not heard his father's request. He then had to avoid his father for the rest of the day in case he asked him again.

The nurse used this opportunity to share a simple formulation of the maintenance cycle of panic. Using John's example, she illustrated the links between thoughts, feelings, physiology and coping behaviours. As she described this, she also drew it very simply on a paper asking John if he recognised this vicious circle. He agreed that it did seem to 'fit' his experience although he could not see how to tackle it, particularly as his fears seem very real at times of high anxiety.

The nurse offered written information about the physical effects of anxiety. She also empathised with his fears and normalised them by explaining that intense anxiety symptoms can be very alarming, and that worries about collapsing are a very common and understandable reaction when a person does not understand what is happening.

She suggested it would be useful to find out more about John's symptoms in order to make a plan to tackle them. Together they discussed how they could do this. They decided upon a simple diary sheet to record specific details. These included, when and where the attacks occurred, what physical symptoms were present and how severely he would rate his anxiety level on a scale of 0–10. The next section asked John to consider what had occurred to trigger the attack; for example, Dad asking me to go out, or thought about having to go to college. The final section then asked John to record what he did to try to cope followed by a re-rating of his anxiety level after he had done this. John expressed concern that he might forget to fill in the diary. It was agreed it would be useful to explain to his parents what was happening so they could assist with the recording. This provided the nurse with the opportunity to share with them the panic formulation of John's difficulties, and allay their concerns about their feared relapse of psychosis.

The nurse visited John the following week and together they looked at the diary sheets. It became clear that a pattern was emerging of triggers arising from requests, or thoughts, about having to leave the house. John typically reacted with an increasing heart rate, breathlessness and common thoughts of 'I'm having a stroke', 'I'm going to collapse', accompanied by an image of him on the floor in the street surrounded by strangers laughing. Each time he coped by staying in his room. He rated this as initially helpful, but the anxiety quickly built-up again when his thoughts returned to having to out.

This diary information was then compared with the early formulation to check that the shared understanding was still accurate. This formulation of the maintenance cycle then provided the basis upon which to target interventions. It became clear that John had two negative automatic cognitions, one articulated as a thought the other as an image. These indicated two unhelpful beliefs. The first relating to negative social evaluation by people outside of his home, and the second catastrophising of the effects physical symptoms of the anxiety he was experiencing.

Using the shared formulation of John's problems the mental health nurse worked with him to use a variety of cognitive behavioural interventions. They devised behavioural experiments to test out John's beliefs regarding collapse and his fears of social humiliation. These involved encouraging him to simulate his anxiety symptoms by vigorous exercise, and the nurse simulating collapse in a crowded place whilst John observed peoples responses. These experiments were combined with a hierarchy of feared situations. John was encouraged to practise these with the help of his family, and thought records where used to monitor and challenge negative automatic thoughts about doing these things.

As John's mastery of his anxiety improved and his activity increased the nurse sat down with him to reflect upon what he had learned from their work together. He identified the vicious circle of anxiety, noticing negative thoughts and finding ways of getting more realistic information as particularly important.

John was encouraged to write these down. They then discussed a plan for continuing to build on this work and constructed a blueprint. This included things John could do himself and things his parents could help him with. They also agreed upon the role that the nurse would have in continuing to monitor and support John. It was decided who would be most helped by having a copy of John's blue print and he decided upon his mental health nurse, the GP and his parents. Finally, a review date for looking specifically at anxiety was set for three months ahead.

Conclusion

The cognitive behavioural model of emotional disorder describes the relationship between thoughts, feelings, physiology and behaviour. The aim of the mental health worker using the model should be to work collaboratively with the client to understand how it applies to their unique circumstances. For the individual suffering from a psychotic illness the picture is particularly complex.

Positive symptoms combined with the negative effects of psychiatric treatments, stressed caring networks and social discrimination will all have influence.

The challenge to the mental health worker is to assess these areas accurately, prioritise target problems, and then create with the client a simple and understandable formulation of their difficulties before going on to identify appropriate intervention strategies.

This chapter has aimed to introduce the mental health worker to the basics of the cognitive behavioural model of depression and anxiety in order that these factors can be incorporated into assessment and treatment plans for individuals suffering from schizophrenia.

Further Reading

Beck, A.T., Rush, A.J., Shaw, B.F. and Emery, G. (1979) *Cognitive Therapy of Depression: A Treatment Manual*, New York, Guildford Press.
Blackburn, I.M. and Davidson, K. (1995) *Cognitive Therapy for Depression and Anxiety*, Oxford, Blackwell Science.
Greenberger, D. and Padesky, C.A. (1995) *Mind Over Mood. Change How You Feel by Changing the Way That You Think*, New York, Guildford Press.
Hawton, K., Salkovskis, P.M., Kirk, J. and Clarke, D.M. (1991) *Cognitive Behaviour Therapy for Psychiatric Problems. A Practical Guide*, New York, Oxford University Press.
Wells, A. (1997) *Cognitive Therapy of Anxiety Disorders. A Practice Manual and Conceptual Guide*, Chichester, Wiley.

References

Baguley, I. and Baguley, C. (1999) 'Psychosocial Interventions in the Treatment of Psychosis', *Mental Health Care*, 21(9), 314–18.
Beck, A.T. (1976) *Cognitive Therapy and the Emotional Disorders*, London, Penguin.
Beck, A.T. and Emery, G. (1985) *Anxiety Disorders and Phobias: A Cognitive Perspective*, New York, Basic Books.
Beck, A.T., Rush, A.J., Shaw, B.F. and Emery, G. (1979) *Cognitive Therapy of Depression: A Treatment Manual*, New York, Guildford Press.
Birchwood, M. and Iqbal, Z. (1998) 'Depression and Suicidal Thinking in Psychosis', in T. Wykes, N. Tarrier and S. Lewis (eds), *Outcome and Innovation in Psychological Treatment of Schizophrenia*, Chichester, Wiley.
Butler, G. (1998) 'Clinical Formulation', in A.S. Bellack and M. Henderson (eds), *Comprehensive Clinical Psychology*, Vol. 8, New York, Elsevier.
Clarke, D. (1986) 'A Cognitive Model of Panic', *Behavioural Research & Theory*, 24, 461–70.
Ellis, A. (1962) *Reason and Emotion in Psychotherapy*, New York, Lyle Stewart.
Hackman, A. (1997) 'The Transformation of Meaning in Cognitive Therapy', in D. Power and C. Brewin (eds), *The Transformation of Meaning in Psychological Therapies*, Chichester, Wiley.

Hawton, K., Salkovskis, P.M., Kirk, J. and Clarke, D.M. (1991) *Cognitive Behaviour Therapy for Psychiatric Problems. A Practical Guide*, New York, Oxford University Press.

Salkovskis, P.M. (1996) 'The Cognitive Approach to Anxiety: Threat beliefs, safety seeking behaviour and the special case of health anxiety and obsessions', in P. Salkovskis (ed.), *Frontiers of Cognitive Therapy*, New York, Guilford Press.

Wing, J., Brewin, C.R. and Thornicroft, G. (1992) 'Defining Mental Health Needs', in G. Thornicroft, C.R. Brewin and J. Wing (eds), *Measuring Mental Health Needs*, Royal College of Psychiatrists, London, Gaskell.

CHAPTER 8

Assessment and Therapeutic Interventions With Positive Psychotic Symptoms

JULIE EVERITT AND RONALD SIDDLE

Introduction

Clients with a diagnosis of schizophrenia commonly exhibit several unusual perceptual and cognitive phenomena such as hallucinations, delusions and thought disorder, which are referred to as positive symptoms of the disorder. These symptoms are often a source of significant distress to patients and have been associated with episodes of self-harm and harm to others (Tarrier, 1987). There is evidence that 10–20 per cent of patients suffering from schizophrenia fail to demonstrate substantial improvements in positive symptoms when they are treated with neuroleptic medication (Kane, 1989) and 60–70 per cent of first episode clients will relapse within two years despite prescription of antipsychotic medication (Ram et al., 1992). Even with good clinical response, side effects can limit drug treatment compliance. As a result researchers and clinicians have sought to develop adjunctive therapies to neuroleptic medication for treating positive symptoms.

This chapter explores a collaborative way of working with clients who experience positive psychotic symptoms. It discusses therapeutic engagement, assessment of positive symptoms, problem identification/formulation and interventions for symptoms that aim to lessen distress and/or disability by producing cognitive, affective or behavioural change.

Background

Many mental health professionals will have been informed during their basic training that talking therapies are of little value in the treatment of positive symptoms of psychosis. However, as early as 1952, Beck reported the successful modification of beliefs using questioning and reality testing in the case of a man with a long history of systematised persecutory delusions (Beck, 1952). Importantly this approach suggested that delusions might be modifiable,

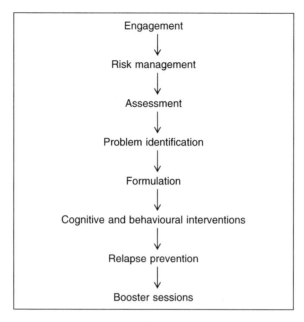

Figure 8.1 Process of therapy

and subsequently a number of small studies provided further evidence to support this hypothesis (for a more extensive review, see Turkington and Siddle, 1998).

During the 1990s several carefully controlled research studies, involving larger numbers of patients have been conducted to evaluate the effectiveness of cognitive behaviour therapy (CBT) in modifying positive symptoms. These studies have provided evidence for the efficacy for CBT in working with treatment resistant symptoms (Kingdon and Turkington, 1991; Tarrier *et al.*, 1993, 1999; Kuipers *et al.*, 1997; Drury *et al.*, 1996; Sensky *et al.*, 2000). The process of therapy described in this chapter has been drawn from the approaches used by therapists working in these studies and broadly follows the stages outlined in Figure 8.1.

Practical/Practice Guidelines

Engagement

Establishing a therapeutic relationship with a client is a essential to the success of any psychotherapeutic intervention with people who have a diagnosis of schizophrenia. The reader is referred to Chapter 4 for a detailed discussion regarding how collaborative working relationships can be developed.

Structure of Sessions

Cognitive behaviour therapy is a structured approach to therapy that aims to offer the client the maximum benefit from the limited amount of time available in each session (Beck *et al.*, 1979). Although it has already been suggested that when working with people suffering from serious mental illness traditional approaches to therapy may need to be adapted (see Chapter 4), therapists should nevertheless still try to adhere to the basic structure of cognitive behavioural therapy. At the beginning of each session an agenda should be established which lists the topics that will be discussed, agenda items might include target problems, assessment or interventions, with the client being actively encouraged to suggest and prioritise items on the agenda. The agenda should include time to review any homework, which was agreed in the previous session. Homework assignments can focus on things that help to generalise lessons learnt in therapy to daily life. If the client perceives therapy as something that makes them feel better then they are more likely to continue with it. The client should be asked for feedback at frequent intervals to establish if they are happy with the way sessions are being conducted, particular attention should be paid to finding out what the clients understanding of the session has been and whether they feel it is relevant to their problems. Eliciting feedback also provides an opportunity to clear up any misunderstandings before they have the opportunity to jeopardise engagement.

Rationales for the Use of CBT

When providing a rationale for the use of CBT the therapist needs to explain the cognitive model notably the relationship between thoughts, feelings and behaviours. It can be emphasised that while our interpretation (thoughts) of situations can trigger powerful emotions at times we are all capable of misinterpreting what is going on. To support this information it is helpful if an everyday example of how our thoughts can effect our emotions and behaviour can be provided. For example, 'imagine that you are walking down the street and you see a good friend coming towards you. You are about to say hello when the friend looks straight past you and carries on walking without speaking'. The patient should then be asked to state the reasons why they might think their friend had done this and how different explanations might effect their feelings and behaviour. Most patients, with help, are able to identify a number of possible explanations ranging from benign ones such as their 'friend was distracted and did not see them' to explanations with more upsetting consequences such as they were 'deliberately ignored'. The aim of the exercise is to demonstrate that what we think can have an effect on our feelings and without additional information we can easily misinterpret a situation. The aim of CBT can be summarised as helping the client to identify thoughts related to situations which cause distress and to explore the evidence which supports these thoughts and to seek to generate alternative explanations. Giving the client something to read about CBT to consolidate the information presented in the session is a good example of appropriate homework.

Normalising Rationales

The use of normalising rationales is an important part of the process of CBT for people suffering from schizophrenia (Kingdon and Turkington, 1991). These rationales aim to reduce the fear generated as a consequence of psychotic symptoms by placing them on a continuum with normal experience. Sleep deprivation, traumatic events, sensory deprivation, hostage situations, solitary confinement and sexual abuse are all examples of stressors that have been shown to have triggered psychotic symptoms in people with no psychiatric history. Clients are encouraged to discuss specific and general stressors that may have contributed to the onset and/or maintenance of their symptoms. By considering symptoms on a continua with normal experiences there is an opportunity to decatastrophise them which will in turn facilitate stress reduction and may also present the opportunity to consider alternative explanations for their experiences.

The use of a normalising rationale helps to establish a rapport with the client based on a collaborative explorative style, it assesses the clients willingness and or ability to explore alternative/contributory explanations for symptoms and it presents an opportunity to use these alternative explanations at a later stage in therapy.

Communication Style

When talking to people about psychotic experiences it is important to show the same level of interest and curiosity that we would hopefully show to anyone who was explaining something of great personal significance. Therefore communication begins with actively listening to the clients experiences and trying to understand and empathise with their meaning to the client. Another useful skill is for the therapist to regularly summarise what they think the client has said to them to check the accuracy of their understanding.

A more advanced skill needed by therapists wishing to practice CBT with this client group is known as guided discovery. Guided discovery (also known as Socratic dialogue) refers to an inquisitive style of questioning that the therapist uses to help the client to explore their experiences and consider the evidence on which they have drawn their conclusions. Where the clients conclusions are not supported by the available evidence they are carefully helped to explore alternative explanations for their experiences (for more in depth explanation and examples of the guided discovery, see Padesky and Greenberger, 1995).

Assessment and Formulation

Assessment of the clients presenting problems provides another opportunity to communicate to them that their difficulties are being taken seriously. The therapist seeks to gather accurate information about the client's background, their current circumstances, the history of their mental health problems, the adverse effects the illness currently has on their life and the strengths and coping strategies they possess to help manage their problems. The results of assessment form the basis of a collaborative problem list, this should be constructed using the clients perception of problems but with the therapist being active in using information from the assessments to prompt the client regarding problem areas. The problem list enables the client and therapist to prioritise areas for further assessment, or to develop a problem formulation.

A formulation represents a collaboratively generated hypothesis of the clients presenting problems. It is essential as an analysis of assessment material, which will serve to guide the client and therapist throughout the therapeutic process. The importance of working with a formulation cannot be overstated. If the formulation accurately reflects the clients experience then when progress is made in one problem area it leads to benefits in other related problem areas. The formulation should also focus the therapists attention on the consequences of symptom modification. This is an important area as it may be appropriate for the therapy to focus on managing the distress associated with symptoms rather than on the removal of the symptoms. For example, a client experiencing auditory hallucinations may at times find the voices comforting and the removal of the voices could lead to loneliness.

Clinical Supervision

Before moving on to describe the specific CBT interventions that can be used to help clients who are experiencing distressing psychotic symptoms: a note of caution. Just as clinicians are advised not to undertake this type of work without the appropriate knowledge base equally, if not more importantly, they should not proceed without an experienced clinical supervisor to oversee their work.

Cognitive and Behavioural Interventions with Psychotic Symptoms

The interventions described in the following paragraphs focus on strategies to help clients alleviate the distress (or other negative consequences) associated with the symptoms, or on techniques to modify the symptoms or the core beliefs (schema) which may underlie the symptoms. The reader is referred to the earlier section on guided discovery for the communication style to adopt with the client.

Coping Strategy Enhancement (CSE)

CSE aims to maximise the client's current resources and ability to cope with their symptoms, it can be used as an approach to help clients experiencing distress associated with either hallucinations and delusions. Following a detailed assessment of the clients mental state CSE begins with the identification of a target symptom which is normally one associated with high levels of distress. The target symptom is then assessed in terms of its frequency, the clients emotional reaction, antecedents, consequences and any coping strategies employed by the client. These can be assessed using a structured interview named the Psychotic Antecedent and Coping Interview (Tarrier *et al.*, 1990). Next the client is encouraged to monitor the target symptom as a homework task to gather more information about antecedents to its onset and factors involved in its maintenance (see Figure 8.2).

The aims of the CSE monitoring is to elicit active coping strategies which can be described as physiological, sensory, behavioural and cognitive. Figure 8.3 lists useful questions to ask when trying to identify coping strategies (Tarrier, 1987).

Once a coping strategy is identified it is important to assess its effectiveness by asking questions such as:

- When you spend time on your own does it always work?
- How effective is it in helping you cope?

It is also important to consider whether a clients coping strategies are positive or negative. Spending time with a friend may help reduce anxiety, auditory hallucinations and enhance self-esteem where as cannabis use may have a

Target problem/symptom:	Hearing voices
Date/time/situation?	Saturday 5 May 10 pm In the pub with Joe
How did you feel?	Tense, frightened, upset
What did you think?	I can't stand this, why is it happening to me again?
What did you do?	Became very quiet Had a double whisky Tried to reason with the voice
How did you cope?	Continued to hear the voices and after 15 minutes told Joe that I was ill and left

Figure 8.2   Example of a client's homework for monitoring a symptom

Physiological:	Do you do anything to relax like take a bath?
	Do you drink alcohol or take any drugs?
Sensory:	Do you block your ears by turning up the TV/Radio?
Behavioural:	Do you do something to change your environment (i.e. increase or decrease social activity)?
Cognitive:	Can you help yourself by thinking in a particular way?
	Do you tell yourself 'its my illness it won't harm me?'
	Do you switch your attention to something new?

Figure 8.3   Questions to elicit coping strategies

Cognitive strategies
- Attention switching/narrowing
- Self instruction
- Rational reconstruction

Behavioural strategies
- Solitary activity
- Social withdrawal
- Engaging in social interaction

Physiological strategies
- Relaxation/breathing exercises
- Pharmacological

Sensory strategies
- Control auditory input

Figure 8.4   Range of coping strategies

Source: Tarrier (1987)

short-term benefit for anxiety but result in a longer-term increase in auditory hallucinations. Coping strategies such as reducing social contact may be useful in the short term but will need to be used as part of an overall treatment plan and not used in isolation as it can lead to social function impairment.

Once the client has been helped to identify the most effective way of coping with a distressing symptom they can be helped to systematically apply this coping strategy whilst monitoring its effect on symptom severity (see Figure 8.4).

Interventions for Working With Delusional Beliefs

When seeking to collaboratively examine beliefs the therapist uses guided discovery (also known as Socratic questions) and asks the client questions which help this process. Some helpful areas for exploration are listed below.

How Did the Belief Develop?

Initial questions should focus on gathering information concerning the development of the belief, for example,

- When did you first notice something was different?
- What sort of things did you notice?
- How long did it last?
- Were there any other people around?
- Did you ask any one what they thought about what you noticed?
- Did you ask anyone for help?

These are questions that the client can generally answer, they will enhance engagement and allow you to move on to consider the evidence for and against the delusional beliefs.

What is the Client's Level of Conviction in the Belief?

The therapist can help the client to consider (as a part of assessment or intervention) the level of conviction they have in a belief. If the belief is anything less than 100 per cent then the doubt can be explored. If a belief is held with a 100 per cent conviction then it may be more beneficial to the therapeutic relationship if interventions are focused on coping strategies before considering strategies to introduce doubt. Importantly good coping strategies can help to modify a patients beliefs that a symptom is uncontrollable.

What is the Evidence for and against the Belief?

By collecting the evidence that supports and challenges troublesome beliefs the therapist provides an opportunity for the client to constructively examine all the evidence relating to strongly held but perhaps distressing beliefs in an atmosphere of collaborative enquiry. It is often the case that simply re-examining all the evidence relating to a belief in an open, honest but also guided way can help to change the conviction with which a belief is held and therefore possibly reduce associated distress or disruption to functioning without a direct challenge. The style of questioning helps to draw the client's attention to matters they may not previously have considered. When a client struggles to generate any evidence that refutes a belief then the therapist may need to provide some prompts, for example 'Has anything ever happened that has made you doubt that X was true?'

Only after attempting guided discovery (even if necessary with prompts) should the therapist give the client direct information, as this misses an opportunity for powerful self discovery. Having collected evidence for and against a belief the therapist and client should consider what is good evidence and what is not this can present the opportunity to consider alternative explanations for the evidence. As a precaution the therapist should ensure that prior to collecting the evidence they have carried out a comprehensive enough assessment to prevent a situation in which the person has a lot of evidence to support their problematic belief and the therapist is unable to generate much in the way of challenging evidence.

What are the Alternative Explanations?

The use of guided discovery will help the client to consider alternative explanations. Guided discovery can help the client to 'step into another persons shoes' and to consider what that person might think if they were in the same situation. The therapist is not asking the client to contradict themselves but is trying to determine if the client can consider or accept that others may view things differently. The careful selection of questions to ask the client may help them to do this. Normalising rationales which were developed in the earlier stages of therapy, may now form part of the formulation and are useful to draw upon as alternative explanations for evidence when seeking to modify delusional beliefs. For example, a client who has not been sleeping due to their perceived need for vigilance may be helped to consider that some of the interpretations they are making about routine situations may be partly due to thinking errors which have been exacerbated by lack of sleep. While clients may not accept that this explains all their symptoms they may be able to see that not sleeping and/or thinking errors is playing a role in the maintenance of their symptoms.

Thinking Errors

In order to illustrate to the client how situations in day to day life may be misinterpreted it is useful to introduce the concept of thinking errors. Thinking errors were first described by Beck *et al.* (1979) in relation to clients suffering from depression. Through the use of guided discovery and homework, the client can then be helped to identify errors in their own thinking and consider the consequences of these errors in the formation and maintenance of their beliefs and other symptoms (see Chapter 7).

What are the Consequences of Thinking in this Way?

For a client who believes that they are being persecuted their response may be, as stated earlier to maintain constant alertness. The client can be helped to explore the consequences of this, that is, a client who is hypervigilant may notice more ambiguous stimuli and run an increased risk of jumping to a wrong conclusion. There is also the risk of being overwhelmed by information increasing the risk of further thinking errors.

How Could the Evidence for the Belief be Tested (Behavioural Experiments)?

Once some doubt has been established the client may be encouraged to carry out behavioural experiments to help collect evidence relating to the belief. Behavioural experiments may also be used to help the client to gather evidence that supports an alternative explanation. For example a client who believed that they were being followed by a person, driving a red car, may collect car registration numbers to test whether it is the same car following them at all times. It is important to consider with the client, alternative ways of gaining this sort of evidence and to consider the pros and cons of such a behavioural test. Behavioural tests can provide powerful evidence be it confirmatory or disconfirmatory. The therapists task is to ensure that the possibility for error is minimised and that the aims of the experiment are achieved.

The overall aim of questioning is to review the evidence for and against beliefs, generate alternative explanations, challenge thinking errors and undertake behavioural tests. The skilled use of a guided discovery/Socratic dialogue delivered when therapeutic alliance has been established is essential to collaboratively and scientifically examine strongly held but distressing beliefs. If the therapist is too direct when challenging a delusional belief psychological reactance may occur where the belief becomes held with even more intensity (Watts *et al.*, 1973). It is important to note that targeting delusional beliefs is only one of many possible strategies of CBT for psychosis and should only be selected as a strategy when informed by the formulation. Modifying grandiose beliefs, for example, without addressing issues such as self esteem may be contra-indicated. The therapist may help the client with grandiose symptoms more by focusing on an intervention package that included interventions to promote self esteem, activity scheduling and problem solving rather than an attempt to reduce conviction in beliefs a client may have about possessing special powers or abilities.

A Cautionary Note: Remember Before Intervention to Consider

- how does the level of distress from the problems/symptoms compare to the level of distress from treatment
- what will the effect be of altering or removing a symptom
- will the outcome of therapy be positive or helpful – the client is unlikely to engage in a treatment which they believe will make things worse for them.

Rational Responses for Voices and Delusions

The client can be helped to develop a healthy 'self talk' in relation to their delusional beliefs or voices. This is known as a rational response. The client is assisted in identifying helpful statements which can include alternative explanations that can be recalled at stressful times. For example a client hearing the voice of an evil spirit may be encouraged to use rational responses such as 'I hear these voices when I'm feeling anxious they can't hurt me and I will feel better if I relax'. To use these effectively the therapist and client will have considered alternative explanations for voices using stress-vulnerability rationales and that the client is developing the rational responses to help them remind themselves of their explanations when they are under more pressure. The responses can be written onto cue cards or recorded on audio cassette to help jog the persons memory.

Interventions for Working With Hallucinations

Researchers have investigated a number of interventions aimed at reducing the distress associated with hallucinatory experiences. Included in the interventions investigated are strategies involving the use of distraction, focusing and collaborative re-examination of a clients beliefs about their hallucinatory experiences. All require the type of assessment we have referred to and a formulation which considers matters such as triggers and maintaining factors. Haddock *et al.* (1996) suggested that a combination of both distraction and focusing would be the most appropriate treatment strategy for many patients.

Distraction Techniques

The therapist can help the client to use a range of distraction techniques (Margo *et al.*, 1981). The use of a personal stereo can be enhanced by encouraging the client to keep a record of its impact on the voices. This combines the use of both distraction and monitoring in the management of voices. Another example of distraction is reading, mental arithmetic and mental games, for example counting backwards from 1,000 in 7s, the aim is to use something that requires concentration but is not so difficult the client feels it is out of their reach.

Focusing Therapy

Bentall, Haddock and Slade (1994) developed a model which viewed hallucinations as occurring when an individual fails to attribute mental events to themselves and instead attributes their presence to external factors. The therapist works with the client to assess the form, physical characteristics, loudness, tone, accent, gender and location in space. The client is encouraged to keep a symptom diary, this can be set as homework and reviewed at the start of therapy sessions.

The therapist encourages the client to focus on the content of the voice and related thoughts and assumptions about the voices. Collaboratively the client is encouraged to make links between the content of the voices and the content of their own thoughts. The therapist and client can then work together to consider alternative explanations and to develop rational responses.

Interventions for Working with Thought Disorder

The presence of thought disorder can be an obstacle to therapy as it disturbs the clients ability to maintain a train of thought. Little research has been carried out on interventions specifically designed to reduce thought disorder but due to the communication problems it presents it can often be a very real threat to engagement. It is important to consider the pace of therapy and to take account of communication problems as moving too quickly will only serve to make therapy more difficult. The more anxious the client becomes the more likely it is that thought disorder will disrupt communication. It is important to keep sessions short, try and identify themes in the patients speech and to ask yourself 'how does this relate to the clients problems'. The accurate use of empathy is important as being able to relate to a clients feeling may be more useful and practical than trying to reflect the actual content of what is being said. Verbal communication can be supplemented by the use of written materials and visual aids, in addition the structure of the CBT session can help by the use of clear agendas and regular summarising and feedback.

Schema Based Interventions/Working with Core Beliefs

At times intervention will focus on the identification and modification of beliefs which are thought to underlie the delusion. These beliefs may be referred to as either core beliefs or schemas. The concept of schema refers to cognitive structures which are relatively stable and enduring and which represent an individual's beliefs about himself and the world (Blackburn and Davidson, 1995). Such beliefs will clearly influence the process of attention and levels of vigilance within an individual at any given moment in time, and lead to particular interpretations of situations and events.

Working with core schema level beliefs may be of particular relevance for grandiose delusions or systematised delusions which are often resistant to other techniques because of the protective function which they may have for a clients self esteem. This type of intervention is generally indicated later in therapy and it has to be acknowledged that the evidence supporting its utility is still developing. To maintain collaboration the client will need clear rationales regarding process and outcomes, and an honest account of the evidence base supporting the intervention. Not all clients will be able to or want to work at this level however schema based interventions may present an opportunity to work with first and second episode clients whose psychotic symptoms have remitted but may benefit from therapy to reduce vulnerability to relapse.

Schemas or core beliefs can be identified by following general themes in cognitions, from questioning around the significance of specific events and from using the downward arrow technique (Kingdon and Turkington, 1991). Cognitions or processes identified in the formulation may help to identify assumptions and core schemas and could be an example of how a formulation can generate a more detailed assessment. The Dysfunctional Attitude Scale (DAS: Weissman and Beck, 1978) can be used to gain a better understanding of underlying core beliefs which may be implicated in the relapse or maintenance of symptoms.

Though the evidence supporting schema based interventions is at this time limited, there are indications (Sensky *et al.*, 2000) that adopting an individualised schema based formulation can be beneficial to clients over the long term. The manner in which this benefit is attained is not known but it is speculated that by attempting to alter the core beliefs or by working on a very individual schema based explanation for symptoms the client becomes more engaged in therapy.

Fowler *et al.* (1995) present five dysfunctional themes that they found occurred frequently in their study:

- The belief that the self is extremely vulnerable to harm
- The belief that the self is highly vulnerable to losing self control
- The belief that the self is doomed to social isolation
- The belief in inner defectiveness
- The belief in unrelenting standards

A person preoccupied with delusional beliefs of a paranoid nature may have a core belief about the self being highly vulnerable to harm as they have a mistrust of others intentions and actions.

General principles for modifying schema have been reviewed in a number of sources (Padesky and Greenberger, 1995) and include

(1) weakening old schemas using continua and historical tests; and
(2) building more adaptive schemas using continua, positive data logs, behavioural experiments and historical tests.

Conclusion

This chapter has described the use of cognitive-behavioural therapy in psychosis and considered the different stages of therapy. It is important to emphasise that engagement takes precedence over all else and if threatened the therapist will need to attend to this for further work to be possible. The aim of the therapy is to help establish a shared understanding along the lines of the stress-vulnerability model with the client, from this point interventions can be collaboratively identified and implemented. Throughout therapy the client has an opportunity to learn a number of coping strategies and techniques which may help to alleviate their distress. The awareness of the consequences of thinking errors may help reduce the chance of further delusional and non delusional catastrophic misinterpretation which can continue to be useful to the client once the therapy sessions have been completed.

Further Reading

Chadwick, P., Birchwood, M. and Trower, P. (1996) *Cognitive Therapy for Delusion, Voices and Paranoia*, Chichester, Wiley.
Fowler, D., Garety, P. and Kuipers, E. (1995) *Cognitive Behaviour Therapy for Psychosis: Theory and Practice*, Chichester, Wiley.
Kingdom, D. and Turkington, D. (1994) *Cognitive Behaviour Therapy of Schizophrenia*, New York, Guildford Press.
Nelson, H. (1997) *Cognitive Behavioural Therapy with Schizophrenia: A Practice Manual*, Cheltenham, Stanley Thornes.

References

Beck, A. (1952) 'Successful outpatient psychotherapy of a chronic schizophrenic with a delusion based on a borrowed guilt'. *Psychiatry*, 15, 302–12.
Beck, A.T., Rush, A.J., Shaw, B.F. and Emery, G. (1979) *Cognitive Therapy of Depression*, Chichester, Wiley.
Bentall, R.P., Haddock, G. and Slade, P.D. (1994) 'Psychological treatment for auditory hallucinations: theory to therapy', *Behavior Therapy*. 25, 51–66.
Blackburn, I. and Davidson, K. (1995) 'Cognitive Therapy for Depression and Anxiety' Oxford, Blackwell.
Drury, V., Birchwood, M. and Cochrane R. *et al.* (1996) 'Cognitive therapy and recovery from acute psychosis: a controlled trial II. Impact on recovery time', *British Journal of Psychiatry*, 602–7.
Fowler, D., Garety, P. and Kuipers, E. (1995) *Cognitive Behaviour Therapy for Psychosis Theory and Practice*, Chichester, Wiley.
Haddock, G., Bentall, R.P. and Slade, P.D. (1996) 'Psychological Treatment of Auditory Hallucinations: focusing and distraction', in G. Haddock and P.D. Slade (eds), *Cognitive Behavioural Intrventions with Psychotic Disorders*, London, Routledge.
Kane, J.M. (1989) 'Schizophrenia: Somatic treatment', in v.H.I Kaplans and B.J. Sadock (eds) *Comp. Textbook of Psychiatry* Baltimore. Williams & Watkins.
Kingdon, D. and Turkington, D. (1991) 'The use of cognitive behaviour therapy with a normalising rationale in schizophrenia', *Journal of Nervous Mental Disease*, 179, 207–11.
Kuipers, E., Garety, P.A. and Fowler, D. *et al.* (1997) 'The London–East Anglia trial of cognitive behaviour therapy for psychosis I: effects of the treatment phase', *British Journal of Psychiatry*, 171, 319–27.
Lancashire, S. (1998) *The KGV(M) Symptom Scale version 6*, unpublished paper, University of Manchester.

Margo, A., Hemsley, D.R. and Slade, P.D. (1981) 'The effects of varying auditory input on schizophrenic hallucinations', *British Journal of Psychiatry*, 139, 122–7.

Padesky, C.A. and Greenberger, D. (1995) *Clinicians Guide to Mind over Mood*, New York, Guildford Press.

Ram, R., Bromet, E. and Eaton, W. *et al.* (1992) 'The natural course of schizophrenia: a review of first admission studies', *Schizophrenia Bulletin*, 18, 185–208.

Sensky, T., Turkington, D., Kingdon, D., Scott, J.L., Scott, J., Siddle, R., O'Carroll, M. and Barnes, T.R.E. (2000) 'A Randomised Control Trial of Cognitive Behavioural Therapy for Persistent Symptoms in Schizophrenia, Resistant to Medication', *Archives of General Psychiatry*, 57, 165–72.

Tarrier, N. (1987) 'An investigation of residual psychotic symptoms in discharged schizophrenic patients', *British Journal of Psychiatry*, 26, 141–3.

Tarrier, N., Harwood, S. and Yussof, L. *et al.* (1990) 'Coping Strategy Enhancement (C.S.E): A method of treating residual schizophrenic symptoms', *Behavioural Psychotherapy*, 18, 643–62.

Tarrier, N., Beckettt, R., Harwood, S., Baker, A., Yusupoff, I. and Ugarteburu, I. (1993) 'A trial of two cognitive behavioural methods of treating drug resistant residual psychotic symptoms in schizophrenic patients: I. Outcome', *British Journal of Psychiatry*, 162, 524–32.

Turkington, D. and Siddle, R. (1998) 'Cognitive therapy for the treatment of delusions', *Advances in Psychiatric Treatment*, 4, 235–42.

Watts, F.N., Powell, E.G. and Austin, S.V. (1973) 'The modification of abnormal beliefs', *British Journal of Medical Psychology*, 46, 359–63.

Weissman, A.N. and Beck, A.T. (1978) 'Development and Validation of the Dysfunctional Attitudes Scale'; paper presented at the annual meeting of the Association for the Advancement of Behavior Therapy, Chicago.

CHAPTER 9

Identifying and Overcoming Negative Symptoms

RONALD SIDDLE AND JULIE EVERITT

Introduction

The symptoms of schizophrenia are commonly described in two broad categories; positive symptoms and negative symptoms. Positive symptoms are considered excesses, that is, go beyond what is considered to be 'normal' behaviour or experience. Negative symptoms, are generally considered to be deficits in normal functioning and include the core negative symptoms such as flattening of affect and poverty of speech (Barnes and Liddle, 1990).

Negative symptoms are important because they can have an effect upon outcome from treatment (Fenton and McGlashan, 1994; Thara and Eaton, 1996) and can have an unhelpful effect upon therapeutic interventions used in treating positive symptoms of schizophrenia. In addition researchers exploring family relationships (see Chapter 11), inform us that it is often negative symptoms which cause irritation and antipathy in family members. This may well result in the expression of higher levels of expressed emotion, a factor which is itself associated with an increase in relapses (Barrowclough and Tarrier, 1992). Treatment of negative symptoms is therefore likely to have benefits for both the individual and family.

This chapter addresses the cluster of symptoms associated with the syndrome of negative symptoms, the psychosocial interventions that target these symptoms, and considers how to minimise the impact of negative symptoms. We examine some of the ways which negative symptoms may be assessed and consider some of the problems negative symptoms can cause. Interventions which address these symptoms are discussed, using case material to highlight some of the issues.

What Are Negative Symptoms?

Some of the interest in the positive/negative symptom distinction comes from the suggestion that they represented two separate disease processes (Crow, 1980). Positive symptoms were attributed to an increase in dopamine receptors while negative symptoms were thought to result from loss of brain cells and structural changes in the brain. Subsequent work has made further categorical distinctions and has resulted in three proposed characteristic symptom clusters (Liddle, 1987). The first, psychomotor poverty, relates to negative symptoms, the second is disorganisation and includes thought disorder and inappropriate affect, finally, delusions and hallucinations were termed reality distortion.

There are two kinds of negative symptoms (Barnes and Liddle, 1990). Primary negative symptoms are thought to be the product of an enduring deficit state, while secondary negative symptoms can be thought of as a consequence of positive symptoms.

Negative Symptoms in Terms of the Stress-Vulnerability Model

This position proposes that negative symptoms of schizophrenia are a response to difficult psychological and social situations – a personal coping strategy against stress. The person's withdrawal from social situations and reduced activity may serve as protective feature against further relapse. For example, distressing paranoid delusions may result in the person hiding in their bedroom for long periods or terrifying hallucinations may be relieved by periods of isolation, that is, a reduction in sensory stimulation.

The secondary negative symptoms are thought to be far more temporary and more easily treatable than primary negative symptoms (Carpenter *et al.*, 1988), although it may be difficult to distinguish between these two types.

Primary negative symptoms include alogia, anergia, anhedonia, and emotional blunting.

Alogia

Alogia, which relates to the impoverished thinking which can occur in patients with schizophrenia and can be characterised by *poverty of speech*. Other symptoms include *thought blocking*, and an increase in the time taken to respond when asked questions.

Anergia

Anergia is a lack of energy or drive. People with anergia may be unable to motivate themselves, possibly resulting in poor hygiene, occupational difficulties and drastically reduced levels of social functioning. People can suffer deterioration in performance and may spend hours without any spontaneous activity. This can have disastrous consequences for people in employment or taking further education.

Anhedonia

Anhedonia is a symptom where people have difficulty in experiencing pleasure or taking an interest in recreational pursuits, sexual matters, or friendships. Several people with these symptoms find it difficult to express a closeness to others and have considerable difficulty developing and maintaining relationships with friends or peers.

Emotional Blunting

Emotional blunting is where the person has difficulty experiencing and demonstrating emotion and can cause difficulty in maintaining relationships. With this symptom people can show unchanging facial expressions and may fail to make appropriate eye contact.

In many cases attention and concentration may also be impaired and the patient may be unable to think in abstract terms, being able only to display a concrete thinking style.

Assessing Negative Symptoms

There are a number of reliable and valid methods of measuring negative symptoms, most of which involve some form of structured or semi-structured interview. However, since absence of a characteristic is often harder to describe and measure than the presence of a characteristic, assessing the degree of a reduction in functioning is problematic. The results obtained can be affected by the familiarity of the assessor with the patient, since it would be unreasonable to expect anyone to demonstrate their full repertoire of emotional and verbal responses, if anxious or suspicious of the assessor.

The results of a global psychopathology assessment, for example the KGV (Krawiecka *et al.*, 1977) may indicate the need to use a more specific assessment. The aim of the assessment process is to elicit assessment information that will inform the formulation, subsequent interventions and evaluation. In the following section a detailed assessment tool for negative symptoms is described; an assessment which measures the consequences of negative symptoms, social functioning and an assessment which informs the intervention process will also be described.

The Scale for the Assessment of Negative Symptoms (SANS) (Andreasen, 1989) provides a more detailed and comprehensive estimation of negative symptoms. The SANS comprises five sub-groups of negative features: alogia, affective flattening, avolition-apathy, anhedonia-asociality and attention. Training assessors is said to produce good levels of reliability across the five sub-scales. Since a number of the individual items relate to symptoms found in other disorders, the issue of confusion between negative symptoms of schizophrenia and other disorders such as depression or the side effects of neuroleptic medication should be borne in mind when evaluating the results of this assessment.

The Social Functioning Scale (SFS) (Birchwood *et al.*, 1990) is useful for recording the extent to which the person is active within their social environment – an important assessment, since reduced functioning is the major outcome of negative symptoms. The SFS measures a variety of dimensions ranging from social withdrawal to employment, social and recreational activities, relationships and ability and frequency of completing domestic tasks. The results of the assessment can be converted to give an estimate of the person's level of social functioning compared to other people experiencing schizophrenia.

Resource assessment is a further assessment which is useful in developing treatment plans. This assessment can be continually updated and focuses on a person's strengths, assets and supports. The person can find the process of generating a list of current and past resources rewarding. It is of benefit to involve family members in this assessment process. It is a useful assessment because people with schizophrenia are often seen as having a number of problems. The individual's problems seem to dominate the perception others have of the person (and may even affect the perception of the sufferer themselves). Positive attributes maybe overlooked. This information can be used in the development of therapeutic interventions and can help to maximise the effectiveness of interventions.

The kind of information collected in this assessment includes:

Strengths What the person can do
What the person likes to do, an interest or hobby
(this section would include the skills and abilities, hobbies and interests the person had in the past)

Assets What material resources has the person got?
For example, a good range of quality clothes, television, secure tenancy

Supports People who have input, relatives, friends, voluntary and statutory workers. People at the photographic club, other students attending further education classes, people who attend the luncheon club, the neighbour who helps with the garden.

People do change. Even if someone with negative symptoms appears to remain static irrespective of the work that is done together, progress will be made, though perhaps at a slower rate than is expected or wanted. This can be very disheartening for the client, family and friends and members of the care team. It is essential, therefore, that detailed assessment, particularly baseline information, is recorded. This can then provide tangible evidence that change is taking place, that effort is being rewarded, and the person, and their family, has the ability to effect progress from their own actions.

Distinguishing Between Negative Symptoms and Other Types of Pathology

Depressive features are commonly found in schizophrenia, particularly during the more florid phases, with depressive features seen in up to one half of patients (Leff, 1990). Although the features of depression and the negative symptoms of schizophrenia can overlap as in the anhedonia and alogia sub-scales of the SANS (McKenna *et al.*, 1989), those depression and negative symptoms are separate and distinct from one another in most areas (Barnes *et al.*, 1989). Any work which targets either negative symptoms or depression in schizophrenia, would benefit from having clear goals and objectives, which take account of these overlaps. Having a clear idea of the symptoms of depression and negative symptoms will help to clarify the two, so that appropriate interventions might be used.

Other phenomena that affect people with schizophrenia and are some-times mistakenly thought of as negative symptoms or depression include neuroleptic-induced deficit syndrome (see Chapter 6) and neuroleptic-induced pseudo-parkinsonism (Barnes, 1994).

The Consequences of Having Negative Symptoms

Negative symptoms can have a profound effect on a person's quality of life. Interpersonal communication is affected which can result in relationships of family members and friends deteriorating. The person reduces their involvement in hobbies, pastimes, work and vocational pursuits so further reducing intellectual stimulation, interpersonal contact and sometimes financial income.

Relatives or friends may complain about the patient's lack of responsiveness. The patient themselves may also notice and be concerned about their own lack of emotional responsiveness. Symptoms such as poverty of speech and reduced content of speech serve to distance the person from normal and rewarding social interactions, while lack of volition limits the opportunity to engage in rewarding or pleasurable activities or of feeling a sense of mastery from tackling successful projects. Reduction in concentration can have an additional and unhelpful effect upon the likelihood of obtaining feelings and thoughts of mastery and pleasure through successful social interaction.

Several other factors can be identified which may exacerbate or contribute to the effects of negative symptoms. A poor self concept may result from the person reflecting on their previous social life, the loss of those aspects of life and the thoughts of personal failure at not being able to sustain these areas of social activity. Institutionalisation has been long considered to contribute to the social withdrawal and poor self care skills found in some patients rehabilitated from hospitals. In addition the stigma associated with schizophrenia and financial constraints could have an effect upon an individuals willingness and ability to participate in social events.

Family studies have shown that people with negative symptoms are a source of distress for carers, with many relatives believing that the person's behaviour is because of laziness (Barrowclough and Tarrier, 1992). Family members can also experience feelings of 'burden' because of the reduction in domestic and self care activity of the client, the belief that they are 'doing more than their fair share' (Fadden *et al.*, 1987). This not only increases their workload but can result in family members reducing their social activities and personal relationships outside the home. This can be an additional source of stress, dissatisfaction and discord within the family unit.

Treatment for Negative Symptoms

Adapt the Style of Work

Working with people who experience negative symptoms can be one of the most challenging areas in which the mental health worker can become involved. Maintaining a balance between an enthusiastic and low-key approach is a difficult therapeutic skill.

On the one hand the worker must convey the belief that positive changes can be achieved and that the person is able to make those changes, and on the other hand, it can be easy to overwhelm the person and give the impression that a high level of work is expected between the client and mental health worker.

Because of the nature of negative symptoms and the work involved in addressing them, a situation can be envisaged where, over time, the worker can begin to feel drawn into a mutual atmosphere of apathy and stagnation as improvement in the client's condition appears to be unchanging, despite high levels of effort on the part of the worker.

Developing a style of working that sustains a positive therapeutic perspective, while moving at a pace which generates change without exerting undue pressure for the client, is the result of understanding the symptoms, the timescales involved in negative symptom work, and viewing the process of work in this area as a therapeutic partnership. The mental health worker's approach needs to be that of a supportive and uncritical helper.

Consider the Structure of the Session

For patients with limited concentration the agenda should be limited to 2–3 items and sessions should rarely last for longer than 30–45 minutes. As each session progresses, it would be prudent to monitor the person's responses and their non-verbal communications such as restlessness and an even more pronounced loss of interest, for indications that the person's concentration span has been exceeded. The session can then be modified to accommodate the current condition of the person. By asking the client for feedback on his involvement in the session the therapist will also gain an early insight into concentration.

Adapt the Style of Interaction

The use of a conversational but focused style can be utilised to maintain engagement when either apathy or poor concentration is evident. This kind of interaction can be less demanding and can allow the person to 're-charge batteries', before returning to the therapeutic topic in hand. The questions asked during therapy will inevitably be varied as the course of therapy progresses. Because of the poverty of speech content, the person should be given time to allow responses or elaboration to questions, however, long pauses to encourage elaboration, could be perceived by the patient as pressure to respond. Pitching the balance between open and closed questions and the pace of interaction is a clinical skill that needs to be mastered. An example of such a dialogue could be:

Mental health worker: 'Tell me about your childhood?'
(Puts the patient under pressure to respond)
A better question would be:
Mental health worker: 'Did you have a good childhood?'
Client: 'No.'
Mental health worker: 'Oh dear, was it bad all the way through?'
(Closed question, which could be followed up, and shows concern)

It should be noted that we are not suggesting that workers only use closed questions. Instead, we are suggesting that therapist gives due consideration to the potential effect of pressuring the person, by strict adherence to open questions only. It would be useful even early in therapy, to ask an occasional open question, particularly once therapeutic rapport has been established.

Maximising involvement in the therapy process can be helpful in assisting the client to overcome apathy or any doubts that they may have regarding his or her treatment and also to set limits and pace the work. By involving the person in agenda setting, by collaborating during sessions, and by asking for feedback openly, the client develops a feeling of control in their treatment and the perception that the therapy is in their interest. By achieving this it is possible that apathy is less likely to be exacerbated by dissatisfaction with therapy. Feedback allows the client an opportunity to discuss matters relevant to the process of therapy. Receiving comments about the session, such as: 'it was too long' is valuable information which guides the structure and length of future sessions. Clients need to be encouraged to voice these opinions both during and at the end of sessions.

Education

Negative symptoms can be as widely misunderstood as hallucinations and delusions. The client and, where appropriate, family members can perceive the lack of activity, emotional blunting and restricted communication as negative personal characteristics rather than illness related symptoms. People with schizophrenia may be described as 'lazy', 'not bothered', or 'negligent of their responsibilities'. These descriptions can attract negative attitudes and behaviour towards the sufferer and reinforce poor self esteem in the person himself or herself.

Information about the symptoms and how they relate to the course of the illness is needed, as well as an explanation of how these behaviours relate to the stress-vulnerability model of schizophrenia.

The long timescale which is likely to be needed to make an impact on these problems needs to be understood. Sensitivity is a critical feature in discussing this information as the prospect of treatment (or lack of functioning) over this time period can be extremely disheartening and may even cause the client (and carers) to give up before work begins.

Behavioural approaches used in the treatment of depression might equally be used in the treatment of some of the negative symptoms of schizophrenia. By increasing activity, it can be possible to increase feelings and thoughts of mastery, pleasure, or both. Assuming that the client has consented to work on these problems, developing a collaborative approaches is essential and following discussion, if it is agreed that a behavioural approach is appropriate a number of techniques can be utilised.

Graded Task Assignment or Goal Setting

Sometimes the activities and tasks faced by a person can be overwhelming and demoralisation can quickly take over. Graded task assignment involves the breaking down of a task or skill into its component parts. For this technique to be of value the task, for example, tidy the lounge, would be broken down into components that were readily achievable and were each possible within the concentration span of the patient, and allowing for breaks and rewards between the component parts.

Activity Scheduling

After identifying the problems of inactivity the mental health worker can explain the three types of activity which seem to characterise most of our day to day activities. These are:

- *Pleasure activities*, which we simply enjoy doing; we enjoy these activities for their own merits. Examples could include; eating chocolates, watching television, having a beer, having a bath, and so forth.
- *Mastery activities* are those which are not usually pleasurable, but the person achieves a sense of satisfaction when the activity is done. This might include; having a bet on the horses, gardening, tidying the room.
- *Chores* can be pleasurable, involve a sense of mastery or can be simply tasks which a person feels obliged to do. They might give no sense of pleasure or mastery. Examples might include taking the kids to school, paying the bills, or washing up dishes.

From this list of activities it can be seen that it would be helpful to have different ratios of activities. Initially the worker might aim to help the patient to increase mastery and pleasure activities. Reducing the perception of an excess of chores while concurrently increasing the mastery/pleasure activities can be a matter of changing attributions, along with increasing actual levels of activity. Setting short-term achievable goals allows for the client to develop a sense of achievement regarding the day's activities and will enhance engagement. Care is clearly needed to ensure the person is not overloaded and that a number of purely pleasurable activities are included for each day, or activity period.

Information gained from the social functioning scale and the strengths and resources assessment can be put to effective use in this strategy for increasing activity. The worker and client can formulate a plan which breaks the day into smaller, sometimes hourly, segments. Tasks, activities, and rest periods are built into the schedule in a way that enables the person to balance their day, which is more likely to result in pleasure or a sense of achievement and accomplishment or both. Where negative symptoms are more severe the aims and objectives should be modest. Workers need to facilitate the client's success, encourage positive experiences and opportunities for positive reinforcement. It is often necessary to set modest goals, which encourage the person, reward success and effort. Some clients may derive some benefit from having a predictable pattern to their day, while others would prefer more variety in their activities from one day to the next. The client and worker's task is to decide how best to achieve this, since for some clients a weekly activity plan might be prohibitively daunting and yet it may not be possible to plan activities day to day. In all cases the ideal situation would be for the person to set these goals and tasks for themselves. This is one area where the relatives or friends of the person could be particularly helpful by encouraging limited but achievable goals, and helping to identify and overcome obstacles such that a sense of accomplishment is achieved. Clearly there is potential for family involvement here. Relatives could be involved in monitoring progress, offering an appropriate level of stimulation or prompting, and most importantly in the giving of reinforcement or rewards for efforts made.

Work Undertaken Between Sessions

Agreeing on work/tasks that the client can undertake between meetings is a component of good cognitive therapy and a key element of graded task assignment and activity scheduling, but care must be exercised when utilising work between sessions with people who have negative symptoms. Where homework is to be used, care should be taken to ensure that the homework is achievable, determined by the client and problems in completing the task are anticipated and discussed.

'What do you think you will learn from doing this?'

'Will you be able to summon up the energy to do this?'

It is important that the person does not feel under pressure to complete the between session work. A technique which can help is to link an infrequently performed task, for example reading a leaflet or thinking about a particular topic with a frequently performed action such as drinking a cup of tea (Premack, 1965). For some clients it would still be appropriate to spend time allowing for the likelihood that between session work will not be achieved, thus minimising any guilt that might occur. It may also be useful to have a written record of agreed work to stimulate recall.

As with all work that clients are given to do in between sessions, this work must be reviewed and appraised early in the session. The nature of these symptoms will indicate how much effort the person has had to commit in order to complete, if only partially complete, activities agreed in the last session. It is vital that this work is positively commented on and, in deed, this activity should be seen, by the worker, as an opportunity to provide the client with encouragement and verbal reinforcement.

Case Vignette

Tom, a 34 year-old client lives with his wife, June. He has had three acute episodes of illness, the last one occurring seven years ago. Tom's level of functioning before the illness was very different to the way he presents now; he had a good 'work ethic', was a hard working builder's labourer and skilled at DIY. He helped around the home and at neighbours and friends, was an 'active' father to his stepson, and a 'good husband' with an active social life. June is a strong, hard working woman who organises the household and fulfils all the practical tasks in the home. She cares for her husband and provides him with substantial support.

June referred Tom to services stating that she was finding it difficult to cope with her husband's low levels of activity.

A wide range of assessments were undertaken with Tom including the KGV, SFS, LUNSERS and resources assessment. These assessments revealed a number of clinically important details which informed the development of a formulation. Tom's mental state examination revealed an absence of positive symptoms but clear signs of negative symptoms; psychomotor retardation, poverty of speech and flatness of affect. Tom's social functioning was also at a low level. He was prescribed one oral neuroleptic at a low dose, LUNSERS assessment indicates a very low experience of side effects. Tom's reduced levels of social functioning were considered to be a result of the negative symptoms of schizophrenia. By utilising the activities and interest identified in the resources assessment in a slow and incremental way Tom and June hope to see an increase in Tom's engagement in activities

Psycho-education – details were given about negative symptoms and treatment options. Each area was covered slowly and encouragement was given to ask questions and clarification. Custom-made handouts were provided covering the areas. Tom and June were encouraged to ask questions at any time in the future and information was revisited in subsequent family sessions.

Goal Setting

Tom's goals, to return to his high, pre-illness, work rate and his active social life were represented in targets he set for himself such as returning to his local for a drink with his friends or decorating the kitchen and living room. However such targets he repeatedly set but failed to even attempt, and Tom would become frustrated by his lack of drive. June's goals for Tom were more down to earth such as housework tasks, gardening, child care duties lots more. A goal setting strategy aims to modify the over ambitious expectations that clients and their relatives make. Putting their need for higher levels of functioning into the context of the education sessions enabled the couple to see the rationale of increasing functioning in small graduated steps.

As identified in the resources assessment in the past Tom used to enjoy a 10p bet on the horses. The initial goal was agreed and stated that he would walk the 100 metres to the bookies on the corner, once a week, to place a bet. He did not anticipate any problems achieving this goal and none were encountered. June was encouraged to take part in the treatment process by providing positive reinforcement when he achieved an agreed activity. When this task was established into a routine, after three weeks, a domestic task was added. When June returned from doing the shopping every morning, Tom would make her a cup of tea. Over the next year, several discrete tasks were added to his routine, for example, washing up after the evening meal, spending an hour gardening every weekend, which he enjoyed and in fact spent much longer in doing.

> ## Box 9.1   Interventions
>
> - Make an assessment
> - Adapt your style of work
> - Organise the delivery of the interventions
> - Consider session structure
> - Adapt the style of interaction
> - Education
> - Graded task assignment/goal setting
> - Activity scheduling
> - Work undertaken between sessions

Compared to baseline data, Tom's level of social functioning has greatly improved. While it is not at the level it was before his illness it has improved since the start of treatment. Tom and June were happy with the results, and it has encouraged them to continue this method of improving social functioning.

An increase was seen in subsequent SFS assessments, but more importantly June commented that she felt that she 'was not running the show single-handedly'. This emphasises that not only are positive changes made in the target behaviours but also an improvement in the dynamics of the relationship can be gained as a by-product of the intervention.

Conclusion

Negative symptoms are likely to have several effects upon a person's domestic and social life. Although there is little evidence as yet for the efficacy of psychological interventions directed at negative symptoms, techniques and strategies can be utilised to minimise and reduce the consequences of these symptoms. A detailed initial assessment together with a collaborative approach is the foundation for successful work in this area. An approach which is non-pressurising and mindful of the need to take a long-term view regarding the resolution of these problems is advocated as it may be possible to help the patient to overcome their difficulties more effectively.

Suggested Further Reading

Hamilton, M. (1978) *Fish's Outline of Psychiatry*, 3rd edn, Bristol, John Wright.
Hogg, L. (1996) 'Psychological Treatments for Negative Symptoms', in G. Haddock and P. Slade (eds), *Cognitive Behavioural Interventions with Psychosis*, London, Routledge.

References

Andreasen, N.C. (1989) 'The scale for the assessment of negative symptoms (SANS) conceptual and theoretical foundations', *British Journal of Psychiatry*, 155, 49–52.

Barnes, T.R.E. (1994) 'Issues in the clinical assessment of negative symptoms', *Current Opinion in Psychiatry*, 7, 35–8.

Barnes, T.R.E., Curzon, D.A., Liddle, P.F. and Patel, M. (1989) 'The nature and prevalence of depression in chronic schizophrenic in-patients', *British Journal of Psychiatry*, 154, 486–91.

Barnes, T.R.E. and Liddle, P.F. (1990) 'Evidence for the validity of negative symptoms', in N.C. Andreasen (ed.), *Schizophrenia: positive and negative symptoms and syndromes*, Vol. 24, Basel, Karger.

Barrowclough, C. and Tarrier, N. (1992) Families of Schizophrenic Patients: Cognitive Behavioural Interventions, London, Chapman & Hall.

Birchwood, M., Smith, J., Cochrane, R., Wetton, S. and Copestake, S. (1990) 'The Social Functioning Scale: The development and validation of a scale of social adjustment for use in family intervention programmes with schizophrenic patients'. *British Journal of Psychiatry*, 157, 853–9.

Carpenter Jr., W.T., Heinrichs, D.W. and Wagman, A.M. (1988) 'Deficit and Non-deficit Forms of Schizophrenia', *American Journal of Psychiatry*, 145, 578–83.

Crow, T.J. (1980) 'Molecular pathology of schizophrenia: more than one dimension of pathology', *British Medical Journal*, 143, 66–8.

Fadden, G., Kuipeβ, E. and Bebbington, P. (1987) The burden of care: the impact of functional psychiatric illness on the patients's family, *British Journal of Psychiatry*, 150, 285–92.

Fenton, W.S. and McGlashan, T.H. (1994) 'Antecedents, Symptom Progression, and Long-Term Outcome of the Deficit Syndrome in Schizophrenia', *American Journal of Psychiatry*, 151(3), 351–6.

Krawiecka, M., Goldberg, D. and Vaughan, M. (1977) 'A standardised psychiatric assessment rating for chronic psychotic patients', *Acta Psychiatrica Scandinavica*, 55, 299–308.

Leff, J. (1990) 'Depressive symptoms in the course of schizophrenia', in L.E. DeLisi (ed.), *Depression in Schizophrenia*, Washington, DC, American Psychiatric Press.

Liddle, P. (1987) 'The symptoms of chronic schizophrenia: a re-examination of the positive-negative dichotomy', *British Journal of Psychiatry*, 151, 145–51.

McKenna, P.J., Lund, C.E. and Mortimer, A.M. (1989) 'Negative Symptoms: Relationship to other schizophrenic symptom classes', *British Journal of Psychiatry*, 155 (suppl. 7), 104–7.

Premack, D. (1975) 'Reinforcement Theory', in A.E. Kazdin (ed.), *Behavior Modification in Applied Settings*, Homewood, IL, Dorsey Press.

Thara, R. and Eaton, W.W. (1996) 'Outcome of Schizophrenia: the Madras longitudinal study', *Australian and New Zealand Journal of Psychiatry*, 30, 516–22.

CHAPTER 10

Relapse Prevention Intervention in Psychosis

ALICE KNIGHT

Introduction

Relapse is defined by 'the emergence or exacerbation of positive symptoms which tends to be preceded by subtle changes in mental functioning up to 4 weeks prior to the event' (American Psychiatric Association, 1987). Relapse prevention interventions therefore offer a way in which these 'subtle changes' can be identified, monitored and acted upon as soon as possible in order to prevent a relapse from occurring. This period prior to relapse is known as the 'prodromal period' and is normally characterised by changes in the person's mood, behaviour and thoughts, which usually appear 2–6 weeks prior to relapse.

Relapse rates in psychosis are extremely high. For example, Robinson *et al.* (1999) carried out a study of relapse in 104 participants with a diagnosis of either schizophrenia or schizoaffective disorder after their first episode. Five years after the initial recovery 81 per cent of the participants had relapsed at least once. They stated that the risk is diminished by antipsychotic drug treatment. The majority of research in this area has focused on the use of antipsychotic medication, however, as highlighted by this article, it clearly has only a limited impact on the prevention of relapse. It is therefore important to explore psychosocial approaches that can be used alongside medication when working with clients in an attempt to prevent relapse. However, there are problems with research in this area. Relapse can be categorised in different ways, for example as the onset of symptomatology or using hospitalisation to illustrate relapse. There has also been a great variability in psychosocial approaches that have been explored in the research literature to date. There is clearly a need for more research using large samples and specific systematic psychosocial approaches to examine the efficacy of such interventions in the prevention of relapse. This chapter therefore draws upon findings from the research to date in an attempt to present a structure to carrying out a psychosocial approach to relapse prevention, which can be used in conjunction with traditional psychiatric approaches.

In the past two decades there has been a growing body of evidence supporting the idea that identifying and monitoring an individual's prodromal

signs, and establishing appropriate action plans in the event of them occurring, can help to prevent relapse or at least reduce the impact of the experience. This would therefore reduce the level of psychological and social
disability resulting from it. In addition, it serves to increase the individual's
understanding of their episode(s) and their sense of control over them, which
in turn decreases fear of relapse.

The first research studies that attempted to identify the common signs of a
prodromal phase in psychosis used a retrospective approach where people were
interviewed to establish if they had noticed any change in themselves prior to
their most recent relapse that might indicate a state of reduced well being
(Herz and Melville, 1980; McCandless-Glincher *et al.*, 1986; Birchwood
et al., 1989). These studies found that the majority of patients and their carers
reported particular changes in thoughts, feelings and behaviours prior to the
episode(s).

Research findings in general have indicated that prodromes in psychosis
appear to be typified by signs such as tension, eating problems, concentration
problems, sleeping difficulties, depression, social withdrawal, anxiety and irri-
tability. They may also include pre-psychotic signs such as suspiciousness and
mild feelings of paranoia. Birchwood (1996) suggests that there are two stages
to the prodromal period: dysphoria (including anxiety, restlessness and blunting of drives) followed by early psychotic symptoms (including suspiciousness,
ideas of reference and misinterpretations). Subotnik and Nuechterlein (1988)
found that these non-psychotic symptoms are sensitive to relapse but not
specific to it but if followed by low-level psychotic symptoms relapse is more
probable.

There is also evidence to suggest that people are often very keen to take
part in activities that may help decrease the likelihood of relapsing. Mueser
et al. (1992) found that patients expressed a strong interest in learning
about early warning signs of the illness and relapse and that it was in fact the
second most important item out of an agenda of over forty topics. In addition McCandless-Glincher *et al.* (1986) found that patients tend to monitor
symptoms and initiate responses, such as engaging in diversionary activities,
seeking professional help, and resuming or increasing their neuroleptic
medication, without being guided to do so.

In light of the findings, Herz and Melville (1980) and Birchwood *et al.*
(1989) both developed specialist measuring instruments with which to assess
small changes in mood and behaviour that might be indicative of prodromal
signs: the Early Signs Questionnaire (Herz and Melville (1980)) and the Early
Signs Scale (ESS; Birchwood *et al.* (1989)). For the purposes of this chapter,
the focus in on using the ESS designed by Birchwood *et al.* (1989) when
describing the identification of early warning signs.

Birchwood *et al.* (1989) used the ESS in a prospective design to follow up
19 patients who had a diagnosis of schizophrenia. The ESS contains of a list
of common prodromal signs from which the client can identify signs that they
experienced mildly, a lot, or did not experience at all in the period(s) prior to

their episode(s). The patients and their carers were asked to complete the ESS every two weeks. Half of the patients relapsed over the course of nine months, and 63 per cent of relapses were predicted using these scales. The use of the ESS rather than a more general measure of psychopathology enabled Birchwood to observe qualitative differences between patients in their early signs and symptoms. It was suggested that the ESS should also help to 'educate the individual, their carers and professionals' and 'promote client's engagement in services, and to share responsibility for prodrome detection between individual and professionals' (Birchwood *et al.*, 1996).

Herz *et al.* (2000) also carried out a prospective study with 82 patients with a diagnosis of schizophrenia or schizoaffective disorder who were randomly assigned to receive either a programme for relapse prevention (PRP) or treatment as usual (TAU). The TAU group received biweekly individual sup- portive therapy and medication management, whereas the PRP group received psychoeducation, active monitoring for prodromal signs with clinical inter- ventions if such signs occurred, weekly group therapy and multi-family groups. Both groups received standard doses of maintenance antipsychotic medication. Over an 18-month follow-up period they found the PRP was effective in detecting prodromal symptoms of relapse early in an episode and they were more likely to identify prodromal episodes before patients met objective relapse criteria or needed hospitalisation. This study therefore highlights the benefits of adopting a psychosocial approach to relapse prevention. It also illustrates that there are a number of ways in which to do this. One such approach was described using a case example by Perry and Tarrier (1995), which presented a general outline which this chapter follows.

The remainder of the chapter guides the reader through the stages of a pos- sible psychosocial approach to relapse prevention which has been informed by the research carried out in the field to date, largely by Birchwood and colleagues. The stages include identifying the early warning signs of a relapse signature; developing action plans; and developing monitoring systems. A case example will then be presented to illustrate this process in clinical practice. This is not the only way to approach relapse prevention but it should be pos- sible from using this chapter and the reading list provided to introduce some of these ideas in your own working area, provided adequate supervision and training is available.

Who Should be Involved in Relapse Prevention Interventions?

It could be argued that anyone who has suffered from psychosis could benefit from doing some relapse prevention interventions, however it is not as straight- forward as this in practice. For example, some people may not want to discuss their psychotic experiences or may have difficulty recalling them. In such cases the client's views must be respected and efforts concentrated on other ways of assisting them. However, this does not mean that relapse prevention work can not be carried out at all. Other people (e.g., carers and other professionals) can play a central role to each stage of the relapse prevention process, and can be used as the informant(s) necessary. Involving people who have regular and frequent contact with the client can help to identify early warning signs and enhance the quality of monitoring by offering another perspective on this process. This can be particularly beneficial if the client has very little insight or loses insight throughout the prodromal period. Even if the carers or professionals have not been involved in the relapse prevention work they may feature in the action plans and therefore it is important that they are made aware of this, understand why and how, and are happy with this arrangement. It is important, however, that the involvement of others is decided upon in collaboration with the client.

There are certain people who are potentially more likely to benefit from carrying out relapse prevention work, such as individuals

- recently recovering from relapse;
- who are particularly fearful of relapse;
- with a history of repeated relapse;
- who have problems with their medication (due to poor adherence or low dosage due to sensitivity to side effects);
- who have experienced psychosis more recently (i.e. in the past 1–6 years);
- living in a highly critical environment.

People will benefit most however, if they are both keen to prevent relapse and willing to take an active role in the process.

The Relapse Prevention Process: Getting Started

The relapse prevention process can be divided into three main stages: the early warning signs of a relapse signature; the action plans; and the monitoring systems. Each of these stages should be dealt with in turn and is described in depth below. Prior to commencing however, and as with all psychosocial interventions, relapse prevention begins with engaging the client in a therapeutic working relationship. Incorporated into this is the psychoeducational component which is important for engaging the client by presenting a rationale for doing relapse prevention interventions, introducing the ideas that will be used and encouraging a need for a collaborative approach to it. In addition, it provides an opportunity for the assessment of any existing explanations that the client may have for their problems and any additional psychoeducational needs, which vary with each individual. It is essential that this is sensitively assessed and the necessary psychoeducational material provided for everyone involved in the relapse prevention process prior to commencement. This will ensure that everyone is approaching it from the same viewpoint.

The rationale should be presented in terms of a stress-vulnerability model (Zubin and Spring, 1977). This model offers a way of understanding the role of psychosocial factors in the onset, maintenance and relapse of psychotic symptoms, and therefore the role that we (the client and people involved in their care) can have in influencing these factors. This role would be to identify such factors and develop monitoring systems and action plans to try to reduce the experience of them and thus in turn reduce the risk of relapse. This information should offer a sense of control over potential relapse and thus a reduced fear of it, which should therefore encourage people to feel motivated towards actively engaging in relapse prevention work.

Identifying false positives (when a prodrome is wrongly identified as occurring) can also cause unnecessary distress and it is therefore important to share normalising information at this stage to explore situations in which early warning signs may occur and not result in relapse. This should help to prevent people from catastrophising about the signs. Similarly it must be explained that relapse prevention interventions do not guarantee that relapse will be prevented, but that it should at least help to reduce the impact of such an experience.

Identifying the Early Warning Signs of a Relapse Signature

Having established a rationale for relapse prevention intervention and engaged the client in the work, the next stage is to identify the clients relapse signature. Each individual has a collection of early warning signs (prodromal signs), some of which are universal and some of which are unique to them. This combination of signs was described by Birchwood *et al.* (1996) as a 'relapse signature' because the collection of signs varies with each individual, like a signature. Establishing an individual's relapse signature can be achieved by exploring any changes they may have experienced before their previous episode(s). This is in relation to their mood, thoughts, behaviour and how they felt in their body before the event, alongside any environmental changes that took place. The more episodes an individual has experienced, the more detail they can add to their relapse signature by pinpointing common signs that occurred across all of the episodes. If somebody therefore does relapse after having already established his or her relapse signature, it can then be defined further. It is extremely important when revisiting prodromal periods with clients to be aware of any distress that recalling such details may cause. Appropriate support should therefore be established prior to doing so.

The universal early warning signs that are appropriate for inclusion in a client's relapse signature can be identified using the ESS. This scale can also be used to establish the client's baseline score. The baseline score is important because the individual may still be experiencing some residual symptoms or some of the signs that have been identified as their early warning signs. In both cases establishing a baseline score allows for more detailed monitoring of both the occurrence of a sign and the level at which it is occurring. This helps to reduce the chances of identifying false positives and also allow for action plans to be adopted immediately for any signs that are being experienced at the time the intervention is being carried out.

As well as being useful for identifying the relapse signature and baseline score, the ESS can continue to be used for monitoring purposes. However, it would be more suitable once the baseline score has been established, to create a monitoring scale that is tailored for each individual. By developing idiosyncratic monitoring scales, which only incorporates the signs of the individuals relapse signature, the process of monitoring would be more specific and simplified. This should therefore encourage monitoring to be carried out.

In addition to identifying universal early warning signs as part of their relapse signature, clients will probably be able to describe signs that are not listed on the ESS that are unique to them. The identification of these unique signs can be done through further clarification of the prodromal period(s) before their episode(s). There are different ways to identify unique signs and it is preferable to use as many as possible in order to gain a detailed description. You could, for example, gain a lot of information through general discussions with the client, their carers or other professionals involved. You can also use the five-factor model created by Padesky and Greenberger (1995) to explain how thoughts, mood, behaviour, physical reaction and environment are interconnected. By placing each early warning sign (both universal and unique) within this model, the client can then link in other factors that are related to it. This provides an opportunity for understanding why signs occurred and how they are interrelated, which also provides a chance to expand on the details of the signs.

Establishing the timing and order of the early warning signs also aids in the understanding of how the signs emerged and could therefore re-emerge in a prodrome. It also provides a further opportunity for more in-depth discussion about the signs. This can be done in different ways, for example, each sign could be written on individual pieces of card and the client could place them in the order that they occurred. Similarly a time line could be drawn and the client could pinpoint where each sign occurred on the line.

Once the early warning signs have been established they can be divided into warning level and danger level signs. Warning level signs appear in the very early stages, signs that Birchwood (1996) termed dysphoria. Danger level signs, or early psychotic experience, appear later and this is the point at which services should be contacted. Dichotomising early warning signs into warning and danger level signs can help to simplify the list further and prevent people from catastrophising over less problematic signs.

Developing Action Plans

Psychological and behavioural action plans need to be developed in order to intervene in the problematic vicious cycles identified (as illustrated by the five-factor model) before they spiral out of control and a relapse occurs. It must be noted that like the relapse signature, the action plans must also take into account the idiosyncratic needs of the individual depending on a number of factors. Such factors include the type of signs in an individual's relapse signature, their interests, their support network involved (both personal and professional), medication arrangements, and any existing coping mechanisms that are already utilised by the individual that could be expanded upon. All of this must be decided collaboratively because it is up to the client to carry out the action plans.

Once identified the psychological and behavioural action plans should help to prevent the warning level signs from becoming any worse and developing into danger level signs, and therefore prevent the need for contacting services. However, it is important for people to be advised to seek help as soon as necessary if the signs do actually worsen. The key is to strike a balance so that services are contacted at the appropriate times. This is a negotiated arrangement with early contact with services advisable in some instances. It is also important to provide the client with necessary contact details and it is crucial that those involved should be consulted prior to being included as a point of contact.

Developing Monitoring Systems

Monitoring systems allow the client and anyone else involved in the relapse prevention process to monitor for the early warning signs. A checklist of these signs allows quick and easy access to the early warning signs and action plans (see Appendix 1). These can be created in various formats to suit the client's needs so that they are likely to use them.

In addition, monitoring diaries provide the opportunity for recording more detail if required (see Appendix 2). This would contain a list of all of the early warning signs, which could be scored daily or weekly and compared to the baseline scores. The diaries also allow a means of providing professionals with more detailed information if contacted by the client. Monitoring systems must be collaboratively agreed upon in order to suit the individual needs of the client, and to ensure that standards set are reasonable and are not too overwhelming, which would be self-defeating in the long term. For example, one person may choose to monitor each day for the first few weeks and then reassess the situation. Another person may decide simply to monitor in times of increased stress.

Creating a Relapse Prevention Manual

A relapse prevention manual provides all those who are involved with a detailed account of all the work that was carried out for quick and easy reference. The contents of a relapse prevention manual should be basic and easy to follow so that it is accessible in times of distress. It should contain a detailed description of their relapse signature, a list of the possible action plans to take in the event of each sign occurring with guidelines on how to carry them out, plus services contact details. It should also include a monitoring checklist and monitoring diaries for use when necessary with instructions. Any additional information that was provided should also be included.

A Case Example of Relapse Prevention in Practice

Sarah had a five-year history of psychosis with a diagnosis of hypermania and had experienced four episodes. She was said to be at increased risk in novel circumstances and had just started a new job, which had caused her some increased stress. She lived with her boyfriend and had regular contact with her parents who had been involved in her care previously. She smoked cannabis and drank alcohol. She had been prescribed stelazine to use if necessary, an arrangement with which she was happy.

Psychoeducational material regarding the rationale for relapse prevention and hypermania was provided and an assessment of Sarah's general mental health carried out. Sarah's early warning signs list and baseline scores were established using the ESS and she was shown how to further clarify each sign of her relapse signature by using the five-factor model. She had experienced difficulties in recollecting the details of her prodromal periods so the model helped her to gain a more detailed understanding of her prodromes by building on the signs she had identified, which resulted in changes to her early warning signs list. This detailed exploration of the prodromal period enabled the identification of new signs that had not been remembered and the elimination of signs that were incorrectly included. The timing of her prodromes was also easier to distinguish with the help of the five-factor model.

Through establishing a baseline score Sarah identified her current preoccupation with certain issues at work, which she also wanted to work on. This related to the relapse prevention work because she had also identified this as an important early warning sign in her relapse signature. For example, before her first episode she was preoccupied with thoughts about the men in her office taking advantage of the young women in the office and prior to the second episode she was preoccupied with thoughts about her brother's baby that had just died during childbirth. This resulted in her experiencing high levels of anxiety on both occasions. In her new job Sarah had found herself becoming preoccupied with worrying that she offended people and found herself becoming slightly anxious as a result. Sarah was therefore shown how to complete a thought record (Padesky and Greenberger, 1995). Through this she learnt to record situations, identify her negative automatic thoughts, generate alternative thoughts, and rate her mood. Examples were provided to illustrate this, and then Sarah practised using thought records in real life situations where she found herself getting distressed by her thoughts.

Having used the five-factor model repeatedly by this stage, Sarah had gained an understanding of how the factors were interrelated. This therefore allowed her to use this knowledge of the gradual process of relapse when developing her action plans. She not only recognised that she could intervene in this process but had some ideas about where, when and how to do this without simply turning to her medication or asking for help. This gave Sarah an increased sense of control over relapse and a reduced fear of it.

Sarah broke down the signs of her relapse signature into sections using the model: thoughts, mood, behaviour, and physiology. This allowed for the development of action plans for each section within this framework. Sarah then broke down the list even further by dividing the signs into 'warning' level and 'danger' level signs to prevent her from catastrophising if warning level signs occurred.

Sarah was able to see by this stage that she had the ability to take some action herself without having to involve services. The action plans that Sarah developed were both psychological and behavioural. Having learnt this skill of completing a thought record she was able to incorporate it into her action plan. She also identified key people with whom she could discuss her concerns. Due to her 'hypermanic' behaviour during episodes she decided to create behavioural action plans that would reduce the number of activities she was involved in and practice methods that she found helpful for improving her relaxation and sleep. She stated that her use of alcohol and cannabis had been influential in the past and therefore reducing her use of these substances if any early warning signs occurred was also incorporated into the action plans.

Having broken down her signs into two levels she was able to manage her medication use effectively by taking it only if danger level signs occurred. The need to contact services if danger-level signs occurred was also highlighted and a procedure was developed, which was tailored to Sarah's needs. This incorporated all her points of contact, with individuals named and contact details provided in order of preference.

Various methods for monitoring were then created that Sarah felt were suitable for her requirements, including checklists and diaries for use in times of increased stress. Examples of this are provided in the appendix. All of the work done in the sessions was recorded in detail in a manual for Sarah to take away for reference. Sarah stated that she found this in itself 'comforting' because it contained all the information she needed and she could put it to one side without worrying that she would forget something.

Six months after completing the relapse prevention intervention Sarah had not relapsed and is much more settled in her job. At the end of the sessions Sarah wrote about her experience for other people who may consider going through the process:

> At first, I was unsure about trying relapse prevention as I was feeling well and wanted to forget about my past experience in hospital. However, I am glad that I chose to go ahead with it. It was an excellent opportunity to examine the causes

of my episodes of illness, and I feel reassured because I will be able to recognise warning signs and take appropriate action, which will hopefully prevent hospital-isation in the future. I would recommend anyone in a similar position to try relapse prevention; there really is nothing to lose and much to be gained.

Despite the success of the relapse prevention work carried out with Sarah, it did not use all the possible approaches that can be taken. For example, nobody else was included in the relapse prevention work. However, the most appropriate approach from the options available with regards to Sarah's needs were, and this is vital. What this case example does illustrate is the benefits in adopting a cognitive framework when doing relapse prevention work. If Sarah had not explored her early warning signs in more depth using the five-factor model, each stage of the relapse prevention process would have looked very different. Her relapse signature and therefore monitoring systems would have included false signs and omitted vital signs. This could have resulted in false positives being reported and causing unnecessary dis-tress. Her action plans would also have been tackling different unrelated problems as a result. Working within this framework thus allows for flexi-bility and makes allowances for the idiosyncratic nature of relapse.

Conclusions

This chapter presented a structured approach to using psychosocial inter-ventions to relapse prevention in psychosis, which utilised the findings to date in the research literature on the area. Prior to carrying out such an ap-proach it is worth noting that 'like psychosis itself, there is likely to be a con-siderable between-subject variability in timing and nature of early symptoms' (Birchwood, 1996). Due to the idiosyncratic nature of prodromes it is not easy to carry out the detailed relapse prevention interventions as described above simply based on the research findings of common universal symptoms. It instead requires a more flexible approach, which can be time consuming. However, this does not mean that no relapse prevention work can take place unless it adopts a flexible and idiosyncratic approach. Some basic relapse pre-vention work could be carried out which would be less time consuming and preferable to no service at all. Providing general information about the nature of relapse and the prodromal period, how common universal and individual early warning signs can be monitored for, and what commonly advised action plans can be adopted would be one such approach.

No matter what approach is used it must be presented in an appropriately sensitive format with support systems in place so as to avoid any unnecessary distress that it may cause. It must be promoted as an empowering tool and therefore a means for reducing stress generated from a fear of relapse. If a less thorough approach is adopted however, it is still important that the relapse prevention plan is tailored to the needs of each individual as much as possible. If carried out properly Birchwood (1996) suggests that 'identifying this individual information is the key to early intervention'. However, whatever approach is adopted, there is a great need for further empirical research to examine the efficacy of such approaches being used in practice.

Appendix 1: Sarah's Relapse Prevention Checklist

Main Early Warning Signs

Warning Level

- I am drinking or smoking cannabis during the day
- I am burning myself out
- My senses seem sharper
- I am not getting much sleep and feel that I do not need sleep
- I am feeling very emotionally high
- I am feeling strong and powerful
- I am living very chaotically
- I am involved in too many projects
- I have a strong interest in sex
- I am being very talkative
- I am spending money more freely

Danger Level – Take Medication and Contact Services

- My thoughts are flowing too fast
- I am suspicious about other people
- I can not separate reality from fantasy
- I think that I am very important
- My behaviour is uninhibited and unpredictable

*If any of the above is happening then I should carry out the most suitable action plans below and begin to **monitor** for all my early warning signs using the monitoring diary (see the manual).*

Main Action Plans

- Talk to my boyfriend and my parents
- Do a thought record
- Do something active (for example, go for a walk)
- Cut down on the amount of things I am involved in
- Cut down on alcohol and cannabis
- Practice some relaxation techniques

Appendix 2: Sarah's Monitoring Diary for Early Warning Signs

Instruction: Write down at the end of every day how much each sign has happened that day. Use the scoring codes below to complete the table and remember also to carry out the appropriate action plan for any of the signs that have happened at all (see the action plans list).

0 = was never a problem
1 = was a little bit of a problem
2 = was a medium problem
3 = was a very big problem

Name: _____
Date: _____
Medication (name and amount): _____

Early warning signs – behaviours	M	T	W	T	F	S	S
My behaviour is uninhibited							
My behaviour is unpredictable							
I have a very strong interest in sex							
I am living chaotically							
I am spending money more freely							
I am being very talkative							
I am not getting much sleep							
I am involved in many projects							
I am drinking during the day							
I am smoking cannabis during the day							

Early warning signs – feelings	M	T	W	T	F	S	S
I am feeling emotionally high							
I am feeling strong/powerful							

Early warning signs – physical reaction	M	T	W	T	F	S	S
I am burning myself out							
I do not feel like I need much sleep							
My senses seem sharper							

Early warning signs – thoughts	M	T	W	T	F	S	S
My thoughts are flowing too fast							
I can not separate reality and fantasy							
I am suspicious about other people							
I think that I am very important							

Further Reading

Birchwood, M. (1998) 'Early Intervention in Psychotic Relapse', in C. Brooker and
    J. Repper (eds), *Serious Mental Health Problems in the Community: Policy, Practice
    and Research*, London, Bailliere Tindall.
McGorry, P. (1998) 'Preventative strategies in early psychosis: verging on reality',
    British Journal of Psychiatry, 175, 33, 1–2.

References

American Psychiatric Association (1987) *Diagnostic and Statistical Manual of Mental
    Disorders*, 3rd edn, Washington, DC, American Psychiatric Association.
Birchwood, M. (1996) 'Early Intervention in Psychotic Relapse: Cognitive Approaches
    to Detection and Management', in G. Haddock and P. Slade (eds), *Cognitive Behav-
    iour Therapy for Psychotic Disorders*, London, Routledge.
Birchwood, M., Smith, J., Macmillan, F., Hogg, B., Prasad, R., Harvey, C. and Bering,
    S. (1989) 'Predicting relapse in schizophrenia: the development and implementation
    of an early signs monitoring system using patients and families as observers. A
    Preliminary Investigation', *Psychological Medicine*, 19, 649–56.
Birchwood, M., Todd, P. and Jackson, C. (1998) 'Early intervention in psychosis, the
    critical period hypothesis', *British Journal of Psychiatry*, 172, 33, 53–9.
Herz, M.I., Lamberti, S., Mintz, J., Scott, R., O'Dell, S.P., McCartan, L. and Nix, G.
    (2000) 'A program for relapse prevention in schizophrenia', *Archives of General
    Psychiatry*, 57, 277–83.
Herz, M. and Melville, C. (1980) 'Relapse in schizophrenia', *American Journal of
    Psychiatry*, 137, 801–12.
McCandless-Glincher, L., McKnight, S., Hamera, E., Smith, B.L., Peterson, K. and
    Plumlee, A.A. (1986) 'Use of symptoms by schizophrenics to monitor and regulate
    their illness', *Hospital and Community Psychiatry*, 37, 929–33.
Mueser, K., Bellack, A., Wade, J., Sayers, S. and Rosenthal, K. (1992) 'An assessment
    of the educational needs of chronic psychiatric patients and their relatives', *British
    Journal of Psychiatry*, 160, 668–73.
Padesky, C.A. and Greenberger, D. (1995) *Clinicians Guide to Mind Over Mood*, New
    York, Guildford Press.
Perry, A. and Tarrier, N. (1995) 'Identification of Prodromal Signs and Symptoms
    and Early Intervention in manic Deressive Psychosis Patients: A Case Example',
    Behavioural and Cognitive Psychotherapy, 23, 399–409.
Robinson, D., Woerner, M., Alvir, J.M.J., Bilder, R., Goldman, R., Geisler, S., Koreen,
    A., Sheitman, B., Chakos, M., Mayerhoff, D. and Lieberman, J.A. (1999) 'Predic-
    tors of Relapse Following Responses From a First Episode of Schizophrenia or
    Schizoaffective Disorder', *Archives of General Psychiatry*, 56, 241–7.
Subotnik, K.L. and Nuechterlein, K.H. (1988) 'Prodromal Signs and Symptoms of
    Schizophrenic Relapse', *Journal of Abnormal Psychology*, 97(4), 405–12.
Zubin, J. and Spring, B. (1977) 'Vulnerability: A new view of schizophrenia', *Journal
    of Abnormal Psychology*, 86, 103–26.

CHAPTER 11

Working With Families

DAVID READER

Introduction

It has been argued that users of publicly funded mental health services should receive interventions which meet their specific needs and are proven by research to be effective (Falloon and Fadden, 1993). Research carried out around the world over the past two decades has provided evidence for the effectiveness of working with families of people who have a diagnosis of schizophrenia (Penn and Mueser, 1996).

However, despite this 'scientific validation', family interventions for people with schizophrenia are largely unavailable in many UK mental health services and in some they are effectively absent (Clinical Standards Advisory Group, 1995). Evidence of efficacy and effectiveness has not been sufficient to enable family interventions to enter the mainstream of mental health service provision.

The aim of this chapter is to provide a brief introduction to the concepts that have led to the development of psychosocial family interventions and to introduce a protocol for their implementation with relatives of people suffering from schizophrenia. The protocol is intended to guide the clinical practice of mental health workers. The chapter concludes with a discussion of the difficulties associated with the implementation of family interventions in routine practice and some suggestions regarding how these difficulties can be resolved, so that a 'place' can be found for these interventions in mental health services.

The Concept of Expressed Emotion in Families

Relatives of people who have a diagnosis of schizophrenia are likely to experience feelings of loss and grief (Miller *et al.*, 1990) and may feel stigmatised and socially isolated (Walsh and Harman, 1989). Relatives may also suffer psychological and economic consequences as they adjust to a new and unexpected care giving role (Clark, 1994). Without help to understand the illness and recognise and respond to its symptoms, family members may develop their own explanations for the affected person's behaviour and cope with it in an instinctual way, according to their own upbringing and experience. Such

responses can be understood as attempts to cope with the impact of an unexpected and disturbing illness. While some responses might be deemed adaptive or helpful, research has shown that critical, over-protective or hostile
coping responses by family members can have a detrimental effect on the
course of the illness. These behaviours collectively known as 'high expressed
emotion' (EE) have been the subject of investigation by studies in many different cultures over the past forty years (Brown *et al.*, 1972; Vaughn and Leff,
1976; Tarrier *et al.*, 1988; Vaughn *et al.*, 1984; Wig *et al.*, 1987).

This research has shown that people with schizophrenia who live in high EE
environments relapse twice as frequently as those that live in low EE environments (Kavanagh, 1992). It has also been shown that carers who have developed high EE coping responses report greater perceived burden of caring
and more psychological distress (Barrowclough and Parle, 1997). Therefore
inadequate information and support for families can be said to have a detrimental effect on both the person with schizophrenia and the carers' well being.
The mechanisms by which expressed emotion affects relapse are not fully
understood, but it is probable that the frequency of relapse for people with
schizophrenia increases because of their sensitivity to the stress in the
household environment (Kavanagh, 1992).

It is important to emphasise at this point that in the context of the present
chapter, high EE coping responses are simply viewed as attempts by families
to cope and do what they think is best for the person. Families are faced
with significant problems and receive inadequate information and support to
enable the development of other ways of coping. Families are therefore viewed
as a valuable source of help to the patient in their recovery and the role
of professionals is to help the family in their efforts to support the patient.
Therefore the role of psychosocial family intervention in schizophrenia can be
summarised as being to

  (i)   provide the family with support;
 (ii)   help them understand the illness and how its symptoms manifest them-
        selves in the patient's behaviour;
(iii)   assist the family to develop ways of coping with problems associated with
        the illness;
 (iv)   help the family strike a balance between encouraging and supporting the
        person while avoiding making critical comments or doing too much for
        them;
  (v)   assist family members to manage their own stress and to look after them-
        selves by not sacrificing all their own interests and activities in an effort
        to care for the person with schizophrenia.

Family Intervention Studies

Many carefully controlled research trials have now been conducted in many
different cultures to test the hypothesis that providing support and information

to families will reduce relapse rates and improve other outcomes. The nature and duration of family intervention provided by research teams has varied but the results of these studies have predominantly been very encouraging and have shown that it is possible to reduce the frequency of relapse for the affected person and reduce levels of psychological distress for carers. We are now beginning to get a clearer picture regarding which interventions are likely to be most effective in relation to the needs of particular families.

In her review of family intervention studies, Fadden (1998) has attempted to identify the key features of successful interventions. In her view, successful interventions share a here-and-now focus, include the family and the person with schizophrenia, emphasise skills acquisition by families, provide information about the disorder and promote positive, non-blaming attitudes by therapists. The protocol which follows has attempted to incorporate these features, under the following headings: engagement, assessment, education, stress management and ending the intervention.

The Research-based Protocol

This protocol describes the content of family intervention based on what have been shown to be the effective components of research studies. The protocol describes phases of the intervention process, beginning with the initial identification of needs and concluding with the ending of the intervention. Elements of the protocol are illustrated with examples from a case study. It is envisaged that the protocol will be used as a framework to guide clinical practice and to complement a programme of training and/or supervision in family interventions for people with schizophrenia.

The Protocol

Practical Considerations

There are many advantages in having two therapists work with a family. Deficits in skills and knowledge in one therapist can be compensated for by the other and the opportunity to reflect upon problems and plan the intervention with a colleague can be extremely useful. The presence of a co-therapist can help re-establish control when one therapist is 'drawn into the emotional vortex in the family' (Leff, 1994, p. 73) and allows good communication to be modelled.

Co-therapists need to work closely together and it is essential that time is dedicated to preparation for and reflection upon sessions. Barrowclough and Tarrier (1992) suggest that one therapist acts as keyworker for each session, organising the agenda and deciding who presents each item.

Consideration needs to be given to the time and location of appointments and it will often be necessary to arrange after hours appointments in the family home in order to include all family members and to achieve better outcomes (Fadden, 1998).

Identification and Engagement

An ideal service would be able to provide intensive help to all families with a relative experiencing schizophrenia. Constraints upon services make this difficult to achieve and it is helpful to consider who is most likely to benefit. There is evidence that input for families of people with schizophrenia may be particularly beneficial (Goldstein *et al.*, 1978). The majority of studies commenced family interventions during an acute episode of schizophrenia, usually when the affected person was admitted to hospital (Fadden, 1998). This does not exclude work with families when the person is in remission and the family is not at crisis point, but it is acknowledged that therapists may need to attend more to alliance-forming strategies in order for such families to change existing coping styles (Barrowclough and Tarrier, 1992).

Practitioners will know that not all acutely ill people are admitted to hospital during a first episode or a relapse, and, indeed, many services are actively developing and implementing intensive home treatment approaches (Marks *et al.*, 1994). A further consideration is whether or not the person is receiving or taking anti-psychotic medication, since the combination of family intervention with medication further reduces the risk of relapse (Vaughn *et al.*, 1976; Tarrier *et al.*, 1988).

Engagement of families can be enhanced by recognising that health behaviour may be influenced by decisions based upon cost-benefit considerations. Thus, the family's participation will depend on the perceived likelihood of the person experiencing a relapse, the perceived efficacy of the intervention in reducing relapse risk and the perceived costs (physical, psychological and economical) to both the person with schizophrenia and family. These cognitive processes need to be acknowledged and assessed and steps taken to maximise the benefits of the intervention and decrease the costs (Barrowclough and Tarrier, 1992).

Clinical Example. Engagement

The potential psychological costs of engaging in family work for relatives will vary according to each relative's relationship to the person with schizophrenia. Parents, siblings, children and spouses are likely to have their own fears and expectations regarding their relative's mental illness. Relatives may react with anger or denial making engagement difficult or impossible. For example, it proved impossible to involve the younger sister of a man with schizophrenia in family work because of her fear that she might be vulnerable to schizophrenia herself. During the first family meeting, the person with schizophrenia's mother raised the question of what had caused her son's illness. She had already expressed fears that he would never be 'normal' again and was clearly experiencing intense grief and loss. One therapist gave a brief answer which included references to genetic and hereditary factors in the development of schizophrenia. The patient's sister did not contribute to the rest of the session and looked worried and uncomfortable. She did not attend the next session and her parents reported that she had been very worried about her own vulnerability to schizophrenia. The mother's question could have been anticipated and a more considered response could have been prepared by the therapists, taking account of each family member's knowledge of schizophrenia. For the person with schizophrenia's sister, it was very difficult and painful for her to discuss these fears with her brother and parents and, therefore, she needed the opportunity to discuss her anxieties individually.

It is helpful to see the affected person and family together for an initial session, when the purpose of the intervention can be explained. The goals of family intervention include enhanced clinical management of the affected person's disorder by supporting the efforts of the family (Barrowclough and Tarrier, 1992), efficient stress management, improved family problem solving and instruction in specific strategies to cope with residual symptoms and problem behaviours (Falloon *et al.*, 1988). This meeting can be used to acknowledge the problems associated with mental illness, both for the person directly affected and for the relatives and to suggest that the therapists would like to interview family members individually in order to understand the family's needs so that they can collaborate with the family in addressing these issues. Information on the style of the sessions should be given, emphasising that the intervention is essentially collaborative and educative, using skills training methods when thought appropriate. Finally, it is important to establish ground rules for sessions, such as the location and duration of sessions, the anticipated number of sessions, and expectations of all participants' behaviour, including therapists and family; for example, confidentiality, punctuality, taking turns to speak and equal opportunities to speak for all (Leff, 1994).

Assessment

Individual assessments should be carried out with all family members, including the person with schizophrenia.

Assessment of the Relatives

The aim of the assessment is to enable the relatives to express their concerns and difficulties associated with the affected person's illness and to identify the relatives' strengths and resources. While it is not the purpose of the assessment to identify EE, it is recommended that therapists take account of such attitudes and behaviours during the assessment and are familiar with the ways in which criticism and emotional over-involvement may become evident (Barrowclough and Tarrier, 1992, pp. 55–7).

The following themes are included in the Relatives Assessment Interview (RAI) (Barrowclough and Tarrier, 1992) and should be covered during the initial interview:

(1)   the relatives' understanding of the illness and its management, noting factors that lead to improvement or exacerbation of symptoms and behaviour;
(2)   the impact of the illness on the relative, including specific examples of burden such as restrictions on social life, financial hardship and distress;
(3)   coping strategies used to deal with positive and negative symptoms and the effects these have on other family members and the affected person;
(4)   the relationship with the person with schizophrenia and examples of dissatisfaction with his or her behaviour;
(5)   areas of strength such as effective coping strategies, social supports or a positive relationship with the affected person.

The RAI can generate a great deal of information which cannot easily be recorded in note form during the interview and, therefore, it is suggested that the interview is audio taped and analysed later.

Additional information relating to the relatives' knowledge about schizophrenia and its management can be obtained using the 'knowledge about schizophrenia interview' (KASI) (Barrowclough and Tarrier, 1992). This assessment can be used to help prepare educational sessions and evaluate changes in relatives' attitudes and beliefs about the affected person's illness following such sessions.

The 'general health questionnaire' (GHQ) (Goldberg and Williams, 1988) is a self-administered questionnaire which can be used to assess levels of psychological disturbance among relatives, while, the 'family questionnaire' (FQ) (Barrowclough and Tarrier, 1992) provides additional information on relatives' distress and coping in relation to a checklist of problems experienced by people with schizophrenia. Both the GHQ and FQ can be repeated at the completion of the intervention to evaluate progress and outcomes.

Assessment of the Patient

The aim of the assessment with the affected person is to identify problems and strengths. In order to measure the person with schizophrenia's symptomatology and social functioning, it is recommended that the following three scales are used:

(1) KGV (Krawiecka *et al.*, 1977).
(2) Social functioning scale (SFS) (Birchwood *et al.*, 1990).
(3) Health of the nation outcome scales, version 3 (HoNOS) (Wing *et al.*, 1996).

These scales can be repeated during and after the intervention to monitor progress and as a final outcome measure.

Clinical Example. Patient and Family Assessment

Alan's diagnosis of schizophrenia was made after his third admission to hospital. During his first two admissions, his psychotic symptoms improved very quickly but re-emerged soon after returning home to his family. At an early stage it appeared that family interventions would be appropriate for Alan and his family but steps to initiate such work were delayed because of uncertainty regarding Alan's diagnosis and concerns that Alan would perceive attempts to engage his family as alienating. On the other hand, his family were finding it extremely difficult to understand and cope with Alan's behaviour. Alan lives with his parents and older sister, Jean. Alan himself had reported tension at home and his mother had referred to 'unhappiness' at home. His mother had given up personal interests in order to be at home with him and was frequently tearful when discussing him. Jean and her father also referred to arguments at home and both tended to blame Alan's mother for his illness, by being too 'strict' and 'nagging'.

Each member of the household was interviewed individually using the RAI and KASI and each was asked to complete the FQ. These assessments confirmed much of what the therapists had observed and assessed informally. Father and daughter tended to blame Alan's mother for his condition, accusing her of being too 'fussy' with her children when they were young and by imposing strict rules of behaviour upon them. Alan's mother felt that there had been a tense atmosphere at home for many years and that her married life had sometimes been unhappy. She felt that her role as mother had disappeared once her children had grown up and that they were now closer to their father. She described this in terms of emptiness and loss and admitted that she felt isolated and unvalued. All three were very concerned that Alan sometimes did not take his medication and they all agreed that his inactivity and untidiness were frequent problems. Information from the KASI showed that none of the family had a good understanding of the causes of Alan's illness, with all of them indicating that they thought a persons upbringing was the most important factor. Although his sister, Jean, believed Alan was suffering from depression and not schizophrenia, she demonstrated attitudes and beliefs which were likely to promote Alan's recovery and help her to cope. His mother's management strategies consisted of making herself available to Alan and 'giving him love' and her answers to the KASI suggested that she would not carry out other strategies which might be more beneficial.

Education

It is important to note that education alone may not reduce EE levels or relapse rates (Tarrier *et al.*, 1988). It is more useful to see the information-giving role in terms of setting the scene for work with families, since acquiring knowledge about schizophrenia and then using that knowledge in management strategies are two different goals (Barrowclough and Tarrier, 1992). The following considerations also need to be borne in mind when preparing and giving information to families: the reading level required for written materials; the presentation of selected information, as only a few items will be retained by recipients; possible variations in assimilation of information between family members; and, the principle that education is a continuing process throughout the intervention (Falloon and Fadden, 1993).

Information obtained from the RAI and KASI will guide preparation for educational sessions, highlighting strengths and deficits in knowledge and potentially helpful and unhelpful strategies. Typically, information is given and discussed over two sessions and would include the following areas:

(1)   the nature of the illness – aetiology, symptoms and prognosis;
(2)   the vulnerability–stress model;
(3)   the role of medication;
(4)   sources of help, advice and information.

Educational Materials

A large amount of published educational material is available. Three sources of information are M. Birchwood and J. Smith (1985) *Understanding Schizophrenia* (Birmingham, West Birmingham Health Authority Mental Health Series); C. Barrowclough and N. Tarrier (1992) *Families of Schizophrenic Patients* (Appendix 6); and G. Wilkinson and T. Kendrick (1996) *A Carer's Guide to Schizophrenia* (London, Royal Society of Medicine Press).

Clinical Example

Two sessions were devoted to giving information about schizophrenia to Alan and his family. During the first session the therapists described what is known about the aetiology of schizophrenia, the positive and negative symptoms of schizophrenia and introduced the family to the stress-vulnerability model. Each relative was given information to take away and read at the end of the session. The second session was devoted to giving information on the origins and causes of schizophrenia and it was planned to introduce a 'normalising' model of symptoms, based on the work of Kingdon and Turkington (1995). The rationale for this session was based on the outcomes of the family assessments which showed that Alan's father and sister were tending to blame his mother for his illness and that she herself believed that Alan would never be 'normal' again. It was hoped that it might be possible to de-catastrophise his mother's view of schizophrenia and facilitate support for her from her husband and daughter by modifying their beliefs about her role in causing Alan's illness.

At the beginning of the second session, the therapists checked with the family if they had read the information on schizophrenia. Each person had read the information and said that they could see similarities between the symptoms described and Alan's symptoms. However, Alan's mother said that she had not been able to read the whole piece because she found it too distressing. She was upset because she felt that there was no hope of Alan making a full recovery. This belief not only seemed to cause her distress but also prevented her from engaging in behaviour which might help Alan towards recovery and maintained her existing self-sacrificing and over-protective behaviours. At the same time, the therapists were aware that it was important that the family were given an accurate and realistic description of the possible course of Alan's illness. One of the therapists then went through the written material with the family to identify those aspects which were worrying and gave a fuller explanation of each aspect in turn.

Stress Management

It is suggested that a transactional model best conceptualises stress: 'stress is best seen as a transaction between the stimulus – in this case, the illness and its consequences – and the individual's response – attempts to cope' (Barrowclough and Tarrier, 1992, p. 86). By identifying a stimulus and a response, the transactional model leads to strategies which aim to alleviate the problem (stimulus), such as individual symptom management for the affected person, and others which aim to modify relatives' appraisals of the problems and ways of coping (response). Therefore, while stress management is a technique in itself, it also encompasses a range of other approaches which may help to reduce stress. Allied approaches are problem-solving, communication training and cognitive-behavioural techniques. The use of these approaches, either in isolation or in combination with each other, will contribute to an overall stress management strategy. Barrowclough and Tarrier (1992) suggest that stress management *per se* should contain the following elements:

- a definition of stress;
- identification of current stressors;
- self-monitoring of stressors;
- details of resources available to the relative (e.g., social supports, interests, successful coping strategies);
- targeting one or two specific situations and the completion of a detailed cognitive-behavioural analysis;
- collaboration on interventions based on the analysis;
- evaluation of the outcomes of interventions.

Problem-solving

Problem-solving training is considered a key strategy in stress management (Falloon and Fadden, 1993) and many of the successful intervention studies have incorporated behavioural goal-setting and problem-solving approaches (e.g. Hogarty *et al.*, 1986; Tarrier *et al.*, 1988). Falloon *et al.* (1988) have proposed a six-point plan for problem-solving and goal achievement:

(1) pinpoint the problem/goal;
(2) generate possible solutions;
(3) evaluate the possible consequences of applying each of these solutions;
(4) agree on a best strategy;
(5) plan and implement;
(6) review the results.

A 'constructional' approach, emphasising positive behaviour change, rather than a 'pathological' approach, which focuses on the elimination of behaviours is more likely to generate successful solutions (Barrowclough and Tarrier, 1992).

In enabling families to become proficient at problem-solving it is important to select a topic for practising the process which is not one of the family's current hot issues. The family can best learn how to problem solve by using neutral, non-emotive examples of 'problems', such as 'where to go for a family day out', or 'what time to have tea'. In these kinds of questions all family members have an equal stake and an equal say and an imaginative example can result in an enjoyable exercise where the family can have a quality experience and learn the principles of problem-solving. Hot issues may tend to focus on a behaviour of the affected person which causes irritation to other family members. Choosing an issue like this does not allow the family to learn and understand the problem-solving method, may cause additional stress within the family, lead to an exclusive and inappropriate alliance between therapists and family members and alienate the affected person. If the family cannot come up with a 'neutral' problem the therapist should offer an example.

Following successive problem-solving exercises the family will be more equipped to address more complex problems.

Clinical Example. Problem-solving

Alan's family agreed to problem solve 'where to go for a family day out'.

1. Pinpointing the problem and setting a goal

It was agreed that the problem could be stated in the following way: To decide where the family should go for a day without limit of money or resources.

2. Generating possible solutions

Many solutions were generated by 'brainstorming'. 'Las Vegas, with un-limited cash we can make a million', 'A day on a beach, with a picnic and Champagne', 'Blackpool, with the pleasure beach and fish and chips'.

3. Evaluating the consequences

Following an evaluation of the pros and cons of the suggested proposals the family came up with a day in Paris, 'It's near to get back if Alan becomes unwell, we can go up the Eiffel Tower, and there's something to do if it's raining'.

4. Agreeing a strategy

It was agreed that Alan's father would book a private jet, for next Monday and a taxi to the airport at 10.30am. The family agreed to meet at the family home by 10.00am.

5. Planning and implementation

The family role-played what to do on their day in Paris.

6. Reviewing results

The family then, hypothetically, reviewed how the day went. This gave the opportunity for humorous banter to take place, while the therapists rein-forced the elements of the process.

Communication Training

Communication training does not appear in all intervention studies, but is a major component in the work of some of the influential figures in family inter-ventions (e.g., Falloon *et al.*, 1988; Leff, 1994). Falloon and his colleagues emphasise the importance of communication skills in reducing stress and facilitating problem-solving. They identify four basic communication skills: expressing positive feelings; making a positive request; expressing unpleasant feelings and attentive listening (Falloon *et al.*, 1988). Training, or re-training, family members in these skills is done using behavioural techniques such as rehearsal, role-play, modelling and constructive feedback. Again, non-hot issues should be chosen for this intervention for the reasons cited above.

Clinical Example. Communication Training

The first stage in this intervention was to express a positive feeling. A ratio-nale was provided which gave a clear understanding of the advantages for this type of communication. Family members were encouraged to generate further reasons for expressing positive feelings. The family and therapist reviewed the current levels of skill and the frequency of this kind of communication. It became apparent that the expression of positive feelings did not happen very often and people felt that their efforts towards others were taken for granted.

The components of the skill were explained:

- looking at the person and using a warm tone of voice,
- explaining what the person did that pleased you,
- and how this made you feel.

Jean was then asked to take part in a role-play where the therapist modelled the components by thanking her for the drink that was offered when they came in. Family members were then asked to think of something that a family member had done for them, in the last couple of days, where they could have said that it had pleased them. Each family member in turn was asked to rehearse the skill by saying to the person what it was that pleased them using the steps indicated. Alan's father looked at his daughter Jean and thanked her for the cup of tea she brought out to him while he was gardening this morning: 'I really needed it – it made me feel that you were concerned for me digging in this cold weather'. Jean was asked to give feedback to her father saying the things she liked about the way he had spoken to her and if she had any suggestions for improvements. Other family members were also asked to comment. The therapist praised the father, addressing each step in the process. Other family members in turn undertook the exercise. The session finished with a summary of the aims and rationale for communication training generally and for today's exercise, expressing a positive feeling.

Cognitive-Behavioural Techniques

Barrowclough and Tarrier (1992) observe that many of the 'thinking errors' found among depressed or anxious people can be found in the relatives of people with schizophrenia. Thus, relatives may make faulty attributions about the affected person's behaviour, catastrophise or jump to conclusions. Cognitive-behavioural interventions may be able to change unhelpful beliefs and modify behaviour (see Chapter 7).

Ending the Intervention and Follow-up

Ending the intervention, or disengagement, should be discussed with the family at the outset of the intervention, when the question of timescale or

number of sessions is negotiated. Falloon *et al.* (1988) suggest that the family
is asked to conduct a problem-solving discussion on the issue of ending sessions towards the end of the intervention, so that they can develop their own
strategies and plans for the future. The final session with the family should
include a review of the work undertaken and positive aspects of the intervention should be identified. Some time should also be devoted to developing an
action plan in the event of problems occurring in the future. To maximise the
benefits of the intervention to the family and avoid dependency, follow this
advice: 'aim to make yourself redundant at the earliest possible time' (Falloon
et al., 1988).

Implementing Family Interventions in Routine Practice

It has been recognised that practitioners trained in family intervention are
failing to engage families in routine practice (e.g., Kavanagh *et al.*, 1993;
Fadden, 1997). Several explanations for this unsatisfactory situation have
been proposed, identifying potential barriers at the practitioner, family and
organisational level.

- In common with other innovations, family intervention may be resisted
  by some practitioners who are not convinced of the need to adopt new
  approaches or for whom it conflicts with established concepts and practices (Backer *et al.*, 1986).
- It has been argued that the observable outcomes from family intervention,
  such as relapse prevention, are not immediately apparent and, therefore,
  practitioners lack immediate reinforcement of their efforts (Kavanagh *et
  al.*, 1993).
- In addition, would-be family work practitioners may need to address issues
  relating to the conceptual validity of the terms 'schizophrenia' and 'severe
  mental illness' (Boyle, 1990) and the role of the family in the aetiology
  and course of schizophrenia (Johnstone, 1999).
- One family intervention service has reported contending with a 'management culture of benign neglect' and 'insidious opposition' from colleagues
  (Hughes *et al.*, 1996), a view reflected in another study which found that
  practitioners were struggling to integrate family work with other clinical
  demands with little or no organisational support, in terms of flexible
  working times and clinical supervision (Kavanagh *et al.*, 1993).

Overcoming these barriers represents a challenge to mental health service
commissioners, service managers, practitioners and educators. For family interventions to be implemented successfully it is essential that practitioners have
access to thorough training and supervision (see Chapter 18). Greater access
to such training is needed to further disseminate family work skills. Primary

healthcare services and in-patient services may be ideally placed to detect difficulties with relatives and assess their needs and problems. In the United Kingdom, government policies such as the National Service Framework may help to direct the organisational changes required to effectively prioritise work with people experiencing severe and enduring mental health problems.

Conclusion

- Randomised-controlled trials of cognitive-behavioural family interventions have demonstrated benefits for both affected people and families, in terms of delayed relapse and reduced family burden.
- The common features of successful family interventions can be identified and have been presented in this chapter as a protocol to guide clinical practice.
- In routine mental health services, family interventions remain the exception rather than the rule. Wider dissemination and implementation requires collaboration between service commissioners, providers and educators.

Family interventions may still be largely unavailable to many people and their families because there remains insufficient evidence from actual clinical practice for their effectiveness. According to one view, 'evidence from dusty journals in an academic library, usually relating to a different country, needs to be supported by evidence from local projects before commissioners of services will be willing to pass from the contemplative stage of change to the action stage' (Hodgson, 1998). Thus, health service commissioners not only need to be convinced of the evidence, they also need to be convinced by the evidence from the implementation of the evidence in real services. In other words, while an impressive body of scientific evidence exists, there is not enough evidence from routine services to convince commissioners and health service managers to act towards implementing family interventions strategies. The challenge now, therefore, is for mental health services to begin to develop such evidence and demonstrate the value and worth of family work to people with schizophrenia and their relatives.

Further Reading

Barrowclough, C. and Parle, M. (1997) 'Appraisal, expressed emotion and distress in relatives of schizophrenic patients', *British Journal of Psychiatry*, 171, 26–30.

Barrowclough, C. and Tarrier, N. (1992) *Families of Schizophrenic Patients: Cognitive Behavioural Intervention*, London, Chapman & Hall.

Fadden, G. (1998) 'Family intervention', in Brooker J. and Repper (eds), *Serious Mental Health Problems in the Community: Policy, Practice and Research*, London, Balliere-Tindall.

Falloon, I.R.H., Laporta, M., Fadden, G. and Graham-Hole, V. (1993) *Managing Stress in Families. Cognitive and behavioural strategies for enhancing coping skills*, London, Routledge.

References

Backer, T.E., Liberman, R.P. and Kuehnel, T.G. (1986) 'Dissemination and adoption of innovative psychosocial interventions', *Journal of Consulting and Clinical Psychology*, 54, 111–18.

Barrowclough, C. and Parle, M. (1997) 'Appraisal, expressed emotion and distress in relatives of schizophrenic patients', *British Journal of Psychiatry*, 171, 26–30.

Barrowclough, C. and Tarrier, N. (1992) *Families of Schizophrenic Patients. Cognitive Behavioural Intervention*, London, Chapman & Hall.

Birchwood, M., Smith, J. and Cochrane, R. *et al.* (1990) 'The social functioning scale: the development and validation of a scale of social adjustment for use in family intervention programmes with schizophrenic patients', *British Journal of Psychiatry*, 157, 853–9.

Boyle, M. (1990) *Schizophrenia: a scientific delusion?* London, Routledge.

Brown, G.W., Birley, J.L.T. and Wing, J.K. (1972) 'Influence of family life on the course of schizophrenic disorder: a replication', *British Journal of Psychiatry*, 121, 241–58.

Clark, R.E. (1994) 'Family costs associated with severe mental illness and substance use', *Hospital and Community Psychiatry*, 45, 808–13.

Clinical Standards Advisory Group (1995) *Schizophrenia*, Vol. 1, London, HMSO.

Fadden, G. (1997) 'Implementation of family interventions in routine clinical practice following staff training programs: a major cause for concern', *Journal of Mental Health*, 6(6), 599–612.

Fadden, G. (1998) 'Family intervention', in C. Brooker and J. Repper (eds), *Serious Mental Health Problems in the Community: Policy, Practice and Research*, London, Balliere Tindall.

Falloon, I.R.H., Mueser K. and Gingerich F. *et al.* (1988) *Behaviour Family Therapy: A Workbook*, Buckingham, Buckingham Mental Health Service.

Falloon, I.R.H. and Fadden, G. (1993) *Integrated Mental Health Care*, Cambridge, Cambridge University Press.

Goldstein, M.J., Rodnick, E.H., Evans, J.R., May, P.R.A. and Steinberg, M.R. (1978) 'Drug and family therapy in the aftercare of acute schizophrenics', *Archives of General Psychiatry*, 35, 1169–77.

Hogarty, G., Anderson, C.M. and Reiss, D.J. *et al.* (1986) 'Family Psychoeducation, social skills training, and maintenance chemotherapy in the aftercare treatment of schizophrenia. I: one-year effects of a controlled study on relapse and expressed emotion', *Archives of General Psychiatry*, 43, 633–42.

Hughes, I., Hailwood, R., Abbati-Yeoman, J. and Budd, R. (1996) 'Developing a family intervention service for serious mental illness: clinical observations and experiences', *Journal of Mental Health*, 5(2), 145–59.

Johnstone, L. (1999) 'Do families cause schizophrenia? Revisiting a taboo subject', *Changes*, 17(2), 77–90.

Kavanagh, D.J. (1992) 'Recent developments in expressed emotion and schizophrenia', *British Journal of Psychiatry*, 160, 601 20.

Kavanagh, D.J., Piatkowska, O., Clark, D., O'Halloran, P., Manicavasagar, V. and Rosen, A. (1993) 'Application of cognitive-behavioural family interventions for schizophrenia in multidisciplinary teams: what can the matter be?', *Australian Psychologist*, 28(3), 181–8.

Kingdon, D.G. and Turkington, D. (1994) *Cognitive Behavioural Therapy of Schizophrenia*, Hove, Psychology Press, Lawrence Erlbaum.

Krawiecka, M., Goldberg, D.P. and Vaughn, M. (1977) 'A standardised psychiatric assessment scale for rating chronic psychotic patients', *Acta Psychiatrica Scandinavica*, 55, 299–308; modified by Lancashire (1998).

Lancashire, S. (1998) *The KGV (M) Symptom Scale Version 6*, unpublished paper, University of Manchester.

Leff, J. (1994) 'Working with the families of schizophrenic patients', *British Journal of Psychiatry*, 164 (Suppl. 23), 71–6.

Marks, I., Connolly, J., Muijen, M., Audini, B., McNamee, G. and Lawrence, R.E. (1994) 'Home-based versus hospital-based care for people with serious mental illness', *British Journal of Psychiatry*, 165, 179–94.

Miller, F., Dworkin, J., Ward, M. and Barone, D. (1990) 'A preliminary study of unresolved grief in families of seriously mentally ill patients', *Hospital and Community Psychiatry*, 41, 1321–5.

Penn, D.L. and Mueser, K.T. (1996) 'Research update on the psychosocial treatment of schizophrenia', *American Journal of Psychiatry*, 153(5), 607–17.

Tarrier, N., Barrowclough, C. and Vaughn, C. *et al.* (1988) 'The community management of schizophrenia: a controlled trial of behavioural intervention with families to reduce relapse', *British Journal of Psychiatry*, 153, 532–42.

Vaughn, C. and Leff, J. (1976) 'The influence of family and social factors on the course of psychiatric illness', *British Journal of Psychiatry*, 129, 125–37.

Vaughn, C., Snyder, K.S. and Freeman, W. *et al.* (1984) 'Family factors in schizophrenic relapse: a replication in California of British research on expressed emotion', *Archives of General Psychiatry*, 41, 1169–77.

Walsh, O.F. and Harman, C.P. (1989) 'Family views of stigma', *Schizophrenia Bulletin*, 15(1), 131–9.

Wig, W.N., Menon, D.K. and Bedi, H. (1987) 'Expressed emotion and schizophrenia in North India', *British Journal of Psychiatry*, 151, 156–73.

Wing, J.K., Curtis, R.H. and Beevor, A.S. (1996) *HoNOS, Health of the Nation Outcome Scales. Report on research and development*, London, Research Unit, Royal College of Psychiatrists.

Part III

Working and Living in the Community

CHAPTER 12

Working and Schizophrenia

JENNY DROUGHTON AND STEVE WILLIAMS

Introduction

This chapter focuses specifically on how the availability or otherwise of paid or voluntary work, and the nature of such work can be a huge source of stress for people with schizophrenia (Warner, 1994) or provide therapeutic opportunity. It argues that mental health professionals should orientate themselves to the occupational needs of people with schizophrenia in a systematic way to improve recovery, provide outcomes valued by sufferers and their families, that is, work and its associated status, and possibly reduce the secondary disabilities associated with schizophrenia. The aim of this chapter to challenge the undue pessimism regarding addressing the vocational needs of people with schizophrenia that is so prevalent among many mental health professionals by reviewing some of the recently published literature in this field. Models of social intervention specifically focused upon employment/vocational needs are described. This chapter also provides a checklist to help grassroots workers ensure that their own PSI practice is appropriately social as well as psychological.

Relationship Between Work and Outcome in Schizophrenia

The relationship between economic downturns in industrial nations and outcome in schizophrenia has been discussed in great detail in an excellent and thought-provoking book by Warner (1994). His attempted meta-analysis of 85 follow-up studies of outcome in schizophrenia stretching over one hundred years has huge methodological problems, many of which are common to this sort of research. His findings should therefore be accepted with caution, but they do suggest that outcome in schizophrenia is better during periods of high employment and worse during periods of high unemployment in industrialised nations. This implies that when jobs are plentiful, people with schizophrenia are in demand as workers (and the focus is on their abilities rather than their disabilities). This increase in work opportunities and positive recognition in turn results in a better quality of life and similar outcomes. Harvey Brenner's (1973) more general research concerning the relationship between economic recession and psychiatric hospital admissions appears to lend further support to Warner's hypothesis.

Work as a Therapeutic Intervention

There is a long history of work as an integral component of institution based mental health services both in the UK and in North America. Space precludes a detailed review of these traditions so interested readers are directed to papers such as that by McGurrin (1994) for an American perspective, and that of Evans and Repper (2000) for the history of British work initiatives. While many earlier work programmes were more custodial than therapeutic and usually in segregated settings, they still at least partly met the occupational needs of people with SMI, as many ex-residents of the large asylums will testify. As the recent transition from institutional to community care has proceeded in Britain, the re-provision of community-based work and employment for those with severe mental illness (SMI) has been grossly neglected. As a result of the current failure to recognise work as an integral component of effective mental health services for SMI, the UK lags far behind many North American and European counterparts in the availability of the necessary skills and service structures. Many clinicians remain ill informed about the evidence base for work and SMI. Table 12.1 highlights some common misconceptions and the research evidence which challenges them.

International Research Evidence

The apparently differential outcome from schizophrenia achieved in developing as opposed to developed countries has been highlighted in an important follow-up study (WHO, 1979). In this study an attempt was made to establish the outcome of schizophrenia across very different countries including developed and developing countries, and to the astonishment of the researchers, outcome appeared to be better in developing as opposed to developed countries. A second study which tried to reduce the number of cases lost to follow up, especially in developing countries was conducted (Jablensky *et al.*, 1992) and this second study had similar results. While many factors could be contributing to the better outcome from schizophrenia observed in developing countries in these studies, it is very evident that employment opportunities for people recovering from schizophrenia were different in developing and developed countries and may have been one of the contributing factors. Work in developing countries was predominantly agricultural and labour intensive, and may very well have been with extended family members as co-workers. While demanding, such work often does not require focused, disciplined, concentration on a repetitive task so typical of low-paid industrial work in developed economies.

Table 12.1 Misconceptions about work and SMI

Myth	Fact
• *Work is too stressful for people with SMI*	• An American longitudinal study of people with SMI found that at follow-up those who were working had fewer symptoms and higher levels of global functioning, self-esteem & financial satisfaction than those who were unemployed (Mueser *et al.*, 1997)
• *Those people with the most severe level of positive and/or negative psychotic symptoms are least suitable for work*	• The extent and severity of psychotic symptoms are *not* significant in determining whether a person with SMI will succeed in work (Pozner *et al.*, 1996)
• *The cognitive deficits associated with SMI are insurmountable obstacles for most users who want to work*	• Cognitive deficits are far more amenable to intervention than previous thought (Wexler *et al.*, 1997)
• *Helping users obtain and sustain work is best left to teams of employment specialists and not an integral part of care packages*	• Outcomes are better when employment experts are part of the CMHT and when work is prioritised for all SMI clients as part of their care package (Torrey *et al.*, 1998)
• *The work attendance of people with SMI is too unreliable to expect mainstream employers to offer them work*	• People with SMI are no less reliable in their work attendance than other people – they just have *different* patterns of absence compared with the general population (Perkins, 1991)
• *Having help to find and keep a job is a low priority for service users*	• Users themselves rate assistance with the occupational and social aspects of their lives as one of the most important care needs they have (Shepherd *et al.*, 1994)
• *Users prefer temporary jobs and schemes rather than permanent jobs in competitive settings*	• Users want real jobs rather than temporary jobs or just 'playing at shop' (Rogers *et al.*, 1991)
• *Competitive employment should not be considered until users are symptom-free or at least well-stabilised*	• Psychotic symptoms are far more likely to improve when people with schizophrenia have paid work rather than unpaid work (Bell *et al.*, 1996)
• *Users have unrealistic and over-ambitious job preferences which they often change*	• Users' job preferences are realistic and remain stable (Becker *et al.*, 1996)

Attempts have been made at vocational rehabilitation in some developing countries utilising simple, low-cost, self-help community solutions which are well-matched to the social and community context. One important example of this more 'low–tech' approach is that of workplace-based sheltered workshops for people with SMI in China, with apparently good results (Luo and Yu, 1994). The role of work in aiding recovery from schizophrenia has also been reported in rural Indian communities (Warner, 1994).

In the west, Wing and Brown (1970) also noted that one factor which distinguished inpatients with schizophrenia who did not improve from those who did was the former group's lack of occupation. There has been little notable British research into work and SMI with the exception of a small randomised trial by Griffiths (1974) which proved inconclusive. No further British randomised control trials of work programmes for people with SMI have been undertaken since, though several are in the pipeline. The majority of recent UK literature is therefore descriptive rather than experimental in nature. However, it has established several important facts:

- Despite employment rights legislation the rate of employment for people with SMI (at 15 per cent) is far less than that for people with other disabilities (Evans and Repper, 2000).
- The majority of people with SMI actually want to work (Perkins and Repper, 1996).
- Job discrimination against people with SMI is widespread (Read and Baker, 1996).
- Initiatives can be implemented to address vocational needs at the local as well as national level (Pozner *et al.*, 1996).

The different initiatives and approaches which aim to enable people with SMI to get back to work are collectively known as 'vocational rehabilitation'. The main types of vocational rehabilitation are summarised in Table 12.2.

For a variety of cultural and economic reasons, the United States is further ahead than Britain in the availability of effective interventions to enable people with SMI to work. In some states there has been widespread change from institution-based interventions such as day treatment to genuinely community based interventions such as 'assertive community treatment' (Stein and Santos, 1998). Reflecting this change, there is a substantial body of recent North American research on interventions for enabling people with SMI to participate in work and arguably far greater political will to enable people to return to work. The American literature and services place considerable emphasis on supporting people with SMI where possible to enter or re-enter competitive employment. This refers to

> . . . employment in integrated work settings among workers without disabilities, for which the client is paid by the employer wages equal to wages paid to other workers doing the same or similar jobs. (Drake *et al.*, 1998, p. 496)

It therefore contrasts markedly with industrial therapy units and sheltered workshops common in British services until recently. The rationale behind promoting work in mainstream settings is not just based on a philosophy of integration and normalisation but also on robust empirical evidence. Users in competitive employment not only have greater income than those in other schemes (Clark *et al.*, 1998) they also experience fewer symptoms. Earlier research from the United States indicated the benefits of the clubhouse model of vocational employment whereby some users were offered transitional

Table 12.2 Models of work, employment or training provision for people with SMI

Model	Description
Clubhouses	Community resources run by users (the clubhouse 'members'). Members are responsible for the upkeep of the clubhouse and take on jobs within it depending on their needs. They can also experience work in competitive employment through Transitional Employment.
Employment services	Dedicated staff team or agency assists users in finding and applying for jobs matched to their needs, abilities and interests.
Employment agency	Similar to 'mainstream' employment agencies though tend to emphasise meeting users' specific work requirements over merely filling vacancies. Jobs often temporary rather than permanent. Jobs may be 'shared' between users.
Local exchange trading systems (LETs)	A community-based, cash-free arrangement whereby a group of local users exchange skills, services, and goods.
Self-Eemployment/user run enterprises	Mainstream businesses run by individual, or groups of, users.
Sheltered employment	Offers paid work within commercial settings which have segregated workforces (i.e. entry is reserved for individuals with specific, or any, disabilities).
Sheltered workshops and industrial therapy units (ITUs)	Offer a variety of usually unpaid work activities within institutional-based, segregated settings.
Social firms/ co-operatives	Community-based businesses (e.g. cafes) often with integrated workforces (i.e. users and non-users) which pay competitive wages, share profits, and involve all workers in commercial and practical decisions.
Supported employment	Involves individualised and on-going input to enable users to identify; apply and interview for; train for; and continue to receive the level of additional support they require for, predominantly competitive jobs.
Supported training and adult education	Provision of community-based or community-linked vocation training and non-vocational education. Course arrangements vary: segregated classes may be offered or access to mainstream attendance may be supported by dedicated project workers or a 'buddy' system.
Transitional employment	Offers time-limited placements in open employment on a part-time basis, as a staged approach to preparing users to return to independent employment. (Usually provided as part of the clubhouse model)

Source: From an article by Evans and Repper (2000) reproduced with permission from Blackwell Science Ltd.

(i.e. time-limited) employment (TE) either in the clubhouse or in competitive settings (Hill and Shepherd, 1997). However, more recent research has indicated, again unsurprisingly, that most users prefer permanent rather than temporary jobs (Rogers *et al.*, 1991). Furthermore, any beneficial effects of TE are not sustained once the job ends.

A promising type of vocational rehabilitation is known as 'supported employment' (SE). SE aims to place people with SMI in competitive employment wherever possible. There are different variants of supported employment though one specific approach has been extensively defined and researched and is known as Individual Placement and Support (IPS). This particular variant of SE involves

> . . . competitive jobs, rapid job searches, continuous assessment, integration of clinical and vocational services, job matching based on consumer choice, and follow-along supports. (Bailey *et al.*, 1998, p. 25)

IPS emphasises rapid placement through a philosophy of 'place and train' rather than traditional 'train then place' approaches. Yet, despite its emphasis on rapid placement, SE/IPS does not result in negative outcomes such as increased symptoms or hospital admissions. Conversely, it appears that SE is more successful precisely because rapid placement and on-the-job support and training are more useful to people with SMI than job training in artificial settings, partly because of poor transfer of learning (McGurrin, 1994). SE is also more preferable to users (Rogers *et al.*, 1991) than prevocational training (PVT). The superiority of SE over PVT in increasing rates of competitive employment for people with SMI was recently confirmed by a systematic review on vocational rehabilitation (Crowther *et al.*, 2001). SE is a well defined intervention, particularly IPS which is clearly described in a training manual that facilitates its implementation in routine services. Supported Employment, in particular IPS, markets itself as a recovery-oriented approach to SMI (Becker *et al.*, 1998).

IPS claims to represent

> . . . a community-based approach to SE that encourages illness-self management and normal, adult roles through its focus on competitive employment and individual choice. (Becker *et al.*, 1998, p. 51)

The main findings of the extensive research undertaken into IPS are summarised below:

- IPS produces superior vocational outcomes than pre-vocational training or day treatment programmes (Bailey *et al.*, 1998).
- Users and their carers report greater satisfaction with IPS as opposed to day treatment (Torrey *et al.*, 1995).
- Even long-term clients of day services can benefit from IPS (Bailey *et al.*, 1998).
- Training and selection of staff for SE programmes is critical (Bailey *et al.*, 1998).
- IPS can result in some financial savings for services (Bailey *et al.*, 1998).

Despite the substantial evidence base, SE and IPS are not without their limitations or critics. The American findings are undeniably impressive but have not yet been replicated in British settings. IPS will not be suitable or acceptable to all so alternatives must be investigated and made available. Also, whilst IPS dramatically increases the chances of someone with SMI acquiring a job, it may be less successful in ensuring their retention of that job over time (Becker *et al.*, 1998) and conversions of existing services to SE may results in 'social losses' for users (Torrey *et al.*, 1998). Given the substantial employment gains SE provides these potential 'social losses' should not be used as a reason for not changing services to SE models, but valued aspects of traditional services will need to be reprovided. IPS and SE are based on particular norms about the role of work, which may be culturally specific and might not be shared by all. Therefore SE might need to be adapted to meet the different occupational norms and needs of different communities.

The Policy Perspective on Work and SMI

In addition to the evidence base confirming the importance of work opportunities for people with SMI, there is a growing emphasis in British government policy on addressing this neglected area, for example the 1998 White Paper *Modernising Mental Health Services: safe, sound, supportive* (DoH, 1998). Since the election of the Labour government in 1997 there has been a focus on tackling 'social exclusion' and the links between it and health inequalities. The commitment to develop occupational opportunities for people with SMI is reiterated in the *National Service Framework for Mental Health* (DoH, 1999). The compelling research evidence associated with employment for people with SMI means it is imperative that the relative unavailability of effective, community-based interventions and services regarding work is challenged.

Models of Work and SMI

The following two models provide useful frameworks for understanding the role of employment for people with SMI, and how it may be achieved and sustained.

The Stress Vulnerability Model

Unemployment and employment can be integrated into several areas of the stress vulnerability model of psychosis (Zubin and Spring, 1977) (see also Chapter 1 in this book). Most obviously, unemployment can be understood as a psychosocial stressor and as such may contribute to acute episodes and future relapses. This relationship is of course bi-directional. Long-term unemployment of people with SMI may also contribute to the development and maintenance of a disorder with a chronic course. A disorder with a chronic course may in turn be further exacerbated by social and hospital policy if it offers ineffective institution-based work or activity programmes with very low expectations. Secondary psychosocial disabilities may also occur partly as the result of the effects of unemployment for people with SMI. While unemployment may act as a psychosocial stressor, it is also true that for some people employment may also be experienced as stressful. Most available evidence indicates that employment is far less likely than enforced unemployment to be experienced by users as a stressor. Nonetheless, Scheid and Anderson (1995) have reported that some users find their experiences of work stressful with fear of relapse a common concern. Interestingly, this study found despite finding work stressful the same people enjoyed their job, had no absences from work due to psychotic symptoms and derived a sense of pride from their role as worker. The following aspects of the work environment were cited as sources of stress by users:

- demanding or critical bosses
- over-concerned (over-involved) supervisors
- work colleagues who gossiped about, or ridiculed them (either about their illness or work performance)
- tasks involving high levels of co-operative effort (e.g. group tasks lasting for long periods of time)
- tasks which were fast-paced (i.e. over-stimulating).

Clearly, these aspects which users found problematic are the characteristics of high expressed emotion (EE) environments (see Chapter 11). The similarities between stressful family environments and stressful work environments have already been highlighted by other researchers (Cook, 1992; Jenkins and Karno, 1992). Work environments may have equal or even greater potential to be toxic than family settings. Certainly there are likely to be less detrimental consequences from removing yourself from a stressful family environment, for instance by going for a walk, than from walking 'off the job'. The Scheid and Anderson (1995) study also identified which work environments users found least stressful and where they fared the best. These were settings characterised by

- 'non-demanding (though not necessarily low skill or concentration) tasks requiring steady but not intense effort to meet expectations' (p. 172);
- very limited interaction with others;
- 'a clearly defined set of tasks which could be completed by the consumer at his/her own pace with little co-operative involvement with others' (p. 172);
- a supportive work environment where employers and fellow workers were aware of the problems the user experienced but did not keep asking about their well-being;

- allowances being made for the need for time off for appointments and even admissions;
- lenient attitudes towards users ability to perform complicated tasks.

Clearly then, the nature of specific work environments is crucial in determining whether any one user will experience them as stressful. This in turn will be mediated, or not, by the intrinsic coping strategies that the individual possesses/utilises.

The Social Disability and Access Model

The Social Disability and Access Model (Perkins and Repper, 1996), advocates changing the community and the work environment, to ensure it meets the needs of the person with SMI rather than assuming that the user has to change first (e.g. become 'symptom-free' etc.) to render them ready for work (Perkins and Repper, 1996). As such this approach is more societal and political in its focus than the stress vulnerability model which is more individual and family focused. Because of this difference in emphasis, both models can be usefully combined to underpin a framework for enabling people with SMI to work.

Aspects of the social disability model can be recognised in the rapid placement philosophy of supported employment. Thus support is tailored to the person's needs in the workplace rather than postponing employment and offering segregated training until the person is deemed 'ready' for work. A Social Disability and Access approach looks at rendering the workplace ready for the person with SMI and not other way round. As such the provision of 'accommodations' is crucial, that is adaptations to either the work setting, routine, or tasks, which will enable users to access and remain in employment. Such occupational accommodations are commonplace for people with physical or sensory disabilities yet in Britain they are still rare for people with mental health problems of any kind. However, considerable progress has been made regarding accommodations to enable people with SMI to access educational courses. Hooper (1996) for instance has suggested the useful analogy of a 'virtual ramp' to enable users to access community education resources and opportunities. The type of 'accommodations' which this ramp needs to encompass include those features identified by users as helpful such as flexible work schedules (Mancuso, 1993).

Interventions to Promote Employment Opportunities for People with SMI

Given the substantial evidence regarding the advantages of work for people with SMI and the effectiveness of SE approaches, clinicians, teams and services need to review their practice to initiate much needed change. Even more important is that professionals' attitudes need to undergo a shift 'from a support and maintenance ideology to a recovery ideology for mental health services' (Torrey *et al.*, 1998, p. 74). Once a recovery-focused philosophy becomes central to practice, the following practical measures can be implemented by all mental health professionals:

- Identifying an 'honest baseline' as to what proportion, if any, of your clinical time and effort is actually spent on interventions which address occupational needs.
- Conducting a training needs analysis regarding work and SMI. What do you and your team know about effective interventions in this area? What is known about local resources, such as benefit specialists, and local needs?
- Formulating a training plan in conjunction with service users, managers and purchasers.
- Accessing relevant information to develop your knowledge and skills.
- Assessing the work needs and aspirations of all users with SMI as a routine part of the Care Programme Approach.
- Maintaining the clinical inputs such as medication management to maximise the chances of the person succeeding in the work environment.
- Taking ownership of the challenge by setting up or becoming involved in a small scale local work initiatives (Perkins *et al.*, 1997).
- Creating and nurturing links with occupational and vocational specialists with a view to skills sharing and reciprocal learning.
- Ensuring users receive appropriate and specialist benefits advice before starting a job.
- Linking with primary care colleagues to raise the profile of work for SMI and to tap into general practices' specialist community knowledge, some primary care teams have themselves taken the initiative and developed work projects for their patients with SMI (e.g. Nehring and Hill, 1995).
- Recognising that users who attain and retain work may have needs concerned with job performance problems and interpersonal or social difficulties as well as needs regarding their mental health (Torrey *et al.*, 1998).
- Instigating regular assessments both before and throughout the course of a job 'to document stressors, reactions, problems and accommodations, and supports as they occur' (Becker *et al.*, 1998, p. 80) and offering a flexible response to fluctuations in users' needs.

Conclusion

For progress to be achieved in our ability and willingness to offer effective work opportunities to people with SMI, a paradigmatic shift in the attitudes of mental health practitioners and services is required. Without such a change in attitudes, training clinicians about the available effective strategies is unlikely to result in a substantial increase in the actual implementation and provision of these approaches. Whilst services and clinicians can draw up action plans now, further research is required to identify

> . . . which types of . . . (work) program are most beneficial for which types of clients and at which stages of their recovery process. (McGurrin, 1994, p. 37)

Research is also required to clarify which particular accommodations are required for people with SMI (Mancuso, 1993) and whether such accommodations increase job tenure. Furthermore, effective methods of adapting the successful family interventions approach to modify high expressed emotion work environments need to be investigated, as do tailoring relapse prevention interventions. Further research underway (Crowther, 2000) aims to explore the benefits of psychological strategies to increase users motivation for work. Finally, research is needed to identify the barriers and the 'enablers' in terms of increasing users access to higher level jobs. This is vital because regardless of their skills and ambitions, people with SMI returning to competitive employment by way of SE or other means generally find it notoriously difficult to move beyond entry-level jobs such as domestic or basic administrative work or manual labour. Changes in the disability benefits system are also required as massive disincentives still remain for most people with SMI who may wish to attempt to work for anything over four hours a week. Legislation must be strengthened to outlaw the widespread discrimination that people with psychosis experience when trying to enter or re-enter the workforce, and to ensure reasonable accommodations are made for employees with SMI. Grassroots mental health staff have a role to play in campaigning for such changes in the law as do users' organisations, health ansd social care managers, employers and national leaders.

Further Reading

Crowther, R.E., Marshall, M., Bond, G.R. and Huxley, P. (2001) 'Helping people with severe mental illness to obtain work: systematic review', *British Medical Journal*, 322, 204–8.

Hill, R.G. and Shepherd, G. (1997) 'Positively Transitional or Unfortunately Permanent? The Status of Work Within Clubhouses in the UK', *A Life in the Day*. 25–30.

Perkins, R.E. and Repper, J.M. (1996) *Working Alongside People with Long-Term Mental Health Problems*, London: Chapman & Hall.

Pozner, A., Ng, M.L., Hammond, J. and Shepherd, G. (1996) *Working it out. Creating work opportunities for people with mental health problems: a development handbook*, London, Sainsbury Centre for Mental Health/Brighton: Pavilion Publishing.

Warner, P. (1994) *Recovery From Schizophrenia: Psychiatry and political economy*, 2nd edn, London, Routledge.

References

Bailey, E.L., Ricketts, S.K. and Becker, D.R. *et al.* (1998) 'Do long-term day treatment clients benefit from Supported Employment?', *Psychiatric Rehabilitation Journal,* 22(1), 24–9.

Becker, D.R., Drake, R.E., Farabaugh, A. and Bond, G.R. (1996) 'Job preferences of clients with severe psychiatric disorders participating in supported employment programs', *Psychiatric Services,* 47(11), 1223–6.

Becker, D.R., Torrey, W.C. and Toscano, R. *et al.* (1998) 'Building Recovery-oriented Services: lessons from implementing individual placement and support (IPS) in community mental health centers', *Psychiatric Rehabilitation Journal,* 22(1), 51–4.

Bell, M.D., Lysaker, P.H. and Milstein, R.M. (1996) 'Clinical Benefits of Paid Work Activity in Schizophrenia', *Schizophrenia Bulletin,* 22, 51–67.

Brenner, M.H. (1973) *Mental Illness and the Economy,* Cambridge, MA, Harvard University Press.

Clark, R.E., Dain, B. J., Xie, H., Becker, D.R. and Drake, R.E. (1998) 'The Economic Benefits of Supported Employment for Persons with Mental Illness', *Journal of Mental Health Policy and Economics,* 1(2), 63–71.

Cook, J.A. (1992) *Outcome assessment in psychiatric rehabilitation services for persons with severe and persistent mental illness.* Prepared for the National Institute of Mental Health, Contract No. 91MF23474902D.

Crowther, R., Bond. G., Huxley, P. and Marshall, M. (2000) *Vocational rehabilitation for people with severe mental disorders (Cochrane Review),* Cochrane Library, 3, Oxford, Update Software.

Crowther, R.E., Marshall, M., Bond, G.R. and Huxley, P. (2001) 'Helping people with severe mental illness to obtain work: systematic review', *British Medical Journal,* 322, 204–8.

Department of Health (1998) *Modernising Mental Health Services: safe, sound, supportive,* London, The Stationery Office.

Department of Health (1999) *National Service Framework for Mental Health,* London, The Stationery Office.

Drake, R.E., Fox, T.S. and Leather, P.K. *et al.* (1998) 'Regional Variation in Competitive Employment for Persons with Severe Mental Illness', *Administration and Policy in Mental Health,* 25(5), 493–504.

Evans, J. and Repper, J. (2000) 'Employment, social inclusion and mental health', *Journal of Psychiatric and Mental Health Nursing,* 7, 15–24.

Griffiths, R.D. (1974) 'Rehabilitation of chronic psychotic patients', *Psychological Medicine,* 4, 316–25.

Hill, R.G. and Shepherd, G. (1997) 'Positively Transitional or Unfortunately Permanent? The Status of Work within Clubhouses in the UK', *A Life in the Day,* 25–30.

Hooper, R. (1996) Adult Education for Mental Health: a study in innovation and partnership, *Adults Learning,* November, 71–4.

Jablensky, A., Sartorius, N., Ernberg, G., Anker, M., Korten, A., Cooper, J.E. Day, R. and Bartelsen, A. (1992) *Schizophrenia: manifestations, incidence and course in different cultures,* Cambridge, Cambridge University Press.

Jenkins, J.H. and Karno, M. (1992) 'The meaning of expressed emotion: theoretical issues raised by cross-cultural research', *American Journal of Psychiatry,* 149(1), 9–21.

Luo, K. and Yu, D. (1994) 'Enterprise-Based Sheltered Workshops in Nanjing: a new model for the Community Rehabilitation of Mentally Ill Workers', *British Journal of Psychiatry*, 165 (suppl. 24), 89–95.

Mancuso, L.L. (1993) *Case Studies on Reasonable Accommodations for Workers with Psychiatric Disabilities*, Sacramento, CA, California Department of Mental Health.

McGurrin, M.C. (1994) 'An overview of the effectiveness of traditional vocational rehabilitation services in the treatment of long term mental illness', *Psychosocial Rehabilitation Journal*, 17(3), 37–54.

Mueser, K.T., Becker, D.R., Torrey, W.C. and Xie, H. *et al.* (1997) 'Work and non-vocational domains of functioning in persons with severe mental illness: A longitudinal analysis', *Journal of Nervous and Mental Disease*, 185(7), 419–26.

Nehring, J. and Hill, R.G. (1995) *The Blackthorn Garden Project: Community Care in the Context of Primary Care*, London, Sainsbury Centre for Mental Health.

Perkins, R.E. (1991) *Access to Work*. Paper presented at the British Association for Behavioural Psychotherapy Annual National Conference, University of Oxford.

Perkins, R., Buckfield, R. and Choy, D. (1997) 'Access to employment: A supported employment project to enable mental health service users to obtain jobs within mental health services', *Journal of Mental Health*, 307–18.

Perkins, R.E. and Repper, J.M. (1996) *Working Alongside People with Long-Term Mental Health Problems*, London, Chapman & Hall.

Pozner, A., Ng, M.L., Hammond, J. and Shepherd, G. (1996) *Working it out. Creating work opportunities for people with mental health problems: a development handbook*, London, Sainsbury Centre for Mental Health/Brighton, Pavilion Publishing.

Read, J. and Baker, S. (1996) *Not just sticks and stones. A survey of the stigma, taboos and discrimination experienced by people with mental health problems*, London, MIND Publications.

Rogers, E.S., Walsh, D., Masotta, L. and Danley, K. (1991) *Massachusetts survey of client preferences for community support services (Final report)*, Boston, Center for Psychiatric Rehabilitation.

Scheid, T.L. and Anderson, C. (1995) 'Living with chronic mental illness: understanding the role of work', *Community Mental Health Journal*, 31(2), 163–76.

Shepherd, G., Murray, A. and Muijen, M. (1994) *Relative values: the different views of users, family carers and professionals on services for people with schizophrenia*, London, Sainsbury Centre for Mental Health.

Stein, L.I. and Santos, A.B. (1998) *Assertive Community Treatment of Persons with Severe Mental Illness*, New York, Wold. Norton.

Torrey, W.C., Becker, D.R. and Drake, R.E. (1995) 'Rehabilitative day treatment vs. supported employment: II. Consumer, family and staff reactions to a program change', *Psychosocial Rehabilitation Journal*, 18(3), 67–75.

Torrey, W.C., Mead, S. and Ross, G. (1998) 'Addressing the Social Needs of Mental Health Consumers when Day Treatment Programs Convert to Supported Employment: can consumer-run services play a role?', *Psychiatric Rehabilitation Journal*, 22(1), 73–5.

Warner, P. (1994) *Recovery From Schizophrenia: Psychiatry and political economy*, 2nd edn, London, Routledge.

Wexler, B.E., Hawkins, K.A., Rounsaville, B., Anderson, M., Sernyak, M.J. and Green, M.F., *et al.* (1997) 'Normal neurocognitive performance after extended practice in patients with schizophrenia', *Schizophrenia Research*, 26, 173–80.

Wing, J.K. and Brown, G. (1970) Institutionalism and Schizophrenia: a comparative study of three mental hospitals 1960–1968, Cambridge, Cambridge University Press.
World Health Organization (1979) *Schizophrenia: An International Follow-Up Study*, Chichester, Wiley.
Zubin, J. and Spring, B. (1977) 'Vulnerability: A new view of schizophrenia', *Journal of Abnormal Psychology*, 86, 103–26.

CHAPTER 13

Neighbourhood Networking – Working With the Community as a Source of Support: A Practical Guide

DOUGLAS INCHBOLD

Who is This For?

This chapter is aimed at those people who have working responsibility for the support of people who suffer from mental health problems. It is directly relevant to workers in statutory or voluntary organisations who have day to day contact with the people who use their services.

It is written as a practical guide showing why it is important to help the people who use their services to form alternative networks of support, how to begin to do so, and some of the problems which may be encountered.

It is also very relevant to policy-makers and service managers as it describes a style of operation that has implications for service structures, management and the allocation of resources.

The chapter may also be of interest to people who are experiencing mental health problems, or their families and carers, since it may raise awareness of a range of support that they can benefit from. It may be also applicable to some 'self help' activities.

It concerns support for people experiencing any sort of mental health problem, but is mostly concerned with people suffering severe mental health problems, including schizophrenia.

What it is About

When a person is undergoing difficulties in maintaining their mental health and find they need to turn to professionals for help, there is a tendency for that help to focus very quickly on to a narrow range of responses. These are designed to overcome any immediate crisis and provide sufficient stability to enable recovery. However, if a service then provides much longer term support, especially to people with the most severe problems, a far broader outlook is necessary. A service that merely responds to crisis and does little to enable a service user to engage with more natural sources of support over the longer term may make little progress in improving the mental stability and quality of life of that person.

What an individual needs in order to enjoy stable mental health and a good quality of life is not located entirely within the internal processes of their mind, or within their family. For most people, there is also a need to feel part of a community, both a community based on a shared interest, or on local proximity.

Nevertheless, for many people, life is becoming increasingly isolated. Individuals and families operate with such self sufficiency that community of any sort is of declining importance. Many people are satisfied with passive leisure pursuits, travelling in isolation and not knowing their neighbours.

But life in relation to wider communities is still vital for everyone in terms of personal identity, for making a living and for maintaining status as a citizen. For many people who have low incomes or are socially disadvantaged and excluded, closer contact with a community of any form is far more vital. People with less personal resources, for example a strong sense of purpose, adequate finances or a supportive family, are more likely to need a variety of sources of practical support and are more likely to depend on wider social interaction to maintain the possibility of continuing social contact. They are more likely to achieve a sense of personal identity from people around them than from wider social conditioning, for example as a professional or as a consumer.

They are also more dependant on maintaining their own social acceptability in local communities as the consequences of being different are more drastic, for example their personal safety may be at stake. People with severe mental health problems are more likely to fall within this part of the population.

So, for many people suffering mental health problems, the ability to feel part of a community and feel accepted and supported is very important, not least to their continuing mental well-being. Yet gaining and maintaining a place within a community of any sort can be one of the most difficult problems to be faced by a person who is likely to be lacking self confidence or may be prone to unusual experiences and behaviour. Is there a role in helping someone to overcome these difficulties? What is the best way to go about it and what are the rewards?

The Current Climate

'Care in the Community' policies of the past thirty or forty years have gradually reversed a long standing policy of isolating and segregating people with severe (and not so severe) mental health problems in institutions. In many ways the large long stay psychiatric institutions were the last remnants of the workhouse system for containing people who, for one reason or another, were unable to earn a living. Despite much effort and progress, there is still much debate about the wisdom of care in the community policies, much of it focusing on the vulnerability or the dangerousness of people who use mental health services. Since 1998, the government has announced the failure of such policies and is publishing proposals for what it sees as a more safe and secure system of care (DoH, 1998). The fact remains, though, that the majority of people with severe mental health problems will continue to live in ordinary or supported accommodation in the community, not in institutions.

Through all of this, there is still as great a stigma about experiencing mental health problems. People who suffer from poor mental health are still subject to prejudice and discrimination. The degree of prejudice prevalent in society as a whole may have lessened or just taken different forms, but it is still a significant factor in weighing up the place of individuals in communities.

The work of helping a person to survive and gain benefit from living in communities should not just focus on the individual. They may require support to increase confidence, develop social skills or know where to go for help, but work with the community is the other half of the solution to the same problem.

The general public needs support in understanding the nature of mental health and illness and in how best to relate to mental suffering or the different behaviour that may result from it. A 'community' is a body of people to whom the individuals, whose support we are concerned with, must relate and with whom we may address these matters.

What is a Community?

In health and social care circles, 'community' simply means 'not in an institution'. Here it is taken in its broadest sense as a body of people with a common interest or purpose. In practice we are concerned with that community of interest which would best serve an otherwise isolated individual were they a part of it. In most cases this may start with a geographically localised community where the common interest is living in the same place, that is, a neighbourhood.

Clearly this covers a vast range of conditions with varying degrees of contact between people living near to each other. Some areas may have the characteristics of communities that we associate with an ideal, where everyone knows each other and is always available to lend a hand. At the other extreme we may think of very alienated or 'atomised' communities associated with the stereotypical suburb or big city centres.

The point here is that everyone, no matter what the nature of his or her local community, is dependent on it to some extent. Everyone learns about their immediate environment even if they have no intention to engage with it. This is what, at the very least, keeps us safe and out of jail. It is the context of the local environment that is mostly discussed here although other sorts of community of interest may be useful to consider, like single interest clubs or societies, associations of people that may be geographically scattered.

A geographical area may have many communities, some of which may interrelate and some of which will not. Some may be rivals to others. Communities may be formed of people with common interest, like some ethnic communities in British cities. With greater mobility and telephones, a community of interest for some people, like some families, may be dispersed over a very wide area.

People who have experienced mental health problems and used mental health services are, for some, a community of common interest in their own right, often developing networks of contact and support, social and leisure activities, and advocacy and campaigning functions.

What Can be Achieved?

The aim here is to find the best means of working to enable people who suffer mental health problems to enjoy life, engaging in their local community and where possible being able to derive some support from it. They may also be able to contribute to such a community and support others. From the point of view of a specialist mental health service, the result should be to decrease dependence on the service for individuals and to improve their mental health through increasing self-esteem and confidence. It is often worth remembering that for most users of mental health services, contact with the service is a very small portion of their life. It is important that there are opportunities to spend some of the rest of the time in positive contact with other people.

It is also worth considering that many mental health services have an evolving function and structure. There are no guarantees that levels of support through such services are sustainable in the longer term. Helping a person to engage with more natural means of support provides them with some insurance against unpredictable change in formal service provision. Those who are the family of people with serious mental health problems, or who are carers in other ways, will also benefit from engagement with alternative sources of support. If the person they care for has a richer social life, for example, it will decrease the burden and stress for them. A carer may benefit from other forms of engagement in their own right, thus enhancing their ability to support someone.

But working with communities to these ends can have other results in the process. It may mean that there is an improved awareness of mental health in a community with the result that there is better tolerance and improved ability of a wider group of people to maintain good mental health. It may mean that some of the formal and informal mechanisms for support are strengthened, for example, personal networks, local advice services, tenant and resident organisations.

Furthermore, many community, voluntary and informal organisations as well as many formal public services that have routine contact with people, will be engaged in dealing with people who have mental health problems of a range of severity. They may well be providing a good 'mental health service' without recognising it as such.

For a specialist mental health service, the results could be an improved public profile, public support, and a more effective service to users and easier access to services by the public. Developing local contact opens up the potential for better public accountability for services. It may also have less predictable results, like improved staff morale and safety.

Some Examples of What Can be Achieved

These practical examples are drawn from work in North Manchester between 1986 and 1998, through a community mental health service. The area covered is an inner city area with levels of deprivation, morbidity and mortality much higher than national averages. Although these examples show success in enabling people with severe problems to derive some support from local communities, it should be remembered that there were also many examples of people being targeted for harassment, assault and theft by local people. Such negative experiences are not unusual for most residents in this area and it is part of the purpose of work with local communities to ameliorate this vulnerability.

Example 1

Mr P was moving to a flat on a council estate in an unfamiliar area after a long period in a psychiatric hospital. He is a shy man in his fifties and was very nervous and uncertain about the move and his own abilities to cope. Prior contacts between the community mental health team and the local residents' organisation meant that as Mr P moved into his flat, some of his new neighbours called to introduce themselves and welcome him to the area. This modest connection clearly called for discretion, but had the effect of reassuring Mr P considerably.

Example 2

A long term relationship between a local community centre and the mental health team had a number of benefits:

● People working in and using the community centre had a better appreciation of the nature of mental health problems and the difficulties facing people who experience them. As a result, many people who were users of the mental health service were welcomed to the community centre and made to feel comfortable turning to them for welfare rights or housing advice, using the luncheon club, attending social activities and so on. For many this was an important alternative to reliance on more formal services many of which, like 'day hospitals', segregate them from society.

- People who used the community centre were able to get access to support and advice about mental health in an easier and less formal way.
- The community centre and the mental health team supported each other as organisations, collaborating, for example, on the recruitment of local people into mental health teams to ensure a more appropriate service and job opportunities for local people. The two organisations were able to provide material facilities to aid each other as well.

Example 3

Mr M is a man in his thirties who lives alone and is very dependent on the support of the mental health services. He likes to drink regularly in a local pub but is prone to extremely unusual, sometimes aggressive, behaviour. He was barred from the pub on several occasions and this threatened to lead to deepening isolation for him. On each occasion, it was the intercession of members of a local tenants' organisation that led to his reinstatement. Members of the mental health team had cultivated links with the tenants' group over a long period, using the opportunity to support the group where possible and to foster their appreciation of the problems faced by people who suffer severe mental health problems.

Example 4

The mental health team developed links with a number of local organisations, offering training, whether formal or informal, on dealing with people who experience mental health problems. Working in this way with, for example, Citizens Advice Bureaux, the police, churches or libraries, was intended to generate more choice for users of mental health services by improving the ways in which they are dealt with by public and community organisations.

How to Begin Working with Local Communities

Can You do it at All?

For many workers employed in the care of people with serious mental health problems, the opportunities to do anything other than face-to-face work with clients are rare. For this reason, it is necessary to be able to argue that time spent in engaging individuals and organisations in local communities is of benefit to service users. That in the long run it may save time and resources for your organisation by encouraging independence and providing alternative means of support which also have the benefit of being more 'normal' and not stigmatising.

Ideally this argument should become a rooted part of the principles and operation of a service. Managers and colleagues should appreciate the value of such work and estimate its impact on service capacity and resources. An open acknowledgement of the value of this work can lead to a discussion on how best to allocate time to it. In doing so, there are a number of points that need to be understood. For example, that there will not be a direct, measurable, relationship between the amount of work dedicated to working with a local community and the benefits for users. Such work is, by its nature, often long term and open ended. In appreciating this, it is worth considering some of the principles of work of people whose profession is community work. Such factors do not mean that evaluation of such work is impossible or unimportant, and this will be dealt with below.

Considering Your Own Role

To engage with a local community on behalf of other people, it is important to have a clear understanding of your role and how other people will see this. To some extent this will depend on the nature of the local area that is targeted. For example, do you wish to be seen as a formal representative of the organisation that employs you? Will you be seen as a figure of authority or as an outsider? How will your motives be interpreted? Self-awareness is an important aspect of preparation, and will need to reflect the wider role of your organisation. For example, consider the common representation of the public view of care in the community policies. How do you respond if challenged on the motivations of your organisation? Are community care policies simply a way of saving money by transferring the burden of care to other public agencies, community organisations and families?

It is also important to be aware of the limits to your role in working alongside local community structures. As mentioned above, the communities you work with derive part of the benefit of this work. In seeking their support for people with mental health problems, something should be offered in return. Contributing to the strength of community organisation and resources will contribute towards your goals. In this reciprocal relationship it is important to have clear boundaries to your involvement, for example,

- It would not be appropriate to assume a leadership role in relation to a community organisation however much that function needs to be fulfilled. The pitfalls here are not just for the viability of your role, but more for the stability and purpose of the organisation concerned.

- You should be prepared for conflicts of interest between community organisations and your own organisation, especially as you may become an important link between them.
- Not all aspects of neighbourhood organisations may be benign. You must be prepared to deal with negative aspects of local attitudes, for example racism or other forms of intolerance. It will be important not to allow yourself to be put in the position of conspiring with such attitudes. It may be important to challenge them whilst still maintaining support for your purpose.

How to Get Started

These are some tips for workers who may appreciate the need to work with their clients in helping them to engage in a wider network of support, but who are constrained by a busy workload.

- Think about the needs of individual clients as a means of directing you to the most likely areas of engagement. What are their more pressing needs? It may be that they need social contact, or the opportunity to talk over particular problems. It may be more urgent that they are able to live safely in their neighbourhood. Make this a topic of conversation and exploration in meeting with service users.
- Discuss these matters with your colleagues and managers. The more team members and associates are involved in generating broader networks, the more effective it is. Having a broader view of the needs of clients can be gained from a collective contribution. A more formal means of assessing the needs of service users for wider sources of support may be required, for example through a specially designed project, an assisted questionnaire or assessment or through the client review system. In a busy service where everyone can only make a limited range of wider contacts, dividing up the task and sharing information is vital.
- Get to know the area in which you are operating. This is especially important for those who do not live in the area where they work. The social segregation between service providers and service users is an increasingly significant feature of professional care, especially in inner city areas. Many community mental health services cover extremely large geographical areas so it may be important to focus on smaller localities of concern to particular service users, or divide the task between several team members.

It is a worthwhile project to undertake a brief profile of a local area, combining a look at some significant census data (e.g. ethnic diversity, wealth/poverty indicators such as car ownership, proportions of people living alone), some local history, a directory of local services and activities and so on.

Often someone else will already have done this who can make a copy available. Local libraries are always a good place to start.

Less formal means might include walking around the area instead of driving in the course of your usual business, using local facilities such as cafes, markets or pubs more often, talking to residents of the area, arranging to visit local organisations to find out what they do.

Setting aside some specific time on a regular basis, say just one hour a week, may provide sufficient opportunity to develop a practical understanding of how best to enhance living in the locality for people who use your service. It will also provide useful range of contacts (who will be just as interested in regarding you as a useful contact) for the future.

Opportunities

Developing knowledge of a local area and contacts with active organisations and individuals, over a period of time, will present a number of valuable opportunities. For example, to

- Discuss mental health issues with a wider group of people. This serves to improve attitudes towards people who experience mental health problems and encourage their acceptance. It also serves to promote a more open general understanding of everybody's vulnerability to poor mental health. In some cases this discussion can be formalised as 'a talk' or a training session. It is an opportunity to discuss some aspects of severe mental illnesses that are often the subject of mystery and fear, for example, what is happening when somebody appears to be talking to a voice in their head? In this context, questions of the dangerousness of people suffering mental illness will always be on somebody's mind. They may raise the matter or may pass over it politely, but it is better to deal with it openly. Introduce people who use your service and who may wish to become more associated with local organisations or specific activities. Prior relationships with the organisations in question mean that this introduction can be as natural as possible, and not like making a formal referral.
- Find out to what extent other organisations and groups are supporting people with mental health problems already, and whether there is scope for additional support to them in this role, for example through training or access to speedy advice from mental health professionals.
- Identify problems in the service you are providing. Taking a view from the outside can be refreshing and challenging. This perspective may demonstrate the need, for example, to make the service more easily accessible or more appropriate to the needs of a particular section of the population.
- Identify gaps in provision. Discussion with local agencies may reveal a need for alternative forms of support in particular areas or to meet a

particular need, for example a self help group or a social and leisure group.

● Work together to provide new forms of support. What is of benefit to your clients, as local residents, will likewise benefit their neighbours. Your collaboration with a range of other local agents may be sufficient to identify how best to meet the needs of a wide range of local people. The support of your organisation may result in the contribution of resources for new activities.

Some Problems

It is important not to underestimate the difficulty of the task of helping people with serious mental health problems to be able to turn to local people and organisations for support. Here are some potential difficulties,

● You are asked directly by a representative of a group, with whom a user of your service has come into contact, to discuss something, which you must regard as confidential. However, the information could be seen as crucial to the ability of the group to accept that person on equal terms.

● Some aspect of a person's behaviour may be unacceptable in a social setting no matter how open minded the company.

● There will often be an expectation that a person with a severe mental health problem encountering a new or difficult social situation will be accompanied. This expectation may come form the participants in the group in question, from the user of the service, or from the support service. To accompany a person in this situation may be to stigmatise their mental health problems further, but could also be seen positively as an opportunity to show how receiving support for a mental health problem can be as socially acceptable as experiencing it.

Evaluation

Service provision in statutory and voluntary services is increasingly subject to evaluation for effectiveness to ensure value for money and adherence to proven good practice. Clearly, activity in developing links and active partnerships with community organisations and informal social networks can be difficult to evaluate, however some suggestions for how these interventions could be evaluated are offered below:

● Goal planning for targeted pieces of work. Where the aim of working with community organisations is sufficiently clear, results may be measured against stated purpose. More often than not, though, the nature of this work is speculative and opportunistic and does not lend itself to such planning unless it is to be a substantial part of your work.

- Goal setting techniques, for use with individual clients. This may detail, for example, the aspirations of someone to be able to go once a week to a social setting that provides opportunities to meet people and make friends. Their progress towards such a goal may be measured over a planned period and subject to review. This process can be linked to regular client review and may provide some means of evaluating the benefit for the individual of a focus on social settings. It does not, however, provide any direct evaluation of the vital background work that facilitates such developments.
- A narrative report, which simply tells how the connection is made between the effort put in to making a constructive relationship with a potentially useful agency and the benefits for individual service users. A number of such reports may be collated to demonstrate the wider benefits of the work. They should, where possible show an involvement of the user in the process of evaluation. There are means by which groups of people are able to use a variety of media to demonstrate how an initiative has had a positive effect for them, for example the use of arts media, such as video.
- Some activities that result from this style of working may be more specific in their scope and lend themselves more to planned evaluation, for example, a group activity may be able to be evaluated by counting the number of people who use it or by measuring their satisfaction.

Conclusion

Recent developments in health and social policy reinforce the importance of this component in mental healthcare. The government's public health policy as outlined in *Our Healthier Nation, Saving Lives* (DoH, 1999a) makes improving mental health a national priority with an emphasis on working in partnership across organisations and across sectors. The overall priority is to lessen inequalities in health through tackling social exclusion. Behind this is recognition, at the heart of current policy, that social exclusion is a major contributor to poor health, especially poor mental health.

The *National Service Framework for Mental Health* (DoH, 1999b) is very clear in this regard, stating, as its first standard, that Health and Social Services should,

- Promote mental health for all, working with individuals and communities.
- Combat discrimination against individuals and groups with mental health problems, and promote their social inclusion.

The style of work discussed above can be an important contribution to meeting this standard while its legitimation through the National Service

Framework should make it easier for service managers to incorporate this perspective into the work of mental health teams. The formation of Primary Care Groups (DoH, 1997) (later to become trusts with responsibility for purchasing services for local populations) has given a more local focus for working in partnership between the statutory services and local communities. There is a stronger recognition that most mental health care is provided in communities and through primary care and that this should be strengthened. In practice it is to be hoped that such changes will provide more opportunities for community services for people with serious mental health problems to become more integrated with the communities in which they live. The participation of those who work in such services at a local level is essential in this process.

Further Reading

Dunn, S. (1999) *Creating Accepting Communities*, London MIND.

Naparstek, A., Biegel, D., and Spiro, H. (1982) *Neighborhood Networks for Humane Mental Health Care*, New York, Plenum Press.

Department of Health (2001) *Making it Happen. A guide to delivering mental health promotion*, London, The Stationery Office.

Sainsbury Centre for Mental Health (2000) *On Your Doorstep: Community organisations and mental health*, London, Sainsbury Centre for Mental Health.

Mental Health Foundation (1997) *Knowing Our Own Minds*, London, MHF.

Mental Health Foundation (2000) *Strategies For Living*, London, MHF.

References

Department of Health (1997) *The New NHS: Modern, Dependable*, London, HMSO.

Department of Health (1998) *Modernising Mental Health Services. Safe, Sound and Supportive*, London, The Stationery Office.

Department of Health (1999a) *Our Healthier Nation, Saving Lives* London, The Stationery Office.

Department of Health (1999b) *National Service Framework for Mental Health*, London, The Stationery Office.

Part IV

Special Considerations

Special Considerations

in Harris et al (2002)

CHAPTER 14

Dual Diagnosis – Substance Misuse and Schizophrenia

MARK HOLLAND

Introduction

It has been estimated that approximately 32 per cent of people who suffer from schizophrenia use illicit substances (Menezes *et al.*, 1996) and up to 16 per cent drink alcohol to excess (Duke *et al.*, 1994). Such prevalence, despite being lifetime, is disproportionate to the general adult population of this country, and similarly the effects of substance misuse are also more pervading and immediate among those with psychosis. Such people, who are commonly referred to as having a 'dual diagnosis', have been shown to be more difficult for traditional mental health services to engage and deliver programmes of care to (Rorstad and Checinski, 1996; Lehman *et al.*, 1994; Smith and Hucker, 1993).

The difficulty in delivering care to this group arises from the combination of their tendency to have a chaotic lifestyle, and the separation of traditional services for people with mental illness from those who misuse substances. This has led to a situation where these people, who are arguably most in need of services, fail to get the care that they require (DoH, 1994).

Recently, concern has been expressed about the inability of services to adequately care for people with a dual diagnosis (Gournay and Sandford, 1996; Holland, 1999) and the need for the development of more effective evidence based approaches has been highlighted. A suitable approach might be one that integrates treatments of known effectiveness for people with a diagnosis of serious mental illness, such as psychosocial intervention (Lancashire *et al.*, 1997) alongside an approach of proven efficacy in helping people who misuse substances (Rollnick, 1995).

This chapter describes how mental health professionals can incorporate standardised psychiatric assessments, clinical drug use rating scales and cognitive behavioural strategies into the planning and implementation of care for clients experiencing co-morbid substance misuse and serious mental illness.

To this end a brief review of the literature concerning the prevalence, aetiology and treatment of people with dual diagnosis will be provided. The remainder of the text will focus upon the development of effective evidence-based care for this client group and issues related to service configuration.

189

Finally a case study to illustrate the core components of effective practice will be presented.

For expediency this text uses the term 'misuse' to denote problematic use, abuse, dependency, addiction or substance use disorder. The abbreviation SMI refers to serious mental illness.

Background

Dual diagnosis cannot be found as a discreet diagnostic category in diagnostic manuals such as DSM IV (American Psychiatric Association, 1994) or ICD 10 (WHO, 1992). The term is used within learning disability services to indicate the presence of both a mental illness and a learning disability. The term in mainstream psychiatry, during the past five years in the UK and for over ten years in the United States, designates individuals who experience simultaneous serious mental illness (usually psychotic) and substance misuse related problems.

People experiencing a serious mental illness (SMI) such as schizophrenia or bi-polar disorder have a stronger likelihood of developing substance misuse compared to the general population (Regier et al., 1990). In addition, the same is true for the incidence of mental illness among the substance misusing population. Therefore, the reports, of both anecdotal and empirical nature, of co-occurring mental illness and substance misuse have surprised few clinicians.

A British review in 1993 (Smith and Hucker, 1993) focused upon the vast literature from the US, in particular the results from the Epidemiologic Catchment Area (ECA) Study (Regier et al., 1990). In this study a sample population of over 20,000 yielded findings of co-morbid substance misuse in excess of 50 per cent among those people with a mental illness. Lifetime prevalence of co-morbidity was 47 per cent in those individuals with a diagnosis of schizophrenia, 84 per cent in personality disorder and 32 per cent in affective disorders.

North American mental health services were the first to respond strategically and operationally (Drake et al., 1993) to the ECA study and its forerunners. Their lead has been followed by services in Australia, Japan, Scandinavia and to a lesser extent the UK. Indeed the influence, in particular, of services in New Hampshire (Mueser et al., 1998a) can be seen in Fife (Mitchell et al., 1992), Dorset (Gibbins, 1998), Birmingham (Graham and Maslin, 1998) and London (Thomas et al., 1999). However, a modicum of caution is advised when importing findings from other countries, not least the States due to medical, economic and cultural differences.

Two themes, in common with the US, have become established as common reference points in the growing British literature concerning dual diagnosis. First, the 'service gap syndrome' (Rorstad and Checinki, 1996) where specialist substance misuse services fail to provide adequately for their clients who also have a mental illness, and where mainstream psychiatric practice does not address the substance misuse demands of its population; and second, the development and application of clinical approaches effective in this client group (see below).

Since approximately one third of the SMI population have a dual diagnosis (serious mental illness and substance misuse combined) research into its aetiology is crucial. Common terms, of questionable clarity but frequent usage, such as drug induced psychosis do more to subvert treatment than generate effective care provision, due to the ease with which they can be applied. Caution must be exercised in diagnosing because of the treatment implications. The trend towards substance misuse causality in SMI has a tenuous evidence base. A useful perspective on substance misuse in SMI is to view the consequences of the substance misuse as environmental stressors. Within a stress-vulnerability model (Zubin and Spring, 1977) clinicians are encouraged to acknowledge the negative consequences of substance misuse rather than focus upon a direct cause and effect relationship between substance misuse and the symptoms of mental illness (Holland *et al.*, 1999).

Theoretical aetiological models have been reviewed recently (Mueser *et al.*, 1998b) and provide factual as well as speculative information that appears clinically useful. Four general models are identified.

(i)   Common factor models that suggest a number of factors may work in concert or individually (e.g. genetic predisposition, a diagnosis of personality disorder) to increase vulnerability to both or either substance misuse and mental illness.

(ii) Secondary substance misuse model that promotes, among other ideas, that SMI sufferers have a super-sensitivity to alcohol or drugs which triggers psychiatric relapse *and* creates an independent substance misuse condition.

(iii) Secondary persistent psychiatric illness model, for which there exists little evidence and

(iv) Bi-directional model which suggests either individual disorder might trigger the other and be maintained by the notion that substance misuse will relieve feelings of dysphoria. Such a belief is commonly found in the substance misusing population.

Why do People with a Mental Illness Misuse Substances?

De-institutionalisation has led to larger numbers of people with a mental illness living in a community setting. The number of long-stay beds has more than halved during the last decade in England and Wales and despite throughput in psychiatric acute admission wards accelerating. Beds remain at a premium. The focus of community-based care will inevitably incorporate the everyday risks faced by the general population such as substance misuse. Also those with SMI are less likely to find employment and often live or gravitate towards areas of low socio-economic status. The increased availability of illicit substances in such areas contributes to the likelihood of substance misuse regardless of psychiatric illness. Subsequently several factors mitigate to increase the vulnerability of the severely mentally ill to misuse substances

The increased opportunity to misuse substances does not alone explain their widespread use satisfactorily. Substance misusers without a mental illness often misuse substances to ameliorate dysphoria; their causal factor for substance misuse is therefore derived from a need to improve their sense of well-being. Since many sufferers of schizophrenia also experience depression and anxiety to clinically significant levels, it appears likely that their substance misuse has the same general causal factors. This again is consistent with the increased prevalence of substance misuse among the mentally ill.

Other theories have been documented concerning the specific psychological and physiological effects of individual substances suggesting that some sufferers might indeed be seeking a particular effect, and therefore exercise considerable choice in obtaining a specific substance (e.g. stimulant misuse to regain a 'high' during depressive phases of bipolar disorder or the initial euphoric effect of alcohol or opiates to alleviate depressive feelings). Evidence contrary to this theory can be observed among those people with depressive symptoms and their continued misuse of depressants such as alcohol or opiates, rather than a stimulant, which would counteract depressive symptoms short-term. Constant stimulant misuse among people with symptoms of mania also opposes the suggestion that substance misuse by the psychiatric population is for specific symptom control, since stimulants will generate increased activity.

It is more likely the choice of a substance is governed by its availability and cost not its specific action. Currently research is limited, albeit growing, concerning cause and course of substance misuse in mental illness.

Caring for and Treating People with a Dual Diagnosis

Clinicians from either substance misuse or psychiatric services need to acknowledge the presence of mental illness among substance misusers, but not necessarily assign a substance induced disorder to them. An initial diagnosis of substance misuse and a mental disorder encourages clinicians and services to address current needs in a holistic manner. It also discourages early causal inaccuracies that could result in far more threatening consequences associated with service exclusion and failure to treat. Anecdotally SMI sufferers assigned a substance induced state have 'slipped through the net' in mainstream psychiatry. They also frequently slip through the net in substance misuse services when the substance misuse is attributed to mental illness.

How Services Can Be Delivered

In general services for substance misuse and services for mental illness are separate. They may both be National Health Service agencies or one, usually, substance misuse, may be local authority.

Importantly, but quite often peripheral to statutory services, are voluntary sector organisations. Voluntary agencies also have substance misuse and mental health distinctions. The adverse result of separate services for the dually diagnosed client is movement from one service to the other. This reduces engagement success therefore diminishing the likelihood of treatment progress. Efforts to address this sequential form of treatment have been made and models of service delivery are best described as:

Sequential Service Delivery

Here existing separate services work with the client, rarely at the same time, usually sequentially. The services have minimal contact with one another. Collaborative approaches between services are not emphasised and delays in communication are common. Clients are in the invidious position of being exposed to two forms of treatment, one after the other or fail to be engaged in either. Treatment programmes for substance misuse and mental illnesses have fundamental differences that can serve to confuse clients and erode consistency.

Parallel Services

Services remain separate organisationally, however formal policy is devised which promotes a working partnership between the two services (Holland, 1998).

This may be operationalised by joint referral meetings, joint assessment procedures and shared client contact protocols. The services continue to provide their specific form of intervention, while enjoying the advantages of good communication and collaborative goal planning. Two agencies with differing skills, approaches, philosophy, buildings and workers can be disadvantageous for similar reasons to sequential treatment.

Services Providing Integrated Treatment

This model of service delivery acknowledges the combined needs of substance misuse and mental health in the client as one. Addressing the combined needs therefore requires an approach that integrates substance misuse and mental health skills. Variations on this theme exist; for example, each service need not jeopardise their specific approach to their 'singularly' diagnosed client group but modify their approach for the dually diagnosed.

Integrated treatment can be provided by either or both services in a locality. However, the main tenet is singular point of contact, that is, the client has one clinician or one team. It is more commonly associated with specialist service provision in the US, which also provide a comprehensive range of facilities for the dually diagnosed.

Summary

Service planning nationally has yet to embrace an individual model of delivery. Nevertheless, a philosophy of collaboration between both types of service does encourage mechanisms essential for good practice, that is, training and communication systems. Thorough communication and an organised approach to care planning would not, in many clients' cases, solve the problems they face. Moreover it will illustrate the need for services to modify their operational strategies while incorporating new skills for a challenging client group with quite complex and tangled needs.

Interventions with People with Dual Diagnosis

Substance misuse services consist of statutory and voluntary sector agencies, both of which usually offer treatment to their clients only if motivation is present. While motivation to address substance misuse related problems is essential, a clients recognition of such problems and the presence of motivation to change, need not necessarily be explicit. The adoption of motivational (Rollnick, 1995) and harm reduction (Carey, 1996) approaches means substance misuse workers enjoy a broad scope to their practice. For example, a client with infected injection sites might accept safe injecting advice. No motivation to stop misusing the substance is apparent in such a client yet the intervention prevents further health deterioration. This illustrates legitimate clinical practice in the absence of motivation to stop or reduce substance intake.

The backdrop to most substance misuse work in psychosis is harm reduction with a longer-term goal of abstinence. This approach, which concerns itself with reducing or ameliorating the detrimental effects of substance misuse, acknowledges that abstinence and rapid intake reduction are not always realistic initial or medium term goals. This mirrors approaches in schizophrenia where symptom management aims to reduce the distress and disruption generated by symptoms rather than obliterate them wholesale.

Motivational approaches of considerable effectiveness have become popular in recent years. The importance of making an accurate assessment of an individuals level of motivation is crucial. Poorly timed strategies to reduce substance misuse can damage future treatment success. For instance, encouraging a client to engage in structured activities (leisure, work, colleges, clubs) when they are only concerned with obtaining their next 'hit', or suggesting a client attend substance misuse counselling when housing, welfare or crisis needs are far more pressing.

An assessment interview should indicate the level of motivation present. One of four stages might be identified: 'precontemplation' – before the person recognises their misuse as a problem; 'contemplation' – thinking around ways of reducing or stopping substance misuse; 'behaviour change/action' concerning practical steps to reduce or stop substance misuse and 'maintenance behaviour' or 'relapse prevention' of substance misuse entirely. After eliciting a client's level of motivation the aim is to assist them in their progress towards 'maintenance behaviour'. At this stage support in consolidation of any motivational factors is necessary. Movement back and forth in stages is not unusual and is not regarded as failure.

The theme throughout motivational approaches is to maintain a long-term view of recovery. Table 14.1 illustrates the lengthy duration of treatment (Drake *et al.*, 1993), and the interventions possible at each motivational stage.

Frequently clients will engage with mental health services but fail to display motivation, remaining pre-contemplative. While continued substance misuse compounds problems of accommodation, relationships, health and financial welfare, each difficulty presents an opportunity for progress. Some clients and most relatives will be more likely to address care needs at times of crisis or deterioration rather than at times of relative stability. This often provides ongoing opportunities to deliver interventions despite motivation being absent.

The needs of clients presenting with substance misuse and symptoms of serious mental illness necessitate the application of skills and strategies from both psychiatric and substance misuse fields. Case management studies (Drake *et al.*, 1996) have shown the delivery of both sets of skills by one worker or one small team (integrated treatment) is more effective than delivery by two separate workers or agencies (parallel treatment).

Current service configuration in the UK encourages a dual co-ordinating and interventionist role for community psychiatric nurses (CPN) and mental health practitioner (MHP). This involves the organisation of several agencies at anyone time. Efforts to limit the number of agencies involved and placing an emphasis upon the interventionist function of a CPN/MHP will provide a consistent approach and encourage success, at least in engagement.

Clinical Skills and Case Illustration

A range of treatments and approaches have been mentioned earlier in this chapter. The effectiveness of specific treatments has not been fully explored either in the UK or elsewhere (Ley *et al.*, 1999). What has been demonstrated,

Table 14.1 Helpful interventions at different stages of motivation: A practical crosswalk between the cycle of change* and stagewise treatment**

STAGE OF MOTIVATION	INTERVENTION
Precontemplation The absence of any thoughts or behaviour concerning substance misuse problems.	**Engagement** Despite absence of motivation the potential to develop a working relationship based on trust is present. At this stage clients have multifaceted problems around issues such as housing, welfare and health. Opportunities emerge immediately whereby a worker can assist with alleviating such problems (e.g. benefits assistance or new accommodation) leading to a therapeutic alliance. Preparatory work is essential for later stages. Successful engagement is the development of trust and acceptance of 'help' however small.
Contemplation The presence of thoughts (not usually behaviour) and ideas concerning reduction/cessation of substance misuse, and/or recognition that some life problems might be derived from substance misuse.	**Persuasion** A variety of strategies encouraging a client to understand the consequences of substance misuse are employed (education, pros and cons of substance misuse). Neither coercion or confrontation is appropriate – they merely compound the substance misuse or undermine the efforts to empathise. The emphasis is upon generating motivation for recovery from within an individual. Persuasion is most effective once engaged; however other appropriate interventions here such as sampling alternative forms of social activity, assertiveness training, structured activities and prescription of specific medication have considerable overlap which suggests that stages of motivation are not entirely discrete.
Behaviour change/action The presence of changed behaviour consistent with (i) reducing the adverse effects of substance misuse and/or (ii) reducing or abstaining from substance misuse.	**Active treatment** The strategies employed to support reduction of substance misuse range from pharmacological adjuncts (e.g. Methadone, Antabuse) and detoxification to psycho-substance education (individual/group) and assertive substance refusal training. Clients at this stage are becoming proactive in their efforts but require constant support and encouragement.
Change behaviour maintenance A stage of consolidation, where reduction or abstinence from substance misuse is established.	**Relapse prevention** Active treatment strategies are equally applicable here. Identifying triggers or predisposing factors of substance misuse are essential. Client and worker collaboration in devising contingency plans in the event of substance misuse relapse or 'near misses' may involve other workers, friends and family. Maintaining strategies of social approval and material/practical benefits reinforces progress. Continued input over a period of years not months will be required for a stable lasting recovery.

Source: *DiClemente and Prochaska (1985) and **Osher and Kofoed (1989).

however, is that mainstream mental health and substance misuse approaches do generally have a positive effect on dual diagnosis clients when they are delivered by a service based on assertive case management principles (Drake and Osher, 1997). Such assertive orientated interventions remain appropriate for traditional services, even in the absence of assertive community treatment. A large Delphi Opinion Survey of interventions for SMI and substance misuse was conducted in the UK recently (Jeffrey and Ley, 1999). Respondents were professionals working primarily with people suffering a dual diagnosis. Consensus emerged that 'training and comprehensive history taking were the best ways of identifying this client group . . . and were central to assessment and treatment'. These findings reflect other efforts to elicit precisely what professionals want and how they might obtain it (Holland, 1999).

This final section describes a single case study and identifies an assortment of assessment and treatment strategies found useful by many professionals working in this field (Holland *et al.*, 1999; Kavanagh *et al.*, 1998).

Case Illustration – Christine Brown

Christine is a 32 year-old woman who works on occasions for her mother in a cleaning agency. She lives with her parents following several unsuccessful attempts to live independently and a recent four month prison sentence. She has one brother aged 29, who lives nearby and whom she visits each day. Both Christine and her brother Theo take street drugs several times a week, usually amphetamine and occasionally cannabis or heroin. Much of their goal-orientated behaviour and social exchanges centre on obtaining and using street drugs.

Christine has suffered three major episodes of paranoid schizophrenia each requiring detention and treatment under the Mental Health Act. She was prescribed neuroleptic medication when first diagnosed and adherence over the six years since onset has been intermittent.

The misuse of street drugs precedes her diagnosis by ten years. Her brother and parents have no psychiatric history. No pre-morbid signs of schizophrenia were reported. Christine was neither poor or achieving at school, she did however mix well, have plenty of friends and was well liked. Her circle of school and early adult friendships diminished rapidly following the development of schizophrenia symptoms. Frequent criminal behaviour, familial conflict and drug seeking behaviour eroded Christine's main sources of support, her parents.

She is living at home and currently experiences significant levels of family stress due to drug misuse and bizarre behaviour associated with her psychotic symptoms. She has been listed for housing with council, private and charitable agencies but none are keen to provide accommodation due in the main to a criminal record. Engagement with her community psychiatric nurse has taken place, however, matters concerning income, frequent drug misuse and symptomatology obstruct attempts to meet her needs despite collaborative treatment planning having taken place.

Assessments

Following Christine's referral from her psychiatrist to the local Community Mental Health Team an initial meeting was arranged. A brief meeting with Christine alluded to a variety of needs described above, however, physical agitation, some suspicions about the CPN's role and poor attention meant little information could be obtained. Several appointments at home were arranged, of which only approximately one quarter were attended by Christine. During the course of six months, baseline assessments were conducted in modified form appropriate to Christine's level of attention, that is, over several sessions, in a variety of settings and during numerous activities:

- Background information – Social, familial and psychiatric history. Present medication and perceived problem.
- Psychotic symptom assessment – Using a validated measure (Kraweicka *et al.*, 1977) this assessment took three sessions. Perceived as intrusive by Christine much of the questioning required careful delivery at opportune moments. Evidence of constant auditory hallucinations, sense of persecution from all her neighbours and formal thought disorder (thoughts being withdrawn) highlighted the need for emphasis to be placed upon positive symptoms.
- Substance misuse assessment – This incorporated assessment of dangers (injecting substances, sites, clean works, reliable dealer), and assessment of amount, types and frequency of drug misuse, including sample analysis. Perceived effects, possible benefits and/or drawbacks of drug misuse.
- Assessment of motivation levels (stage of treatment) and effects of substance misuse (problem/diagnosis) were conducted using purpose designed clinical rating scales (Mueser *et al.*, 1995).
- Peripheral information gathering – The recording of other information such as parents opinions, other agencies views, observations of behaviour at sessions, medication adherence and aspects relating to risk to self or others took place.

Case Comments

Substance misuse was regarded as Christine's major problem by her parents whereas Christine regarded paranoid ideas and feelings as the main area of concern. Assessment demonstrated that both opinions were valid, the overlap of symptoms and the tangled causal effects of illness and substance misuse discouraged emphasis on one or the other.

Table 14.2 Identified needs and intervention with Christine and family

NEEDS IDENTIFIED	INTERVENTION
Reduction of family stress	Cognitive – behavioural family intervention (i.e. education regarding substance misuse and schizophrenia). Ameliorating stress using stress management strategies. Reducing the causes of stress and tension using problem solving and goal setting.Delivered on a weekly basis, issues relating to Christine's behaviour and her parent's response were addressed. Mutually designed plans to reduce family tension improved their intra-family communication. Christine's parents attributed bizarre behaviour, from psychotic illness more accurately. This reduced their expression of blame towards Christine. Christine felt she was viewed as less 'problematic' and her parent's felt 'supported'.
To inject safely, avoid infections and maintain personal safety when pursuing substances.	Risk assessment of drug misuse. See substance misuse assessment above. Provision of literature from credible sources (e.g. Lifeline) and opportunity to discuss salient issues around drugs. Objective information concerning substances physiological and psychological effects, both adverse and positive. Establishing safe injecting procedure was addressed at a local needle exchange where lessons, needles, syringes and sharps bin were available. The absence of site infection and missed veins since demonstrated good effectiveness. Personal safety was discussed, and obtaining substances at night or in isolation discouraged. Self-administration in a secure place (e.g. at home) was encouraged.
To find suitable independent accommodation.	Advocating on behalf of Christine for mainstream housing was prioritised. A plan of intensive home support, available 24-hours/day and addressing practical needs of daily living skills was devised. Securing local housing and incorporating family support without over involvement ensured neighbourhood and parental links would not be severed.
To budget carefully, and avoid pursuit of drug purchasing money by criminal means.	Practical measures such as income and expenditure monitoring. Drug misuse cost analysis and measures to 'pace' drugs until next pay day, such as dividing doses into days and recording on calendar clearly in view. Discussion regarding previous sentence in prison and disadvantages of criminal behaviour. Pursuit of alternative forms of income generation such as work and maximising benefits.
Develop social network away from substance misuse friends and activities.	Motivational interviewing largely reflecting self-motivational statements such as 'I've found myself short of money since I bought my gear', 'my mum always irritates me more after I've just used'. Introducing alternative pastimes and sampling constructive social and recreational activities. Taking an interest in and providing practical assistance restarting the guitar and collecting CDs.

Table 14.2 *Continued*

NEEDS IDENTIFIED	INTERVENTION
Management of paranoid beliefs and auditory hallucinations to reduce their disruptive effect on Christine's life.	Establishing agreement on the nature, extent, and effect of symptoms. Paranoid ideas required reality testing and modification using a variety of cognitive behavioural approaches in tandem. Accompanying on trips to shops and other activities whilst exploring Christine's evidence of persecution.
	Education concerning physiological arousal in schizophrenia and difficulties in processing information. Delivered in a formal and informal manner using diagrams, flow charts and basic text. Application of distraction techniques to reduce effects of voices. That is, if at home, take out newspaper and discuss current issues with parents. Wearing headphones helped when out and appeared discreet and tolerable.
	Support and encouragement to receive depot neuroleptic injection. Provision of neuroleptic information and management of side effects (dystonia mainly) helped adherence. Monthly side-effect assessment using LUNSERS (Day *et al.*, 1995) provided added consistency to the monitoring process.
To reduce feelings of anxiety.	Applied relaxation.
	Education around substance misuse expectancies (e.g. Christine regarded cannabis as an anxiolytic despite its anticholinergic and longer-term paranoid effect). Since her anxiety correlated with paranoid feelings and ideation cannabis served to reinforce and trigger anxiety.

The role of the CPN here was to facilitate goals consistent with both Christine's and her parent's needs. Carrying this out in a collaborative manner required patience through numerous setbacks, especially regarding substance misuse relapse and behaviour.

As Christine expressed no motivation to stop or reduce substance misuse (pre-contemplative) strategies were harm reduction in nature. The goal of establishing a working relationship can be defined by the amount of contact between client and clinician. Since Christine's goals did not include substance misuse reduction, initially interventions were orientated upon practical assistance (housing/benefits), dealing with crises and psychiatric symptoms. Carried out in an assertive (patient, flexible, creative and tenacious) manner, engagement builds a foundation of trust and familiarity necessary for persuasion or motivational work.

While enjoying renewed interests Christine was sensitively drawn into looking at the discrepancies existing between her substance misuse and her desire to pursue her other interests. Conducive with social orientated work is psychological preparation for changes in lifestyle that Christine might undertake should substance misuse reduction goals be agreed upon. Pursuing interventions indirectly associated with substance misuse served as the foundation for future substance related work.

Motivational focused work in pre-contemplation will not, by definition, be an agreed approach. However, motivational strategies such as the listing of advantages/disadvantages of substance misuse and abstinence can be applied in both pre-contemplation and contemplation, provided they are carried out in an empathic, non-confrontational manner. Using open-ended questioning and the eliciting of self-motivational statements provide opportunities to make reinforcing and encouraging comments and gives the client opportunity to hear themselves saying encouraging things. Supporting a client's self-confidence and belief in their ability to make even minor changes successfully promotes a sense of self efficacy prerequisite for longer term stability. The use of rating scales for levels of use (clinical drug use scale) and level of treatment (substance abuse treatment scale) (Mueser *et al.*, 1995) can provide structure and guidance and were particularly useful because of Christine's sustained pre-contemplative period.

Conclusions

It appears likely that dual diagnosis as a term to describe mental illness and substance misuse will become less favoured by clinicians in the future. The term is already attracting stigma and negativity from professionals working in mental health or substance misuse services.

However, it is probable that substance misuse, or detection of misuse, among the seriously mentally ill will increase. Identifying specific interventions with a sound success rate will become increasingly necessary and clinicians in both substance misuse and psychiatric fields will need to develop their repertoire of skills accordingly. Planners and purchasers should note the growing research in dual diagnosis concerned with designing and re-configuring services to best suit effective intervention.

It is anticipated that cognitive-behavioural approaches, including motivational interviewing (Holland *et al.*, 1999; Kavanagh *et al.*, 1998; Graham, 1998), will continue to demonstrate reasonable levels of success with this client group since they can be, and frequently are, applied by mental health workers from a variety of backgrounds or disciplines in a range of care settings.

The effects of problem overload and complexity of needs in the dually diagnosed on professionals should not be underestimated. Indeed the powerful effect generated by some client's condition is responsible for strong feelings of despair and frustration among staff. A feeling of pessimism and an attitude influenced by the perception of poor prognosis in the dually diagnosed will inevitably drain the professional's sense of optimism. This single ingredient, optimism, is key to the successful implementation of care which is likely to endure many years.

The account of Christine illustrates an approach which incorporates core skills from substance misuse and psychiatric services. It does not provide an exhaustive list of interventions or give detail to their implementation.

Essentially, though the case study outlines new boundaries which are legitimate to reach in our effort to devise safe, responsible and realistic care for clients with a dual diagnosis.

Further Reading

Heather, N., Wodak, A., Nadelmann, E. and O'Hare, P. (eds) (1993) *Psychoactive Drugs and Harm Reduction: From Faith to Science*, London, Whurr.

Keene, J. (1997) *Drug Misuse: Prevention, harm minimization and treatment*, London, Chapman & Hall.

Miller, W.R. and Rollnick, S. (1991) *Motivational Interviewing: Preparing People to Change Addictive Behaviors*, New York, Guildford Press.

Rorstad, P. and Checinski, K. (1996) *Dual Diagnosis: Facing the Challenge*, Kenley, Wynne Howard.

Seivewright, N. (2000) *Community treatment of drug misuse: more than methadone*, Cambridge, Cambridge University Press.

Tyler, A. (1988) *Street Drugs: The Facts Explained, the Myths Exploded*, London, Coronet.

References

American Psychiatric Association (1994) *DSM- I*, 4th edn, Washington, DC, APA.

Carey, K.B. (1996) 'Substance Use Reduction in the Context of Outpatient Psychiatric Treatment: A Collaborative, Motivational, Harm Reduction Approach', *Community Mental Health Journal*, 32(6), 291–306.

Day, J., Wood, G., Dewey, G. and Bentall, R. (1995) 'A Self Rating Scale for Measuring Neuroleptic Side-Effects. Validation in a Group of Schizophrenic Patients', *British Journal of Psychiatry*, 166, 650–53.

Department of Health (1994) *Report of the Inquiry into the Care and Treatment of Christopher Clunis*, London, HMSO.

DiClemente, C.C. and Prochaska, J.O. (1985) 'Processes and Stages of Change: coping and competence in smoking behaviour change', in S. Shiffman and T.A. Wills (eds), *Coping and Substance Abuse*, New York, Academic Press.

Drake, R.E., Bartels, S.J., Teague, G.B., Noordsy, D.L. and Clark, R.E. (1993) 'Treatment of Substance Abuse in Severe Mental Illness Patients', *Journal of Nervous and Mental Disease*, 181, 606–11.

Drake, R.E., Mueser, K.T., Clark, R.E. and Wallach, M.A. (1996) 'The Course, Treatment and Outcome of Substance Disorder in Persons with Severe Mental Illness', *American Journal of Orthopsychiatry*, 66(1), 42–51.

Drake, R.E. and Osher, F.C. (1997) 'Treating Substance abuse in patients with severe mental illness', in S.W. Hengeller and A.B. Santos (eds), *Innovative approaches for difficult to treat populations*, Washington, DC, American Psychiatric Press.

Duke, P.J., Pantelis, C. and Barnes, T.R.E. (1994) 'South Westminster Schizophrenia Survey; Alcohol Use and Its Relationship to Symptoms, Tardive Dyskinesia and Illness Onset', *British Journal of Psychiatry*, 164, 630–36.

Gibbins, J. (1998) 'Towards Integrated Care for Patients With Dual Diagnosis. The Dorset Healthcare NHS Trust Experience', *The Mental Health Review*, December, pp. 20–24.

Gournay, K. and Sandford, T. (1996) 'Double Bind,' *Nursing Times*, 92(28), 28–9.

Graham, H. (1998) 'The role of Dysfunctional Beliefs in Individuals who Experience Psychosis and Use Substances: Implications for Cognitive Therapy and Medication Adherence', *Behavioural and Cognitive Psychotherapy*, 26, 193–208.

Graham, H. and Maslin, J. (1998) 'Introduction to a New Service: COMPASS Programme', *Dual Diagnosis Network (MICAA) News*, 2 (Summer), p. 2.

Holland, M.A. (1998) 'Substance use and mental health problems: meeting the challenge', *British Journal of Nursing*, 7(15), 896–900.

Holland, M.A. (1999) How Substance use affects people with mental illness, *Nursing Times*, 95(24), 46–8.

Holland, M., Baguley, I. and Davres, T. (1999) 'Hallucinations and Delusions 2: A Dual Diagnosis Case Study', *British Journal of Nursing*, 8(16), 1095–102.

Jeffrey, A. and Ley, A. (1999) *Delphi Opinion on Intervention for Severe Mental Illness and Substance Misuse. Participants Report*, Torquay, South Devonshire Healthcare Trust.

Kavanagh, D., Young, R., Boyce, L., Clair, A., Sitharthan, T., Clark, D. and Thompson, K. (1998) 'Substance Treatment in Psychosis (STOP): A new intervention for dual diagnosis', *Journal of Mental Health*, 7(2), 135–43.

Kraweicka, M., Golberg, D. and Vaughan, M. (1977) 'A Standardised Psychiatric Assessment Scale for Rating Chronic Schizophrenic Patients', *Acta Psychiatrica Scandinavica*, 55, 299–308.

Lancashire, S., Haddock, G., Butterworth, T., Tarrier, N. and Baguley, I. (1997) 'Training Mental health Professionals to use Psychosocial Interventions with People who have Severe Mental Health Problems', *Clinician*, 14(6), 32–9.

Lehman, A., Myers, C., Dickson, L. and Johnson, J. (1994) 'Defining sub-groups of dual diagnosis patients for service planning', *Hospital and Community Psychiatry*, 45, 556–61.

Ley, A., Jeffrey, D.P., McLaren, S. and Siegfried, N. (1999) 'Treatment programmes for people with both severe mental illness and substance misuse' in *The Cochrane Library*, Issue 2, Oxford, Update Software.

Menezes, P.R., Johnson, S., Thornicroft, G., Marshall, J., Prosser, D., Bebbington, P. and Kuipers, E. (1996) 'Drug and Alcohol Problems among Individuals with Severe Mental Illnesses in South London', *British Journal of Psychiatry*, 168, 612–19.

Mitchell, G., Robertson, S. and Weber, G. (1992) 'A Care Management Project for young adults with dual diagnoses of severe mental illness and substance abuse. A service for people with dual diagnoses', *Journal of Mental Health*, 1, 363–6.

Mueser, K., Drake, R., Clark, R., McHugo, G., Mercer-McFadden, C. and Ackerson, T. (1995) *Toolkit for Evaluating Substance Abuse in Persons with Severe Mental Illness*, Concord, NH, Human Services Research Institute.

Mueser, K., Drake, R. and Noordsy, D. (1998a) 'Intergrated Mental Health and Substance Abuse Treatment for Severe Psychiatric Disorders', *Journal of Practical Psychiatry and Behavioural Health*, May, pp. 129–39.

Mueser, K., Drake, R. and Wallach, M. (1998b) 'Dual Diagnosis: A review of aetiological theories', *Addictive Behaviours*, 23(6), 717–34.

Osher, F.C., Kofoed, L.L. (1989) 'Treatment of patients with psychiatric and psychoactive substance abuse disorders', *Hospital and Community Psychiatry*, 40, 1025–30.

Regier, D., Farmer, N. and Rae, D. (1990) 'Co-morbidity of mental disorders with alcohol and other drugs of abuse: results from the epidemiological catchment area. (ECA)', *Journal of American Medical Association*, 264, 2511–18.

Rollnick, S. (1995) 'What is Motivational Interviewing?', *Behavioural and Cognitive Psychotherapy*, 23, 325–34.

Rorstad, P. and Checinski, K. (1996) *Dual Diagnosis: Facing the Challenge*, Kenley, Wynne Howard.

Smith, J. and Hucker, S. (1993) 'Dual Diagnosis Patients; Substance Abuse by the Severely Mentally Ill', *British Journal of Hospital Medicine*, 50(11), 650–54.

Thomas, M., Brazier, C. and Ferguson, G. (1999) 'The CASA Multiple Needs Service: Perspectives on Multiple Needs', *National Dual Diagnosis (MICAA) Network News*, 4, (Winter 1999), 4–13.

World Health Organization (1992) *The ICD-IO Clarification of Mental and Behavioural Disorders: Clinical Depression and Diagnostic Guidelines*, Geneva, WHO.

Zubin, J., and Spring, B. (1977) 'Vulnerability: a new view of schizophrenia', *Journal of Abnormal Psychology*, 86, 103–26.

CHAPTER 15

Risk and Serious Mental Health Problems

GED McCANN AND MICK McKEOWN

Introduction

The needs of individuals with serious mental health problems are complex and usually of long duration, often affecting all aspects of their lives, and the lives of those relatives and friends who are involved. This complexity may be further heightened where there is risk involved, either to the individual or to others or even where offending behaviour is present. The additional problems that are presented because of risk factors, the involvement of statutory services and powers, and perhaps the criminal justice system, are further exacerbated by the attention of the media. Their intense interest often serves to inflame and complicate problems, rather than resolve them, and together add to the burden experienced by the individual, their carers and professional staff.

This chapter aims to discuss the issues involved for individuals with a serious mental health problem which presents a risk to the safety of others, particularly those with a forensic history. The needs of relatives will be highlighted and discussions will provide some guidance as to how to minimise levels of risk using psychosocial interventions, and how, by involving families the stresses associated with caring for individuals with complex needs can be reduced. To illustrate these discussions examples from clinical practice will be described which will enable practitioners to begin to implement some of these approaches.

Risk and Dangerousness

There is an enduring representation of the mentally ill among the general public and sustained by a mass media hungry for sensationalist storylines. This stereotype equates mental illness with violent or murderous behaviour. These stigmatising images are specifically associated with schizophrenia, though media versions often disregard the complexities of diagnosis in particular stories. Research into the actual incidence of homicide, for instance, has shown that the actual rate of murders committed by mentally disordered offenders has not increased in the time since such records have been kept, and may even

205

have decreased in recent years (Taylor and Gunn, 1999). These statistics are an important refutation of the psychosis-violence stereotype because they relate to a period of time, which has seen a massive retraction in inpatient beds, and the policy of care in the community.

The power of the media to misrepresent the actual risks posed by the over-whelming majority of people with serious mental health problems shows inter esting differences when compared to other examples of information distortion. The Glasgow Media Group (Philo *et al.*, 1994) found that almost universally the public will disregard a media story if its content is at odds with the authen-ticity of their own personal experiences. However, the exception to this is that even people who have immediate and uneventful experience of mental illness, perhaps within their family or close social network, continue to be fearful of violence from the mentally ill.

Perhaps influenced by such attitudes, the dominant form of risk presenting in mental health services is often assumed to be the risk of aggression or violence and the degree to which individual service users are perceived as dangerous. Yet, though these concerns merit serious and considered attention from policy makers and practitioners alike, the issue of dangerousness needs to be placed in perspective in the domain of mainstream psychiatric services. In this context, the notion of risk in relation to mental health is best conceived of in terms of a diverse spectrum of hazards, only one of which is the risk of violence enacted by service users. Indeed, the vulnerability of service users is more typically what is at stake in a more sophisticated appraisal of risk (Ryan, 1998; Stanley *et al.*, 1999).

People with serious mental health problems are proportionally more likely to be the victims rather than the perpetrators of violence and are also much more vulnerable to other threats to their safety and well-being, many of which arise specifically in clinical environments. There is a profoundly elevated risk of suicide in this client group, with the likelihood of other forms of self-injury also increased. Self-neglect is another important category of risk, which, though acknowledged as significant by most observers of mental health services, has received scant coverage in the research literature (Morgan, 1998). Inequalities and inefficiencies in service provision are also notable. Despite being relatively frequent attenders at GP surgeries, standardised mortality rates for the seriously mentally ill are roughly twice those for the general popula-tion, with treatable physical disorders making a significant contribution to these figures (Allebeck, 1989; Burns and Kendrick, 1997).

Once admitted to services in the hospital or community a new range of hazards emerges to which the status of service user confers access to special dimensions of vulnerability. There are the possibilities of assault by other dis-turbed patients within the confines of a ward, or in certain circumstances from abusive members of staff. A requirement to consent or submit to psychotropic medication regimens carries the risk of untoward, and possibly serious, side effects (Chapter 6). Unfortunately, recognition as a user of psychiatric services can elicit hostile or discriminatory responses from communities or neighbourhoods, exacerbating people's health and social problems.

Families

The families of individuals with a mental illness also have many problems to contend with. Not only do they have the problem of coping with a relative with mental illness, but they often have the added burdens associated with their compulsory detention or even, a history of behaviour associated with risk or offending. 'Aftermath', a charitable organisation set up to support the families of serious offenders, also recognises the needs of relatives:

> The relatives of murderers and rapists are often deemed guilty by association, suffering ostracism, abuse and sometimes physical violence . . . they are in their own prison cells. . . . (Groocock, 1989)

They recognise that often the close family of an offender is also deeply affected but find themselves without support, perhaps receiving a hostile reaction from society. They are left to cope with police, the courts and judicial system, media publicity and reactions from the local neighbourhood. For the families of the mentally ill, whether or not there is a history of risk or offending, societal views regarding their culpability are similarly confused and mixed.

Families initial experiences of the psychiatric system, or indeed, the criminal justice system, can have damaging and enduring effects, at a time when their need for personal support and guidance is at its height. More worrying is the fact that many relatives report with disturbing frequency that their own informal assessments of the risk presented by their relative, fall on the deaf ears of disinterested, or ineffective professionals (McKeown and McCann, 2000). For many relatives, the stigma of mental illness is devastating which has repercussions throughout all family members, particularly children (Hughes and Hughes, 2000). Media interest and scrutiny by neighbours and friends can lead to a withdrawal from social contacts and even ostracism from local communities. This barrier to support and guidance by non-professionals is matched only by the lack of information and involvement in the care of their relative by the psychiatric system.

> . . . we very soon came to realise how little we knew about the aetiology or pathology of James's illness, or the long term treatment methods used . . . the worst of it was that nobody within the hospital seemed at all anxious to enlighten us on these matters. (Hughes and Hughes, 2000)

A study by McCann (1993) within a high security hospital, noted that relatives had many worries and concerns that were not being addressed.

They were ignorant of ward routines, hospital procedures and about mental illness and treatment. They had anxieties regarding medication and the seclusion of patients, often fuelled by adverse publicity about the hospital. Relatives continue to experience stress if not provided with support from professionals, and much of this stress results in mal-adaptive coping strategies, such as social withdrawal, hostility toward their relative or others, or even stress related behavioural problems.

Psychosis and Offending Behaviour

Despite the fact that psychiatric service users are more likely to be victimised than perpetrate violent crime, a significant minority does pose a risk of such behaviour and may, eventually, become involved with forensic services. It is for this group that issues arise in services relating to the practicalities of effective risk management, or ethical dilemmas around the degree to which services balance consideration of such risks with concern for the civil liberties of service users. Corollary attention has to be afforded to staff training needs and the relevant expertise to engage with risk management, and where to turn if the specific issue or clinical case lies outwith the experience or competencies of the team. Effective mechanisms for referring and treating people who pose varying degrees of risk in an environment most suited to their particular needs at the appropriate level of security are required. Conjecture would allow us to contemplate a proportion of this group whom, if their potential for violence, or certain precursor behaviours or risk factors could be detected early on, might have their needs managed successfully in mainstream contexts avoiding a forensic trajectory altogether. This possibility is often raised retrospectively by clients or families who commonly relate tales of key practitioners or services failing to act upon pleas for early intervention or support when they identify escalating risk.

The research into mental disorder and dangerousness is unequivocal and contested, perhaps not surprisingly given such complex subject matter. The evidence base is further complicated by variability in the use of crime statistics, with many researchers failing to adequately distinguish between different categories of offending or violence. Broadly speaking, the extent to which mental illness has a causative link to violence or wider criminality is disputed by criminological and psychiatric researchers. The criminological perspective plays down the contribution of mental disorder in this context, emphasising instead the significant influence of various social factors as the best predictors of criminality. Psychiatrists, however, working with smaller more focused samples, have explored the relationship between certain key dimensions of the experience of mental disorder, especially psychosis, and violence. In a review of this literature Wessely (1997) accepts that factors beyond psychiatric remediation are most robustly associated with criminal behaviour and that mental disorder alone is a poor predictor in comparison. However, within these broad demographics men diagnosed with schizophrenia compared with those for any other condition have double the conviction rates for violent crime. There is also some evidence that conviction rates are an underestimate of the actual amount of violence exhibited.

The raised incidence of violence noted in men with schizophrenia has led various researchers to study the role of specific psychotic symptoms in the supposed genesis of violent behaviour. These investigations have identified key symptoms or groupings of symptoms proportionally more likely to be found among violent offenders with schizophrenia compared to non-violent groups. Such symptoms include delusions (Hafner and Boker, 1973), persecutory delusions, especially those eliciting angry reactions (Cheung *et al.*, 1977), organised delusions (Nestor *et al.*, 1995; Taylor, 1993), thought disorder (Gardner *et al.*, 1996) and command hallucinations (Bartels *et al.*, 1991).

Command hallucinations have been an important focus for this research, with Bartels and colleagues (1991) linking them to expressed hostility. The vocabulary of such voices has been remarked upon as qualitatively different from other auditory hallucinations with pertinent themes disclosed, linking commands to aggression, dependency, and self-punishment (Rogers *et al.*, 1990). Honig (1991) suggests that the typical resistive coping strategy of ignoring voices can decline in efficacy over time when faced with prolonged or repetitive exposure to such commands. Juninger (1991) argues that other factors may need to be taken into account if we are to identify which people may act upon command hallucinations. An apparently increased risk of this is associated with circumstances where the voice is identified as a known person, or where delusional ideas have developed associated with the voices.

Link and Steuve (1994) developed such themes in their work that stresses the importance of subjective interaction with psychotic symptoms, especially the ways in which individuals attempt to make sense of their experiences. In short, it seems to be the interpretation and responses to key symptoms, which are crucial in mediating the risk of violence. This line of inquiry has led to the identification and description of a complex of risk factors referred to as threat/control override symptoms. The notion of threat/control override (TCO) is employed as a conceptual framework for linking symptoms to violence where personal factors with the potential to inhibit or resist violent expression are overridden in the presence of certain psychotic phenomena. These include psychotic experiences, which lead to ideas of vengeance, a sense of being threatened, and a lack of self-control. Studies by Swanson and colleagues (1996, 1997) support this reasoning and found a twofold increase in violence if the research subjects described various TCO symptoms.

Service Interventions

The range of services that care for forensic clients with serious mental illness have characteristics, which set them apart from general mental health, provision. First, they tend to be philosophically isolated because of the emphasis placed as much on empowering individuals, as on their control and limitation in terms of the risks that they present. Second, they tend to be physically isolated, either because they provide a regional rather than a local service, or because access to them is restricted. Third, they are exposed to the scrutiny and glare of a number of interested parties, either within the criminal justice system, the medico-legal system, or the public media.

There are few services that manage these complex, competing agenda's unscathed, and fewer still clients or their carers who remain unmoved, or unaffected. Each has their own effect on the services provided, and ultimately the effectiveness of the care delivered. The introduction of a model of clinical practice is needed, which is able to bridge these complexities, is able to meet the needs of clients and carers, and is able to fit comfortably within nursing, psychological, social and medical models of care delivery. Two broad themes inherent within the psychosocial interventions approach are particularly important in enabling this to happen.

The first, is the stress – vulnerability model of schizophrenia (Zubin and Spring, 1977; Zubin et al., 1983) which provides a sound basis for conceptualising the experiences of clients and their carers, as well as providing a framework for multidisciplinary interventions (Chapter 1). When placed within the context of case management the model enables the organisation of care to be effective and monitored closely, both of which being prerequisites for managing risk, and of fundamental importance within forensic settings.

The other important theme is the problem focused approach to the identification, prioritising, and achievement of client goals and needs. Very specific assessments which are reliable and valid are important elements of PSIs, as are the cognitive-behavioural interventions designed to engage, collaborate and empower clients and their carers to manage their own problems.

This problem focused approach within the simple framework provided by the stress-vulnerability model, therefore draws together the individual and their significant others, recognises symptoms within the context of the environment, and forges a clearer relationship between professionals and clients. These significant factors alone provide a sound rationale for the introduction of PSIs in the management of forensic clients. But there are more important reasons.

A further rationale for the development of these approaches is in the area of psychological management of symptoms. Recent research has indicated the benefits of cognitive behavioural therapy in the reduction or amelioration of the positive symptoms of schizophrenia (Sellwood et al., 1994). This work highlights: the importance of patient education regarding their illness; self-monitoring of symptoms; assessment of antecedents and behaviours associated with symptoms; the development of specific, behavioural coping strategies; the use of focusing techniques with auditory hallucinations; and the use of belief modification strategies with delusions (Chapter 8).

These approaches emphasise the need for patients and their families, to gain more control over their experiences, and to consider the effects of the environment, their thoughts, feelings and behaviours, in limiting the negative impact of symptoms. Being able to place their experiences within the context of internal and external events, and being able to exercise some control over them, is of particular relevance for a forensic client group. Often it is a lack of insight, which determines the level of risk associated with problem behaviours.

Insight and Psychoeducation

A patient's failure to acknowledge their illness and need for treatment is often termed 'lack of insight' (McEvoy *et al.*, 1989). In a study completed by the World Health Organization (1973) a 'lack of insight' was the most prevalent feature of a diagnosis of schizophrenia (97 per cent). As a concept it is used in almost every context and appears to have a direct bearing on treatment and medication compliance, dangerousness, suicide and prognosis (Birchwood *et al.*, 1994). For individuals who present a risk to others the level of insight is often the 'key' consideration in terms of risk assessment and management. The less insight individuals display, the more likely they are to remain within the forensic system or to have restrictions imposed on their liberty. Treatment interventions which aim to reduce levels of risk consequently focus on improving insight, as a lack of it is seen as a likely indicator of poor outcome, or of re-offending.

The concept however, although used widely by nurses and other professionals alike, has no commonly held definition, and the research determining its significance is wholly inadequate (Greenfield *et al.*, 1989). For example, 'insight', could be equated with sharing the clinicians views rather than holding possible alternative viewpoints. Depending upon which model of mental health you are in a position to adopt might determine the degree of insight afforded to the patient. Those patients that can express the accepted and more commonly held views about their illness might be assessed more favourably than a patient who holds a more personal explanation of their experiences.

Several studies have attempted to assess and define the term 'insight' (McEvoy *et al.*, 1989; Greenfield *et al.*, 1989). They noted that although a lack of self-awareness was assumed, few systematic evaluations of the views of psychotic patients are undertaken. This has led to the lack of a clear definition of what insight is, and hence its variety of meanings.

Characteristics relevant to a concept of insight fall into five main categories, which are:

- the patients views of their symptoms;
- whether they were experiencing an illness or not;
- possible causes of their experience;

- their views about a recurrence of symptoms;
- and whether any treatments they had received had been beneficial.

In summary, the assessment of insight is complex and is in fact influenced greatly by the relationship between patient and clinician. Educating patients about their illness, and an exploration of the concepts surrounding insight should underpin and inform effective clinical practice.

Greenberg *et al.* (1988) outlines the benefits of their psychoeducation programme for patients:

> The goals of the process are to impart information and to enhance understanding of the illness, needed treatment resources, and supportive services . . . and to create a more productive alliance between patients, families and mental health professionals. (p. 280)

The overall aims therefore go beyond raising insight but attempt to impact on patient functioning and their perceptions of services.

One programme which has been implemented and evaluated within a forensic setting is a group programme within Ashworth High Security Hospital in Merseyside. Two psychoeducation programmes were provided to relatives and patients, over a period of approximately six months. The patients programme was provided seperately from relatives, and delivered within a central rehabilitation unit away from the ward areas.

The programme was conducted over a twelve-week period, with two hourly sessions, provided to a group of up to ten patients. The aim of the programme was to raise knowledge and understanding about schizophrenia, develop more effective coping strategies, and focus on individual offence specific behaviours which increased the level of risk of re-offending. The programme therefore had three stages:

- an initial trust building educational stage;
- a more focused coping strategy enhancement stage;
- and a more individualised stage which focused on specific behaviours.

The programme was evaluated in terms of impact on levels of social functioning, patient symptoms, and a self report qualitative evaluation of the whole programme.

For patients within a forensic setting the most important initial aspect of a programme is to encourage patients to discuss their experiences openly. Several considerations mitigate against this, most notably, the fact that discussing symptoms openly may lead to a lengthening of the patients detention within secure care. The other notable fact is that many patients have committed very serious offences. Being able to discuss these events, in the company of other patients, some of whom they may not know, is very stressful. Therefore, it was felt that initial sessions should be devoted to developing trust between group members, and discussing broad subject matter, which did not focus on individuals. Initial sessions dealt with the subject of schizophrenia as a concept, discussing the different perspectives of its management, and outlining the medical model of symptoms and treatment. An emphasis was placed on the fact that many interpretations of schizophrenia exist, and that although nobody actually knows what causes it, there are certain facts that are known about its management. In this way patients who held a view about schizophrenia which was inconsistent with medical opinion were not challenged, but rather their view accepted as one alternative explanation. Emphasis was placed on the aims of the programme being about sharing experiences in an effort to cope more effectively, rather than about teaching patients about schizophrenia.

The programme used group discussions within either a large or small group context; role play exercises; brainstorming sessions to generate themes; written, audio and video information; and weekly assignments to be completed on the group participants respective wards. The programme content included:

Psychoeducation
- What is schizophrenia?
- Media images and misconceptions about schizophrenia
- Causes of schizophrenia
- Symptoms of schizophrenia
- Treatments for schizophrenia
- Medication

Stress and schizophrenia
- The stress-vulnerability model of schizophrenia
- What is stress, what stressors are there within a forensic setting?
- What stressors occur as a result of events outside of a forensic setting?
- What influences stress
- Coping with stress
- Communicating more effectively
- Institutional life and its problems

Coping with schizophrenia
- Problem solving
- Coping with hallucinations
- Coping with delusions
- Coping with negative symptoms
- Recognising early warning signs of relapse
- Adapting to long-term effects of symptoms

In the final sessions of the educational programme the group participants were encouraged to focus on their own symptoms and experiences, and how they currently cope with them. This involved recalling events before the offending behaviour and constructing a scenario of how those events could be prevented in the future. This also involved the recognition of early warning signs of an impending relapse (Chapter 10), or identifying skills which the individual needs to develop to prevent stress from becoming unmanageable, and reducing the risk of re-offending.

The programme has highlighted the importance of providing information about schizophrenia to patients, and to discuss their experiences with a view to enhancing their ability to cope. Historically, nurses are trained not to focus upon a patients symptoms, and are actively encouraged to divert patients attention on to other subjects in an effort to reduce their anxiety. This programme has encouraged patients to talk in depth about their psychotic experiences. It has allowed them to put their experiences into perspective by raising their knowledge, and understanding the experiences of others. In effect, it has enabled them to assert more control over their own experiences, rather than rely solely on treatment by health professionals. The rationale for this work is supported by other research which has looked at the psychological management of schizophrenia (Sellwood *et al.*, 1994). Nurses perhaps could be focusing more on these approaches, rather than on the current, established nursing interventions.

Case Example

Bill was diagnosed with schizophrenia over twenty years previously and had spent fifteen years of this time within a secure hospital. His family consisted of three brothers, all of whom were married with families of their own. Bill had contact with one of his brothers, and his family, however two brothers and their families did not want anything to do with Bill, and did not want him to be transferred out of the hospital setting.

Bill had killed his mother while experiencing psychotic symptoms and had since been tormented by derogatory auditory hallucinations, many of which were voices he interpreted as his brothers. These voices led Bill to become verbally and physically abusive, and continue to present a serious risk to others.

Individual sessions with Bill had focused upon assessing these auditory hallucinations in much more depth using structured assessment tools and simple diaries which Bill used to record the frequency of his voices, the circumstances surrounding them, and his thoughts and feelings at the time. This assessment work with Bill fostered a close collaborative relationship, as Bill began to discuss his experiences in more detail, together with his own thoughts and beliefs. This work highlighted the fact that Bill's voices were associated with his own guilt and grief regarding his mother, and his beliefs concerning his brothers as he believed he had ruined their lives, and they despised him for it. Further sessions then focused on these thoughts and beliefs concerning his brothers. Contact was made with Bill's brothers to see if they would become involved in his care, and arrangements were also made for Bill to receive grief counselling. In time one of Bills brothers made contact and became a regular visitor, as well as becoming involved in structured psychoeducation sessions. As a result of a focus on Bill's beliefs, emotional support, and the involvement of his brother, Bill's voices began to reduce and he became less distressed by them. Over time he began to interpret them in relation to his own feelings and thoughts, and the level of risk associated with these experiences diminished substantially.

Following this care and treatment which had included psychoeducation, cognitive – behavioural assessment, coping strategy enhancement, and atypical neuroleptics, Bill was now able to be transferred out of the hospital into a more local psychiatric unit. In all of the fifteen years little contact had been established however between Bill's brothers and professional staff, which had resulted in a negative response for involvement in Bill's planned transfer, apart from one of his brothers. In fact, correspondence had been received from the families of two brothers which stated that they would involve local MPs should their brother-in-law ever leave the hospital.

It was at this point that further family involvement was seen as a priority and initial arrangements were made to see the family members as a group, with the help of one of the brothers. The initial meeting was very emotional for each of the family members. It was clear that the family had not been given the chance to express their thoughts and feelings to professionals before. Stress and emotional upset which had resulted from the offence, the court case, the consequent admission to the secure hospital, the break up of family relationships, and the stigma, and lack of knowledge associated with serious mental illness within the family, were vented within the meeting. It was evident that some family members had coped over the years better than others, and some had continued to have flashbacks and other behavioural problems as a result of the offence for many years later. Family members had also coped with these emotions in a variety of ways. Some had coped by eliciting emotional support from other family members, some had used alcohol to reduce the effects of anxiety, others had become irritable or hostile with other family members, the psychiatric system and Bill. Others had not discussed their thoughts and feelings at all and had actually not informed their offspring of where their uncle was, and why he was there. This presented other difficulties as this subject had recently been discussed with the children and had resulted in further emotional upset.

This initial meeting was a chance to hear their stories and to provide any support the family members wished. Effort was focused on engaging with the families and in identifying any further support the hospital could offer. Initially, a further meeting was arranged to provide the family with information about Bill's proposed transfer arrangements, about the care and treatment he had received and would receive within the new unit, and to provide some basic information about the symptoms Bill experienced in the past and presently. All family members demonstrated a lack of knowledge about schizophrenia, and about care treatment. Each were concerned about risks to themselves and their children, and the repercussions from the local community. All were fearful about the prospect of reliving their own individual ordeals, and confronting painful memories from the past.

Despite the difficulties associated with this initial meeting a further meeting was arranged at which each family member again attended. More detail was provided about the circumstances relating to risk management in an attempt to alleviate some of the worries and concerns the family members presented. Having a brother who had maintained some contact with Bill became very influential in persuading the family about changes in Bill, and the reduction in potential problems for them as a family. Some psychoeducation was also provided at this meeting in terms of what symptoms Bill experienced, what they were, and how they could be managed. Bill's brother had also attended the psychoeducation programme for relatives held at the hospital, at which relapse prevention and the recognition of early warning signs was discussed. This also helped in moving the families towards considering that the level of risk presented by Bill could be managed.

Following one further meeting the family members agreed to the transfer of Bill, but did not want any further involvement from professional staff. They wanted to be kept informed of the whereabouts of Bill, but felt that they could not cope with meeting him, or having any closer contact in the near future. Several of the older children involved did wish to visit Bill, and were more open to the notion of developing a closer level of support with him. Bill's brother agreed that he would discuss this with Bill in the near future. Several months later Bill was successfully transferred out into a local psychiatric unit.

Reflection

This case example raises a number of significant issues by illustrating the difficulties for professionals and families if appropriate care is not provided:

First, the early involvement of relatives in the care of individuals with serious mental health problems is important, particularly when there are associated risk behaviours. Involvement should take the form of providing information about the care and treatment of the individual, and the assessment and management of risk either to the individual or family members. Close relatives can provide an enormous amount of accurate, important information for the benefit of enhanced risk assessment. They are sensitive to subtle changes in the individual and are able to provide identifiable relapse warning signs. If knowledge is shared they can become important allies in providing support to the individual, or in taking a more active role in specific coping strategy enhancement.

Often however forensic patients have complex needs, a history of poor family relationships and offending, and may well have experienced mental health services without the resources to adequately address these challenging circumstances. Frustration on behalf of relatives and patients can therefore result, with associated problems of poor engagement with services, anger and hostility toward professionals, burnout and a lack of motivation toward any therapeutic endeavours. These need to be sensitively overcome, and the needs of relatives recognised as an important component of the care provided.

Second, the needs of relatives should be addressed in their own right. Many relatives suffer from the effects of stress, associated with living with an individual with complex problems and needs. The burden of care and the resulting reduction in social functioning can lead relatives to develop minor mental health problems of their own, and in some cases, behavioural problems which can then affect the care of children. Emotional support should be provided as should interventions aimed at increasing the support networks of family members.

Third, education about the management of serious mental health problems has been demonstrated to assist in engaging relatives, and reducing the distress associated with particular symptoms. Enabling relatives to cope more effectively and assist individuals in this process requires good information tailored to the families needs. The patient too requires information and education in order to reduce the effects of their mental health problem, and to return the responsibility back to the patient for their own care. A patient should, ideally, request continuous outpatient care on a voluntary basis, based on a knowledge of their mental health needs and associated problems (Lindqvist and Skipworth, 2000).

Fourth, the symptoms of schizophrenia should be explored with the individual in a collaborative, structured way, which has a focus upon detailed assessment, discussion of associated thoughts and feelings, discussion of beliefs, and a move toward interpreting these experiences in order to reduce distress and associated risk.

Conclusion

Static risk variables such as personal demographics and personality characteristics are uncommon targets for rehabilitation, yet they form the core of all risk assessment tools (Lindqvist and Skipworth, 2000). The assessment of risk needs to be linked to effective management strategies which focus on risk factors that can be changed, rather than immutable factors that provide a risk score. It is these dynamic risk variables that need to be targeted and the care and treatment provided evaluated in order to understand what, in forensic psychiatry, works.

According to Lindqvist and Skipworth (2000), risk assessment and management can be linked to four dynamic features of the individual:

- The disorder itself, particularly where active psychotic symptoms can create dangerous situations.
- Family interactions, and interactions with peers.
- Substance misuse, particularly resulting in impairments of judgement, empathy, anger and impulsiveness.
- Anti-therapeutic environment including the mental health service in which the individual interacts.

Therapeutic work needs to focus on changing these features if risk is to be managed effectively.

Specific training in psychosocial interventions appears to address many of the training implications associated with this view of managing risk. Important aspects of such a training programme appear to be:

- Providing a foundation in the theory and research underpinning the involvement of families and the effects of the environment on symptoms
- Training in current perspectives on schizophrenia and cognitive/behavioural interventions
- Role play and practise of working with groups of patients or families, or with mental health systems and professionals
- Emphasis on facilitating groups rather than leading them
- Need for educational programmes that build on knowledge rather than attempting to replace it.
- Interventions aimed at working with individuals and families as early as possible

Incorporating an understanding of how care and treatment relate to the individual, and the dynamic features of risk management, are also important. The assessment and management of risk, together with training in a range of effective interventions, which actually work, will have an impact on reducing the risks for individuals, families, and society.

Further Reading

Hughes, J. and Hughes, C. (2000) 'Family and Friends', in D. Mercer, T. Mason, M. McKeown and G. McCann (eds), *Forensic Mental Health Care: A case study approach*, London, Churchill Livingstone.

References

Allebeck, P. (1989) 'Schizophrenia: A Life Shortening Disease', *Schizophrenia Bulletin*, 15(1), 81–9.

Bartels, J., Drake, R., Wallach, M. and Freeman, D. (1991) 'Characteristic hostility in schizophrenic outpatient', *Schizophrenic Bulletin*, 17, 763–71.

Birchwood, M., Smith, J., Drury, V., Healy, J., Macmillan, F. and Slade, M. (1994) 'A self-report insight scale for psychosis: reliability, validity and sensitivity to change', *Acta Psychiatrica Scandinavica*, 89, 62–7.

Burns, T. and Kendrick, T. (1997) 'The primary care of patients with schizophrenia: a search for good practice', *British Journal of General Practice*, 47, 515–20.

Cheung, P., Schweitzer, I., Crowley, K. and Tuckwell, V. (1997) 'Violence and schizophrenia: role of hallucinations and delusions', *Schizophrenia Research*, 26, 181–90.

Gardner, W., Lidz, C., Mulvey, E. and Shaw, E. (1996) 'Clinical versus actuarial predictions of violence in patients with mental illness', *Journal of Consulting and Clinical Psychology*, 64, 602–9.

Greenberg, L., Fine, S., Cohen, C., Larson, K., Michealson-Bailey, A., Rubinton, P. and Glick, I. (1988) 'An interdisciplinary psychoeducation programme for schizophrenic patients and their families in an acute care setting', *Hospital and Community Psychiatry*, 39(3), 277–82.

Greenfield, D., Strauss, J., Bowers, M. and Mandelkern, M. (1989) 'Insight and interpretation of illness in recovery from psychosis', *Schizophrenia Bulletin*, 15(2), 245–52.

Groocock, V. (1989) 'The sins of the children visited upon the parents', *The Independent*, 16 March.

Hafner, H. and Boker, W. (1973) 'Mentally disordered violent offenders', *Social Psychiatry*, 8, 220–29.

Honig, A. (1991) 'Psychotherapy with command hallucinations in chronic schizophrenia: the use of action techniques within a surrogate family setting', *Journal of Group Psychotherapy, Psychodrama and Sociometry*, 44(1), 3–18.

Hughes, J. and Hughes, C. (2000) 'Family and Friends', in D. Mercer, T. Mason, M. McKeown and G. McCann (eds), *Forensic Mental Health Care: A case study approach*, London, Churchill Livingstone.

Juninger, J. (1991) 'Predicting compliance with command hallucinations', *American Journal of Psychiatry*, 147, 245–7.

Lindqvist, P. and Skipworth, J. (2000) Evidenc-'based rehabilitation in forensic psychiatry', *British Journal of Psychiatry*, 176, 320–23.

Link, B. and Steuve, A. (1994) 'Psychotic symptoms and the violent/illegal behaviour of mental patients compared to community controls', in J. Monaghan and H. Steadman (eds), *Violence and Mental Disorder: developments in risk assessment*, Chicago, University of Chicago Press, pp. 137–59.

McCann, G. (1993) 'Relatives' Support Groups in a Special Hospital: An Evaluation Study', *Journal of Advanced Nursing*, 18, 1883–8.

McEvoy, J., Apperson, J., Appelbaum, P., Ortlip, P., Brecosky, J., Hammill, K., Geller, J. and Roth, L. (1989) 'Insight in schizophrenia. Its relationship to acute psychopathology', *Journal of Nervous and Mental Disease*, 177, 42–7.

McKeown, M. and McCann, G. (2000) 'Psychosocial Interventions', in C. Chaloner and M. Coffey (eds), *Forensic Mental Health Nursing, Current Approaches*, Oxford, Blackwell Science.

Morgan, S. (1998) 'The assessment and management of risk', in C. Brooker and J. Repper (eds), *Serious Mental Health Problems in the Community*, London, Bailliere Tindall.

Nestor, P., Haycock, J., Doiron, S., Kelly, J. and Kelly, D. (1995) 'Lethal violence and psychosis', *Bulletin of American Academic Psychiatry and Law*, 23, 331–41.

Philo, G., Secker, J., Platt, S., Henderson, L., McLanghlin, G. and Burnside, J. (1994) 'The impact of mass media on public images of mental illness, media content and audience belief', *Health Education Journal*, 53, 271–81.

Rogers, R., Gillis, J., Turner, E. and Frise-Smith, T. (1990) 'The clinical presentation of command hallucinations in a forensic population', *American Journal of Psychiatry*, 147, 1304–7.

Ryan, T. (1998) 'Perceived risk associated with mental illness: beyond homicide and suicide', *Social Science and Medicine*, 46(2), 287–97.

Sellwood, W., Haddock, G., Tarrier, N. and Yusupoff, L. (1994) 'Advances in the Psychological Management of Positive Symptoms of Schizophrenia', *International Review of Psychiatry*, 6, 201–15.

Stanley, N., Manthorpe, J. and Penhale, B. (eds) (1999) *Institutional abuse: perspectives across the life course*, London, Routledge.

Swanson, J., Borum, R., Swartz, M. and Monahan, J. (1996) 'Psyhcotic symptoms and disorders and the risk of violent behaviour in the community', *Criminal Behaviour and Mental Health*, 6, 309–29.

Swanson, J., Estroff, S., Swartz, M., Borum, R., Lachiotte, W., Zimmer, C. and Wagner, R. (1997) 'Violence and severe mental disorder in clinical and community populations: the effects of psychotic symptoms, comorbidity, and lack of treatment', *Psychiatry*, 60, 1–22.

Taylor, P. (1993) 'Schizophrenia and Crime: distinctive patterns in association', in S. Hodgins (ed.), *Crime and Mental Disorder*, Newbury Park, CA, Sage, pp. 63–85.

Taylor, P. and Gunn, J. (1999) 'Homicides by people with mental illness: myth and reality', *British Journal of Psychiatry*, 174, 9–14.

Wessely, S. (1997) 'The epidemiology of crime violence and schizophrenia', *British Journal of Psychiatry*, 170 (Suppl. 32), 8–11.

World Health Organization (1973) *Report of the eighth seminar on the standardisation of psychiatric diagnosis, classification and statistics*, Geneva, WHO.

Zubin, J., Magaziner, J. and Steinhauer, S. (1983) 'The metamorphosis of schizophrenia; from chronicity to vulnerability', *Psychological Medicine*, 13, 551–71.

Zubin, J. and Spring, B. (1977) 'Vulnerability: A New View of Schizophrenia', *Journal of Abnormal Psychology*, 86, 260–66.

CHAPTER 16

Psychosocial Interventions in Institutional Settings

MICK MCKEOWN, GED MCCANN AND JOE FORSTER

Introduction

One of the most pressing issues facing mental health services is how to systematically and comprehensively introduce demonstrably sound interventions, like psychosocial approaches, into real-life, everyday practice. Concern has also been raised over the extent to which different sectors of the whole service may be relatively favoured with progressive developments, resulting in pockets of disadvantage elsewhere. One such demarcation divides community practitioners from inpatient staff (SNMAC, 1999). Anyone interested in psychosocial interventions typically finds a body of work dominated by a focus on community activity. For various reasons, however, a persuasive case can be made for their translation and adaptation into institutional settings.

Whenever novel service developments are proposed staff training is usually at or near the top of the agenda. Healthcare training, however, is seldom a straightforward affair. Of crucial importance is the thorny issue of the relative failure of traditional models of training to result in substantial or enduring changes in clinical practice. Hence, although it is vital that training delivers high quality subject material, and is as thoroughly grounded in evidence as is possible, the training process itself is just as significant. In this chapter we marshal arguments for the introduction of psychosocial interventions in hospital settings and consider which specific interventions could be most effectively applied by in patient staff. We also examine the potential barriers to the implementation of psychosocial interventions in hospital settings and present a clinically based model for training which we feel is suited to realising the desired individual and organisational changes in practice. The advocated approach targets the learning needs of whole teams together, and the training takes place directly in the clinical environment within which any changes to practice have to occur. It is intended that training and practice development are enacted simultaneously, synthesising the different forms of expertise embodied in the trainers and the clinical staff. Essentially, the approach is geared toward achieving an 'organic' process of transformation, with substantive changes to practice more likely to endure.

Background

Research over the past twenty years has provided considerable evidence that people with a diagnosis of schizophrenia can benefit from psychosocial interventions designed to reduce environmental stressors, to enhance people's abilities to cope, and to ameliorate psychotic symptoms. Much of this work has focused on reducing relapse rates through interventions with families (Chapter 11). More recent studies have also indicated the effectiveness of psychological interventions targeted at positive symptoms, specifically hallucinations and delusions (Chapter 8). Interestingly, two trials have evaluated cognitive behavioural therapy for people with schizophrenia cared for in acute in-patient settings (Drury *et al.*, 1996; Tarrier, 1999). The Drury study showed significant reductions in the length of stay for patients who received CBT, and Tarrier and colleagues' SOCRATES project has reported promising preliminary data. A third strategy has been to use psychological techniques to enhance compliance with neuroleptic medication (Kemp *et al.*, 1996).

In this context psychotic symptoms are conceived of as resulting from an interaction between inherent, personal vulnerability and environmental stress. Such stress-vulnerability models have improved professional understanding of the complexity of psychotic disorders, without necessarily claiming to explain their cause (Zubin and Spring, 1977; Nuechterlain and Dawson, 1984). Central to the application of psychosocial interventions is a conceptual shift away from dealing with individuals in therapy in isolation from others. Psychosocial interventions are essentially about treating people as part of a wider social network, typically with respect to close family relationships. Hence, high expressed emotion interactions are a significant source of psychosocial stress, and the required intervention targets the social network to reduce the impact of stress for everyone. If we are to consider translating the extant community psychosocial interventions into in-patient settings we must pay attention to the sources of stress within such environments.

Given that for many individuals admitted to hospital wards, their level of contact with family members is diminished in proportion to the amount of time they spend with professional carers, then the focus shifts toward staff assuming a significant place in the social network. The rationale for proceeding with psychosocial approaches would be enhanced if there was evidence that staff relationships with service users at ward level shared some common features with research into family contexts.

Staffed Care Environments

Expressed Emotion was first directly measured in staff in full-time contact with service users by Moore *et al.* (1992). They made minor adaptations to the Camberwell Family Interview (CFI) (Brown and Rutter, 1966) to make it appropriate for use with professional carers. Sixty-one interviews about different service users were conducted with 35 staff. Twenty staff were rated as low EE and four were high EE in all their interviews, eleven were rated differently for different clients. It was concluded that the proportion of staff rated as high EE (43 per cent) was similar to the proportion of informal carers shown in the family EE studies (Leff and Vaughn, 1985). Scores for criticism, hostility, positive remarks and warmth were all obtained but emotional over-involvement was not shown by staff.

In a further study, Ball and colleagues (1992) compared levels of EE in staff working in two residential hostels with outcomes for the people they cared for. In hostel A, four out of seven staff (57 per cent) rated as high EE compared with only one of the five staff (20 per cent) in hostel B. The relapse rates for residents in each hostel were similar but hostel A had a much higher turnover of residents. During the follow-up period, two residents from hostel B were re-admitted to hospital twice but returned to the hostel, and one resident was discharged to a lower-dependency setting. These outcomes appeared more favourable than those for residents from hostel A, where two residents were readmitted to hospital and did not return to the hostel and seven residents were discharged for negative reasons such as breaking house rules. In summary, the turnover of residents for negative reasons was greater in the higher EE hostel, although the level of relapse measured by hospital readmission was, on the face of it, similar.

Moore and Kuipers (1992) investigated the affective style of staff interacting with patients and compared this with levels of EE, rated using the adapted CFI. Low EE staff were found to appear more supportive, dwelt less on negative feelings and elicited more self-affirmation from their clients, seeming to mirror attributes of EE in relatives. Snyder and colleagues (1994) studied fifteen family-style board-and-care residences of seven or less residents in Los Angeles. Two residents from each home were randomly selected, and the homes' operators were interviewed about them. Two measures were used to rate EE, the CFI and the Five Minute Speech Sample (FMSS) (Magana *et al.*, 1986). High EE ratings were associated with poorer results on a residents' quality of life measure, and with greater hostility and suspiciousness on the part of the residents. Symptom severity appeared to be associated with high EE, suggesting this as an area for further research. Again, emotional over-involvement did not feature in the results.

In a Netherlands study of hospital, ward-based staff (Finnema *et al.*, 1996), a sample of 29 nurses were rated by their service users on a perceived EE Scale and the FMSS. The results showed that perceived EE ratings were lower than the corresponding FMSS ratings (a third of which were high EE). This suggests that there may be factors within the social environment in hospital that mediate perceived EE in a way not yet explained.

In summary, research suggests that professional staff do exhibit high EE responses in their interactions with patients similar to those exhibited by informal carers. Of the in-patient staff studies the mean number who rate as high

EE is 31 per cent (range 13–43 per cent, SD 9.8) which compares favourably with the mean 54.4 per cent high EE found in relatives in the family studies, suggesting lower EE levels in staff. It has also been shown that high EE responses in staff may be exhibited towards specific patients and not all patients in a particular unit (Moore *et al.*, 1992). Staff are also more likely to rate as critical or hostile than informal carers but not emotionally over-involved in their interactions. An expected relationship between low EE in staff and improved outcome is suggested, although direct comparison with the relative studies is not feasible due to lack of standardisation in operationalising outcome in the staff studies.

Interventions With Staff to Reduce Expressed Emotion

Intervention to reduce high EE and so improve outcome, central to the family intervention literature, has yet to be replicated in nurses. Nurses undergo an initial training and further in-service and post-basic educational programmes, and therefore might be expected to be receptive to such a programme. However, operationalisation of the EE construct in nurses remains incomplete, and further work is necessary to disentangle the interaction of many different relationships that exists within staffed settings. Staff studies have used some way of selecting a nurse to be measured, usually using the named keyworker for the service user concerned. There is a danger that other important relationships contributing to EE might be missed. In studies of families with more than one member present, the existence of one high EE relative is sufficient for a high EE rating, while the presence of one or more low EE relatives might fail to mediate a high EE environment (Kavanagh, 1992). In the same way, the EE profile of other staff members might confound the rating of EE in a selected keyworker. Only in small settings might it be possible to rate all of the staff for each individual, unless the point of measurement was moved from the staff member to the service user by measuring perceived EE (Forster, 2000).

Perhaps the major difference between a notion of staff EE and that in family relationships is the expansion of the social network, albeit with key individuals having less total face to face contact. Kavanagh's (1992) interactive model suggests any single pair of individuals engaged in a high EE relationship must exist within the context of the ambient EE of other relationships within the ward environment. As might be expected, emotional involvement seems to be an area where staff EE does not mirror relatives' EE. Reasons for this might include professional relationships lacking the strong emotional bonds that exist between family members, and staff being unlikely to have known people as their past selves before the onset of illness. However, some individual staff and institutional routines lend themselves to a disposition of protection, or a tendency to do things for people, or make decisions for them, which, though unlikely to be rated as emotional over-involvement on the EE scales, may contribute to similar effects.

The finding that staff are more likely to respond positively to clients who are more obviously ill, resonates with the hypothesis that critical and hostile responses from relatives are associated with attributions about the cause of a person's behaviour. That is, high EE responses are more evident when the relative cannot easily attribute the origin of a specific behaviour to illness, and instead explains things in terms of a personal trait. For this reason much tension and stress in families is associated with reactions to negative symptoms, for example thinking motivational difficulties are really laziness.

Although the evidence for staff EE is far from comprehensive, and is replete with methodological problems which probably arise from the lack of a measuring tool sensitive to the complexity of the phenomenon under investigation, there is one consistent finding which mirrors the family EE studies. Low staff EE results in comparatively better outcomes for service users. It seems to make sense then to seek developments which are aimed at incorporating a low EE style of interaction combined with a range of proven effective interventions into routine practice with this client group in inpatient settings.

Critique of Services

Arguably, despite the research evidence regarding the efficacy of psychosocial interventions they are used sporadically even in the community, and more rarely again in institutional settings. Fadden (1997) has remarked upon the extent to which practitioners trained in behavioural family therapy are frustrated in their attempts to deliver this intervention in routine practice. Attention to the quality of psychiatric services has coincided with an increase in media and public interest, largely because of a number of well-publicised incidents in the community, provoking a series of formal inquiries. Typically, the service user at the centre of these tragic events has been identified as suffering a psychotic illness. Somewhat ironically, at around the time this client group achieved such prominent attention from the media, even though they exercise the greatest potential demand on care provision, services were being criticised across the board for failing to give their needs sufficient priority. More general criticisms of services are to be found in a number of government sponsored reviews from this period (Clinical Standards Advisory Group, 1995; Department of Health, 1994).

Evaluations of inpatient services have been especially barbed in their critique (Mental Health Act Commission and the Sainsbury Centre, 1997). In general terms, standard ward care and treatment has been censured for being of a poor standard and almost exclusively focused on the delivery of medication (Clinical Standards Advisory Group, 1995; SNMAC, 1999). Systematic psychological interventions are rarely provided within hospital settings, so that clients frequently complain about the poverty of the therapeutic environment

(Rogers *et al.*, 1993). This critique is usually accompanied by commentary upon staff skill-mix and levels of, or appropriateness of, training. For example, the report on the National Visit to acute psychiatric wards (Mental Health Act Commission and the Sainsbury Centre, 1997) concluded that:

> Many nurses were trained at a time when a number of patients on acute wards had less severe forms of illness, such as depression, where counselling skills could be employed. As the patients on acute wards now have more severe forms of illness, such as schizophrenia and manic-depressive psychosis, different interventions are required. Nurses will therefore need . . . to learn some of the more recent therapeutic psychological interventions for these problems.

The overwhelming recommendation to be found in the various official reviews and reports is that services must become more systematic and focused in their delivery of care. There is a consensus that appropriate assessment and treatment is of paramount concern, and should include the delivery of a range of psychosocial interventions under the aegis of sound case management principles. To this end, meeting the needs of the severely mentally ill has become a national priority and the National Service Framework (Department of Health, 1999) suggests a serious attempt to iron out regional discrepancies in the effective delivery of quality services.

Delivering Psychosocial Interventions in In-patient Environments

It is entirely possible to conceive of as full a range of psychosocial interventions within institutional settings as may be employed in the community. In many respects this will not involve substantial or fundamental adaptations to particular approaches or therapies, such that, essentially, the intervention at ward level is more or less identical to that delivered in the community, it being simply the setting or context which changes. On the other hand, certain interventions, or key aspects of them, need to be shaped to better suit the changed circumstances presented by a clinical rather than domestic environment. A point worth making here is that it is better to think about the implementation of psychosocial approaches in a way which integrates developments across both in-patient and community services. In this way, unhelpful discontinuities between the two sectors can be anticipated and planned against, ensuring continuity of care and professional practice from ward to community.

The establishment of any novel service development, whatever the context, needs to take into account both constraining and supporting factors that exist in the particular environment (see Table 16.1). The implementation of psychosocial approaches must meet the challenge of various barriers to their uptake in in-patient environments, and these will be as varied as there are different types of provision. In contemplating necessary changes to the

Table 16.1   Factors influencing the uptake of PSI in in-patient environments

Constraining factors	Supportive factors
Pressures on staff time. Time taken up in administration or routinised activity.	Concentration of professional personnel in one space. Better if ward has access to full multi-professional team.
Ineffective multidisciplinary teamworking.	Effective multidisciplinary teamworking. Full participation of all members in care planning and case management. Shared responsibilities and accountability among team.
Low staff morale for various reasons.	Pro-active ward management and clinical leadership results in better morale. Efforts to involve staff and value their expertise and contribution to developmental change can improve morale.
Relatively rapid turnover of clients in acute ward contexts.	Continuity of care, especially the case in rehabilitation, forensic, or residential settings.
Limited access to families. Complicated by formal visiting arrangements.	Possibility to access key worker for considerable portions of any day (shift) or week.
Possible severity and volatility of symptoms or behaviour in acute settings militate against effective engagement in therapy.	Acute relapses afford the opportunity to take advantage of expressed need (from service user or family) and establish therapeutic alliance.
Hospital wards can be stressful environments, antithetical to PSI approach. This can result in viscious cycles of stress.	Staff can work collectively to minimise ward stress as much as possible. This can result in virtuous cycles of stress minimisation.
It can be difficult for some service users or staff to view the ward environment as a centre for therapeutic activity.	The establishment of a range of therapies and corollary cultural shifts can engender a therapeutic feel to the ward space.
Inadequate built environment can mean lack of space set aside for therapy, or heavy pressure on the use of limited space.	A good built environment, or better use of available accommodation can create the setting for effective therapies.
	Possibilities for therapeutic group-work.

interventions themselves the organisational realities of ward-based care in modern psychiatric services will be influential in determining the extent to which they can become established into routine practice. This may be especially the case with regard to resource-poor acute wards with heavy pressures in terms of bed occupancy and staffing levels. Of all these organisational issues, perhaps the one most referred to is the pressure on staff time, with the lack of time spent in therapeutic activity being critically raised in various independent reviews of in-patient care. While this is undoubtedly contributed to by the vexed question of resources, it is unlikely to be the sole contributory factor to a complex problem. This raises the possibility of arguing for some solutions based upon more adequate funding of inpatient staffing establishments, with particular attention to training and skill-mix, but also to make more effective use of the given staffing resource by paying attention to specific constraints on staff time which can be identified (usually quite simply by the staff themselves).

Certain aspects of institutional settings, such as the concentration of professional personnel on a single site or the availability of accommodation, equip-
ment and other materials designed for the purpose of supporting therapy, may
afford enhanced opportunities for delivering effective psychosocial interventions. Ward-based keyworker relationships can be established which can either
(or both) set aside dedicated time at agreed intervals for individual therapy,
or, opportunistically, take advantage of key moments of interpersonal contact
as and when these arise to enact supportive psychosocial techniques. Furthermore, especially in the context of medium, longer-term, or residential in-
patient facilities there is the opportunity to achieve high quality therapeutic
relationships which may be more difficult to achieve for some busy community practitioners. The variety of different contingencies which may exist is one
of the reasons we advocate service developments to be undertaken in the
context of interactive training. In this way the authentic requirements of each
ward or setting can be tackled directly.

Whatever the particular circumstances of any in-patient setting some
common issues are important to address. A brief summary of these follows:

- *Engagement of service users and families.* The usual processes and interpersonal skills involved in therapeutic engagement pertain regardless of
  setting. That is not to say that setting is unimportant, and ward-based staff
  will have to attend to issues of timing and the availability of quiet and
  private space, free of interruption, for the duration of therapeutic contact.
  Timing is especially important with respect to relatives, as ward visiting
  arrangements can complicate efforts to meet with key family members. For
  families who have never received systematic support or family therapy,
  especially important in the case of first episodes, the ward staff can play a
  vital role in recruiting families to such initiatives, even if the intervention
  may eventually be delivered by community staff.
- *Use of structured assessments.* The effective employment of a range of
  systematic assessment tools can have many benefits at ward level. These
  include the obvious improvement to care planning and case management
  that should ensue from collecting objective clinical data. Other benefits
  flow from the implicit therapeutic effect of routinely engaging people
  in systematised exchanges about the nature of their experiences, and
  improvements in staff morale due to extensions to their clinical role.
  Important issues for teams include the choices they face about which
  assessment tools they wish to employ in standard practice with all service
  users, and which others they may choose to use more selectively. They will
  also need to establish how their assessment activity supports wider activity in care planning, paying attention to congruence with whichever conceptual framework and philosophy they are using to inform their care.
  Possibly the best thing to do is to develop a ward philosophy grounded
  in principals of normalisation of psychotic experiences and a conceptual
  framework based on stress-vulnerability theory. An individualised care

approach ought to determine the appropriate frequency with which certain assessment tools are administered.

- *Identifying problems and goals.* The most effective care planning is fully participatory, involving service users and family members as appropriate in the construction of the care plan. This ideal is not always achievable, and the written record may well have to record where practitioner and client views differ. Given the complexity of problems and needs exhibited by this client group, it is best to keep problem and goal setting as simple as possible, sticking to behavioural (measurable) wording and clarity of language. It is also useful to prioritise problems and needs and attempt to work on a manageable number at any one time. We have found the use of a simple formulation effective, and this is described elsewhere in this chapter.

- *Psychoeducation.* Education for service users and families can begin on admission to the ward. Most service users and families will need a variety of information, some quite general, some specific to this admission. Information needs can be split into three categories: Practical information about the hospital, ward, staff disciplines and roles, procedures, routines and rules, rights, complaints systems, advocacy, and issues around the administration of the Mental Health Act if necessary; clinical information about psychotic symptoms and ways of understanding them; treatment information about various interventions with a substantial requirement for accurate material relating to medication and side effects.

- *Individual psychosocial interventions* can be delivered in the course of ward based keyworker relationships or by specialist practitioners attached to the ward team. In this context appropriate competencies are important, as is an effective system of clinical supervision. Specific protocols for CBT, arising from the relevant research studies, will likely be available to be drawn on by in-patient staff. Depending on individual need, a range of therapies can be attempted including the assessment of prodromal signs and development of relapse plans, coping strategy enhancement, alliance approaches to medication management, and a broad range of measures to manage stress and promote healthier lifestyles.

- *Group psychosocial interventions.* Because wards often contain a number of service users with similar needs or problems at any one time it is also possible to consider the delivery of group psychosocial interventions. These may be simply organised along psychoeducational principles or can be used to initiate cognitive-behavioural work such as coping strategy enhancement, techniques in the management of positive symptoms, or recognition and management of the early warning signs of psychotic relapse. Family support groups or group psychoeducation for families can also be initiated. The effective use of group work, preferably supported by individual work can be an especially economic use of staff time, and can also help in establishing certain areas of the ward 'space' as a recognised therapeutic environment.

- *Collective ward stress.* The introduction of a psychosocial ward culture must also attend to the aggregate levels of stress in the whole ward, and specifically in interpersonal relationships. Here, the whole team can make efforts to offer a low EE environment and deploy consistent and constructive techniques of positive feedback for observed progress.

The Training and Development Process

Corrigan and McCracken (1995) detail three main barriers to implementing and developing improvements in inpatient environments. These comprise of bureaucratic constraints, accessibility of effective treatments, and, relatedly, insufficient numbers of well-trained personnel. Our favoured approach to working with teams of staff to implement psychosocial interventions aims to directly tackle such impediments (McKeown *et al.*, 2000). This 'organic' process of training and development shares certain philosophical and theoretical features with Corrigan and colleagues' (1995, 1997) 'Interactive Staff Training' and the 'Appreciative Inquiry' approach to organisational change (Cooperrider and Srivastva, 1987).

The Interactive Staff Training model was designed for training teams of staff in behavioural techniques for psychiatric rehabilitation. Whole teams of staff are trained together, with the learning taking place in the actual clinical environment. Research into the effectiveness of the approach has been undertaken (Corrigan *et al.*, 1997) with a large trial currently underway. Appreciative inquiry has been undertaken in various contexts including community projects in the developing world, modern businesses, and the UK prisons service. This model for change is grounded in action research methods. Future studies of whole-team training afford the possibilities of eclectic use of both action research techniques and experimental research designs within single projects.

All of these approaches have in common the fact that process issues are emphasised, drawing on various theories of organisational change. Of course, the content of any training input is important, but how learning is associated with changing practice is paramount. There is a synthesis of any new knowledge brought by the trainers/facilitators with the grass-roots expertise held by the individual participants. Essentially, new practices emerge from a collaborative effort to shape and adapt what is learnt to better fit the actual environment. The ultimate aim is for any positive developments to be self-sustaining. Any changes to working practices are then more likely to last after the trainers leave and become incorporated into daily routines.

The focus is on collective groups, rather than seeing learning as the province of individual students. There is a similar concern with collective outcomes, and ownership of these. As such, whole teams of staff or community groups are targeted, with collaborative working proceeding directly in the environment wherein specific developments are sought. The philosophical starting point is to understand, rather than condemn, any visible faults or difficulties within the host group, and, most importantly, to highlight the positive aspects. Given the often beleaguered situation which typifies inpatient mental health units this strategy is most timely. Interestingly, from a psychosocial perspective, there is an analogue here with behavioural family therapy, wherein the therapists seek to understand the challenges faced by families and foster an affirming style of feedback and interaction, and eventual autonomy in effective problem solving.

Particularly if we think of modern health services, the principles of organisational psychology tell us that ownership of ideas and practice developments is vital. However, it is often the case that ready-made blueprints for practice change are imposed on staff, with predictable and disappointing outcomes. The alternative allows for a style of service development that grows 'organically' towards individual, collective and organisational improvements to services that may not have been anticipated in advance. This process has been described as organic because the practice developments have their origins in the team themselves, and must turn out to be suited to the practice environment because they have been shaped to that end.

Organic Training and Development: A Case Study

We piloted the organic training approach to implementing psychosocial interventions in a inner-city secure rehabilitation unit (McKeown *et al.*, 2000). The client group cared for on the unit would have a serious mental illness diagnosis, typically, schizophrenia, and more often than not would be thought of as treatment resistant. Relying on a stress-vulnerability model enabled us to pay attention to the sources of stress within the ward environment, with a particular focus on the nature of interpersonal interactions. Various members of the multidisciplinary team were actively involved in the project, with the most numerous group being nurses.

In the first six months of the project participating team members attended six small-group teaching sessions held in consecutive blocks on the ward. These introductory sessions comprised a broad introduction to psychosocial interventions and the reliable use of various assessment tolls. Each block culminated with a brainstorming activity generating ideas for implementing psychosocial approaches into routine practice at ward level. In the next stage of the project the facilitators met on the ward with members of the team on two afternoons each week to take the initiative forward. Attendance at these meetings depended on which staff were rostered on the days in question. These development meetings quickly evolved so that one strand focused on strategic issues in the implementation of psychosocial approaches and the other became a multidisciplinary forum for reviewing cases and care planning.

Staff-focused outcome measures were taken at baseline, at six months, and at eighteen months. Significant increases in relevant staff knowledge and reductions in staff stress were found between baseline and the 18-month interval. Although there were positive trends in the data at six months (on

Table 16.2 Practical consequences of organic ward training and development

Innovation	Effects
• Establishment of a ward based model of psychosocial care.	• Structured approach to care. • Attention to sources of stress on ward. • Concern with low EE communication.
• Use of the systematic assessments in routine practice.	• Better quality clinical information. • Authoritative contribution to care planning and decision-making.
• Improving care plans.	• Greater clarity in the documentary record of care.
• Monthly care summaries.	• Assists in longitudinal reviews. • Avoidance of repetition of ineffectual interventions. • Enhanced tracking of individual progress. • Aids risk management.
• Increasing the degree of participation of service users and families.	• Improved therapeutic alliances.
• Developing multidisciplinary case formulation.	• Improved satisfaction with services.
• Establishing a unitary, multidisciplinary system of case notes.	• Improving teamworking and communication.

immediate completion of the taught element) these did not achieve statistical significance. Interestingly, the significant changes emerged following the consolidation and adaptation activity in the intervening period. This time was spent collaboratively developing and implementing changes to working practices. Some key outcomes of this work are listed in Table 16.2.

Conclusions

Arguably, psychosocial interventions and associated training initiatives have neglected in-patient settings. Given the legitimate policy focus on community care and an evidence base dominated by research undertaken in the community this state of affairs is understandable. Nevertheless, inpatient services, the staff who work in them, and the people who make use of their services are left at a distinct disadvantage. Unsurprisingly, the quality of in-patient care has come in for much criticism. Whatever solutions are found, they are unlikely to succeed alone unless the training needs of the staff expected to deliver care in such environments are addressed.

We propose that further work needs to be undertaken to establish which particular aspects of psychosocial interventions are most relevant for the care of individuals in hospital settings, and that their effectiveness in these settings is thoroughly evaluated. Finally, there is an urgent need to develop innovative models for training and dissemination that will ensure the practice of psychosocial interventions by in patient staff so that this is recognised as routine, rather than specialised care.

Further Reading

Cooperrider, D.L., Sorensen, P., Whitney, D. and Yaeger, T. (eds) (1999) *Appreciative inquiry: rethinking human organization toward a positive theory of change*, Champaign, IL., Stipes Publishing.

Corrigan, P. and McCracken, S. (1995) 'Psychiatric rehabilitation and staff development: educational and organisational models', *Clinical Psychology Review*, 15, 699–719.

Fadden, G. (1997) 'Implementation of family interventions in routine clinical practice following staff training: A major cause for concern', *Journal of Mental Health*, 6(6), 599–612.

McKeown, M., Mercer, D. and Finlayson, S. (2000) 'Targeting: the role of training', in L. Cotterill and W. Barr (eds), *Targeting in Mental Health Services: A Multi-Disciplinary Challenge*, Aldershot, Ashgate.

References

Ball, R., Moore, E. and Kuipers, L. (1992) 'Expressed Emotion in community care staff: A comparison of patient outcome in a nine month follow-up of two hostels', *Social Psychiatry and Psychiatric Epidemiology*, 27, 35–9.

Brown, G.W. and Rutter, M. (1966) 'The measurement of family activities and relationships. A Methodological study', *Human Relations*, 19, 241–63.

Clinical Standards Advisory Group Committee on Schizophrenia (1995) *Clinical Standards Advisory Group: Schizophrenia*, Vol. 1. Report of a CSAG Committee on Schizophrenia. London, HMSO.

Cooperrider, D.L. and Srivastva, S. (1987) 'Appreciative inquiry in organizational life', in R. Woodman and W. Pasmore (eds), *Research in Organizational Change and Development*, Vol. 1, Greenwich, CT, JAI Press.

Corrigan, P. and McCracken, S. (1995) 'Psychiatric rehabilitation and staff development: educational and organisational models', *Clinical Psychology Review*, 15, 699–719.

Corrigan, P., McCracken, S., Edwards, M., Kommana, S. and Simpatico, T. (1997) 'Staff training to improve implementation and impact of behavioural rehabilitation programs', *Psychiatric Services*, 48, 1336–8.

Department of Health (1994) *Working in Partnership: A Collaborative Approach to Care. Report of the Mental Health Nursing Review Team* [Butterworth Report]. London, HMSO.

Department of Health (1999) *The National Service Framework for Mental Health*, London, The Stationery Office.

Drury, V., Birchwood, M., Cochrane, R. and MacMillan, F. (1996) 'Cognitive-behaviour therapy for acute psychosis', *British Journal of Psychiatry*, 169, 593–607.

Fadden, G. (1997) 'Implementation of family interventions in routine clinical practice following staff training: A major cause for concern', *Journal of Mental Health*, 6(6), 599–612.

Finnema, E., Louwerens, I., Sloof, C. and Van den Bosch, R. (1996) 'Expressed emotion on long stay wards', *Journal of Advanced Nursing*, 24, 473–8.

Forster J. (2000) 'A patient perceived measure of staff expressed emotion'. Unpublished MPhil Thesis, University of Liverpool.

Kavanagh, D. (1992) 'Recent developments in expressed emotion and schizophrenia', *British Journal of Psychiatry*, 160, 601–20.

Kemp, R., Hayward, P., Applewhaite, G., Everitt, B. and David, A. (1996) 'Compli ance therapy in psychotic patients: A randomised controlled trial', *British Medical Journal*, 312, 345–9.

Leff, J. and Vaughn, C. (1985) *Expressed Emotion in Families: Its significance for mental illness*, London, Guildford Press.

Magana, A., Goldstein, M., Karno, M., Miklowitz, D., Jenkins, J. and Falloon, I. (1986) 'A brief method for assessing the expressed emotion in relatives of psychiatric patients', *Psychiatric Research*, 17, 203–12.

McKeown, M., Mercer, D. and Finlayson, S. (2000) 'Targeting: the role of training', in L. Cotterill and W. Barr (eds), *Targeting in Mental Health Services*, Aldershot, Ashgate.

Mental Health Act Commission and the Sainsbury Centre (1997) *The National Visit*, London, The Sainsbury Centre for Mental Health.

Moore, E. and Kuipers, E. (1992) 'Behavioural correlates of expressed emotion in staff-patient interactions', *Social Psychiatry and Psychiatric Epidemiology*, 27, 28–34.

Moore, E., Ball, R. and Kuipers, L. (1992) 'Expressed Emotion in Staff Working with the Long-term Adult Mentally Ill', *British Journal Psychiatry*, 161, 802–8.

Nuechterlein, K.H. and Dawson, M. (1984) 'A heurisitic vulnerability-stress model of schizophrenic episodes', *Schizophrenia Bulletin*, 10(2), 300–12.

Rogers, A., Pilgrim, D. and Lacey, R. (1993) *Experiencing Psychiatry: Users' views of services*, London: Macmillan, in association with MIND Publications.

Snyder, K., Wallace, C., Moe, K. and Liberman, R. (1994) 'Expressed emotion by residential care operators and residents symptoms and quality of life', *Hospital and Community Psychiatry*, 45, 1141–3.

Standing Nursing and Midwifery Advisory Committee (SNMAC) (1999) *Mental Health Nursing: Addressing Acute Concerns*, London, The Stationery Office.

Tarrier, N. (1999) *The SOCRATES study*, Presentation to the Third International Conference on Psychological Treatments for Schizophrenia, Oxford.

Zubin, J. and Spring, B. (1977) 'Vulnerability: a new view of schizophrenia', *Journal of Abnormal psychology*, 86, 103–26.

Part V

Changing Service – Keeping Going

CHAPTER 17

Involving Service Users

RACHEL PERKINS

Introduction

The involvement of users in mental health services is now a requirement of government policy (Box 17.1) but such 'user involvement' cannot simply be viewed as an 'add-on' to existing ways of working. It involves significant changes in attitudes and practice at all levels:

- *Individual*: user participation at a direct care level in the planning and delivery of individual care, treatment and support.
- *Operational*: user involvement in determining the practices and operation of individual teams, units and services.
- *Strategic*: involvement of the recipients of services in strategic planning and the development of services.

Most providers now make a commitment to involving service users – working in partnership with the recipients of their services – and opportunities for user participation have undoubtedly increased. Yet there remains a gap between rhetoric and reality at all levels. Many service users continue to express doubts about the willingness of mental health services to give users

---

Box 17.1 Government policy and service users

'Patients, service users and carers will be involved in their own care and in planning services.'

(*Modernising Mental Health Services: Safe, Sound and Supportive*, DoH, 1998, p. 7)

People with mental health problems can expect that services will: involve service users and their carers in planning and delivery of care.'

(*National Service Framework for Mental Health*, DoH, 1999, p. 4)

'Services will . . . involve users and carers in planning developments . . .'.

(*Modernising the Care Programme Approach*, DoH, 2000, p. 2)

237

decision-making powers (Campbell, 1997). And such concerns are reinforced by the results of a number of studies. Bowl (1996) found

> Considerable confusion about the meaning and purpose of involvement, little evidence of power-sharing with users and limited commitment of resources to make further participation possible. (p. 302)

Onyett *et al.* (1994) found that only 8 per cent of Community Mental Health Teams involved service users in a decision-making capacity in the operation of the service. Perkins and Fisher's (1996) audit reinforces doubts about the extent of user involvement in care plans.

Barker and Peck (1996) have described a continuum of user involvement running from the passive feeding into the agendas of others to actively pursuing their own agenda. Most mental health services remain at the level of passive end of this continuum.

The aim of this chapter is to review the history and present state of user involvement in mental health services; some literature about what users want from these services; barriers to effective involvement; and challenges facing professionals in dismantling them.

Ten Miles Behind Us and Ten Thousand More to Go: The Development of User Involvement in Mental Health Services

The consumerism which permeated the National Health Service in the 1980s resulted in increased attention to the voices of recipients of mental health services. With actual or quasi 'internal markets' introduced into UK public services, 'the consumer' was accorded much greater influence:

> Such approaches were intended to lead to greater choice, more responsiveness to complaints and service developments based on consumers' wishes. (Barker and Peck, 1996, p. 5)

Shortly before Alan Langlands became Chief Executive of the NHS he told the Health Select Committee of Enquiry into Mental Health Services that 'We are listening to carers and users, the people whom we think know best about services' (Health Select Committee, 1993).

Although 'Survivors Speak Out' and the 'UK Advocacy Network' were founded in the mid 1980s, it would be a mistake to assume that 'user involvement' was simply a creation of NHS consumerism (Campbell, 1996a). The user activism which developed in the context of the USA civil rights movement in the 1970s (following the lead of black, women's, gay/lesbian groups) is described in Judi Chamberlin's ground breaking work *On Our Own*

(Chamberlin, 1997). Although this book was not published in the UK until 1988, the UK Mental Patients Union was active in the 1970s and from the early 1980s there existed campaigning groups such as the British Networks for Alternatives to Psychiatry and the Campaign Against Psychiatric Oppression. However, the history of protest by people designated as 'mad' stretches back to the second half of the nineteenth century (Campbell, 1996a; Sayce, 2000) with the Alleged Lunatics' Friend Society and the work of early feminists – such as Georgina Weldon in her book *How I Escaped the Mad Doctor* and Rosina Bulwer-Lytton in the *The Bastilles of England; or, The Lunacy Laws at Work* (cited in Showalter, 1985, p. 126) – who critiqued the role of psychiatry as a powerful means of social control.

Within service user movements two distinct trends can be distinguished (Perkins and Repper, 1998):

- A radical, anti-psychiatry movement that is concerned with the right to reject psychiatric services and provide user-run, user controlled alternatives outside the existing psychiatric enterprise.
- A reformist user/consumer movement that focuses on improving within existing psychiatric services and campaigning for more involvement and control within these.

Both are important. While most people with mental health problems come into contact with mainstream services, work to improve these is important. But, when users become involved in existing services, they become bound up with traditional models and practices. It is difficult, if not impossible, to both work within existing services and simultaneously sustain the independent and critical stance that may be necessary to bring about more substantial changes. A separate, radical movement is important in providing the independent critique of services and develop innovative alternatives.

The change in political climate of the mid 1980s enabled the small independent action groups of users and survivors, especially those with a less confrontational/separatist approach, to flourish and grow into thousands strong national, regional and global networks (Campbell, 1996a). Users/survivors have been involved in service planning both locally and nationally with, for example, the Department of Health's Mental Health Task Force and in the External Reference Group on whose work the *National Service Framework for Mental Health* (DoH, 1999) was based. Numerous 'community' groups and 'users forums' exist within individual services. Various methods have been developed for enabling service users to take a more active role in the planning of their own care. Alan Leader's *Direct Power* (1995) is 'A resource pack for people who want to develop their own care plans and support networks' (p. 1).

The *Avon Measure* (Avon Measure Working Group, 1996), was developed to help service users to 'Assess your own strengths, wants and needs. Express your views to mental health workers. Have more control over the help you receive' (p. 1). *CUES* (Carers' and Users' Expectations of Services; NSF, 2000) reflects issues defined as important by service users and is designed to help them to become more involved in individual care planning and evaluation over time.

There are UK mental health services where recipients of mental health services are employed as workers in clinical teams (Perkins *et al.*, 1997; Perkins, 1998) and as consultants. Users are involved in staff selection and training (NHS Executive Mental Health Task Force, 1994; Sainsbury Centre for Mental Health, 1997), in research (e.g. Rose, 1996; Faulkner and Layzell, 2000) and service monitoring/evaluation (e.g. East Yorkshire Monitoring Team, 1997; Rose *et al.*, 1998). Chamberlin's (1997) idea of creating user-run alternatives to mainstream psychiatric services has been realised in numerous user-led projects within the United States and to a lesser extent in the United Kingdom (Lindow, 1994; Barker and Peck, 1996).

Despite these developments, the majority of 'user involvement' remains essentially 'tokenistic': rarely do users have the power to significantly influence the development of services or their own care and support within them. For example:

- Users may be given copies of their care plans and asked to sign them, but they typically have little control over their content which remains largely determined by professionals.
- Many 'community meetings' or 'users forums' within mental health teams/facilities do little more than decide upon the destination for the next 'outing' or provide a forum for staff to explain why they cannot or will not respond to the requests of service users.
- The one or two 'user representatives' in planning meetings full of senior professionals, managers and purchasers typically have to operate within the agenda and priorities set by these service providers. Typically, they are ill placed to 'represent' other service users because little attention has been paid to ensuring that resources are available to support parallel independent user groups who can inform their contributions. As user/survivor Edna Conlan (1996) describes:

There are times when, as someone . . . trying to work within mental health services to empower service users, I feel as though I am shaking hands with the devil. This feeling tends to be strongest when I find myself sitting on a high powered committee which is intent on sending out signals that the mere presence of people using services is evidence of its goodwill and obvious commitment to delivering user-centred services. (p. 207)

While the credibility and respectability of users in services may have increased, there has been little increase in choice in the use of services and control over treatments received (Campbell, 1996a).

What Users Want From Mental Health Services

A century of mental health service user action has provided accounts of the things that people want from mental health services. Back in the late 1800s, the Alleged Lunatics Friend Society believed that 'Each patient should have a voice in his or her own confinement and care, and access to legal representation' (cited in Sayce, 2000, p. 25).

As Sayce (2000) points out, the language may have changed, but the demands have not radically changed – a reflection of the limited progress that has been made in the intervening one hundred years.

Read (1996) draws on the numerous more recent service user accounts (e.g. Rogers *et al.*, 1993; Tanzman, 1993; Lindow, 1996; Campbell, 1996b) to describe the eight things that service users most want from mental health services:

- *Information.* Without full information, meaningful choice and involvement is impossible. Most of all, users want information on the effects and side-effects of medication, alternatives to medication, the range of supports and services available, and rights, especially those to receive or refuse treatment. But if people are given information about treatments and services, they may wish to use them, and this challenges professionals' power to decide what is 'best' for 'their' patients (Perkins and Repper, 1998).
- *Choice.* 'Someone who can't sleep may benefit from yoga, sleeping pills, meditation or counselling, but which of those do mental health workers offer? . . . Above all, time and time again, people say that the choice that is missing is someone to talk to' (p. 176).
- *Accessibility.* People want services which are near their homes and that are open when they need them. 'Mental health crises do not conveniently occur between 9.00 and 5.00, and for us, Christmas can be the loneliest time' (p. 176).
- *Advocacy.* 'Generally, service users are scared of mental health workers. Professionals might not feel very intimidating but there's something about the relationship that we have with you . . . It's not easy for us to say . . . what we want . . . especially if we fear that what we want to say is not what the mental health workers want to hear' (p. 176). Advocacy is the process through which individuals and groups express their own rights and concerns (Sang and O'Brien, 1984), and four types of advocacy have been described (Bingley, 1990; Perkins and Repper, 1998):
  - ○ Self advocacy where people represent their own interests and concerns.
  - ○ Peer advocacy where someone who has experienced similar problems assists the person to represent their interests and concerns.
  - ○ Citizen advocacy where a lay volunteer represents someone's interests as if they were their own.
  - ○ Professional advocacy where lawyers or other trained professional assist people in defending their rights.

The National Service Framework for Mental Health (DoH, 1999) says that services must ensure that users have access to advocacy. In involving service users in decisions about their own care, the aim must be to enable people to speak for themselves. When they have difficulty in doing this, people who have experienced similar difficulties and situations – other service users in the form of peer advocates – are probably in the best position to assist them to express themselves. Such self and peer advocacy has been developed and promoted by the UK Advocacy Network: a user-run network which provides training, advice and support in independent, individual, peer advocacy as well as group advocacy (through the development of, for example, user-run patients councils, Conlan *et al.*, 1994). Leader and Crosby (1998), in their resource pack of the development of peer advocacy programmes, argue that these have an important role to play in improving partnerships between service users and mental health workers.

To be effective, advocacy must be independent of the services to which the individual must represent their interests and concerns: mental health workers cannot act as advocates within mental health services. Other professional advocates, such as lawyers and welfare rights experts, may be necessary in assisting people to defend their legal rights.

- *Equal opportunities.* Race, gender, lesbian/gay, class, age . . . all of these are important: people want access to those who will understand their experiences as well as privacy, security and freedom from harassment.
- *Income and employment.* 'Please do close down the big institutions but don't dump us in special needs ghettos where we go to day centres . . .' (p. 177). Despite evidence that, with appropriate support, around 50 per cent of people with serious ongoing mental health problems can successfully gain and maintain open employment (Bond *et al.*, 1997) professionals typically remain pessimistic about employment prospects (Chapter 12). A recent survey indicates that some 44 per cent of people with mental health problems who *have* jobs had been told by mental health workers that they would never work again (Rinaldi, 2000).
- *Self-help.* 'This is not about mental health services on the cheap – it's about unleashing our desires and abilities to support one another and to come up with new and imaginative solutions' (p. 178). For example, the Hearing Voices Network enables voice hearers to share experiences, explanations and ways of coping and benefit from mutual support.
- *Self-organisation.* 'Service users have a lot to contribute to the design and implementation of services, but our experience, knowledge and abilities remain locked away unless we have opportunities to meet together to find common ground and to think about what we really want and how to go about getting it. For that, properly funded and supported patients' councils, local service users' forums and national networks are needed' (p. 178).

Cutting across all of these *respect* is paramount. A continuing lack of respect can be seen in the continued existence of 'separates': 'staff only' toilets, cutlery, crockery . . . Can there be anything more degrading than being 'unfit' to use the same toilet as staff? And if the toilets are not clean enough for staff to use them, how can these staff be fulfilling their duty of care by allowing clients to use them?

'They never listen' is one of the most persistent complaints from service users (Lindow, 1996). The words of service users are too often heard only in order to diagnose.

> I can talk, but I may not be heard. I can make suggestions, but they may not be taken seriously. I can voice my thoughts, but they may be seen as delusions. I can recite my experiences, but they may be interpreted as fantasies. To be an ex-patient or even an ex-client is to be discounted. (Leete, 1988, p. 1)

If mental health professionals cannot accord recipients of their services the respect of listening to, hearing and taking seriously what they say then user involvement, at any level, is impossible.

Seen But Not Heard: Barriers to Participation

Among the many 'stakeholders' involved in the mental health enterprise, the people who themselves have mental health problems – the recipients of mental health services – remain the least powerful. Although many professional groups may feel powerless, such powerlessness is relative.

> The psychiatric system is founded on inequality. By and large, the user is at the bottom of the pile. Our unequal position is symbolised by the compulsory element in psychiatric care . . . the fact of its existence has repercussions for all service users, and these must be recognised. That an individual can be compelled to receive psychiatric treatment affects each patient regardless of whether his [or her] stay is formal or informal. It is hardly possible to be unaware that you are being cared for within a legal framework which allows for treatment against your will. (Campbell, 1996c, p. 59)

Clearly, mental health legislation underpins power relationships within services, and the implications of this cannot be ignored. However, there are other ways in which this power imbalance is maintained.

Ridgeway (1988) argues that the reasons why users' perspectives are often ignored lies at the level of basic attitudes: the pervasive presumption within and outside mental health services that incompetence inevitably accompanies the label of mental illness (Chamberlin, 1977; Leete, 1988). Such assumptions of incompetence not only underpin mental health legislation, but also many day to day practices within services.

Nowhere is the assumption of incompetence more pronounced than in relation to those with a diagnosis of schizophrenia.

Assuming that someone with schizophrenia is capable of making intelligent decisions about his or her own needs is like assuming that a person with heart disease has normal cardiac function and can run a marathon. (Torrey, 1986, p. 95)

Although there are probably few mental health workers who would actually admit to sharing this psychiatrist's extreme perspective, the assumption of diminished ability to make, and take responsibility for, decisions is widespread.

Assumptions of incompetence mean that, if a person has a mental health problem, their views, beliefs and ideas are cast into doubt and the idea that other people may speak for them is endorsed. Mental health workers see their role as acting as some kind of 'benevolent parent' and 'surrogate decision maker' for the 'poor unfortunates' who cannot make decisions for themselves.

Based on such assumptions, there are a variety ways in which the views of service users are routinely disregarded which operate at all levels: individual, operational and strategic (Perkins, 1996; Perkins and Repper, 1998).

Dismissing what service users say as a manifestation of their psychopathology is very powerful, and it is not restricted to psychiatrists and 'medical models'. All the major mental health professions have developed theories – organic, psychological, psychoanalytic, behavioural, systemic – through which the utterances of people with mental health problems are interpreted. When a person says something, such models give the professional carte blanche to interpret what the person *really* means and therefore what they *really* need. Any real involvement is impossible if professionals accord themselves the power to interpret what people mean in this way.

This process is bolstered by the concept of 'insight' on which mental health workers have long relied (Lewis, 1934; David, 1990). Basically, a person is deemed to have insight if they agree with the professional about the existence, nature and treatment of their malaise. If someone's views do not accord with those of the professional then they are all too often deemed to 'lack insight' and their views can therefore be legitimately disregarded. Concepts of insight are extremely prevalent in relation to those with 'psychotic' diagnoses, especially schizophrenia and 'lack of insight' is frequently cited as a justification for compulsory treatment.

The concept of insight – perhaps lack of insight would be most appropriate from the psychiatric perspective – is one of the most powerful and insidious forces eroding our position as competent, creative individuals. (Campbell, 1996c, p. 57)

Participation and involvement is impossible if dissent is viewed as pathology.

You don't understand. (. . . we who are in possession of the full facts must therefore make a decision for you)

It is often implicitly assumed that if a service user does not agree with professionals then they must lack the information necessary to reach the 'correct' conclusion.

When mental health workers give information to clients it is often prompted by their decision to do something with which the professional does not approve. For example, when someone refuses to take their medication, it is common for the mental health worker to respond by giving them a great deal of information about the benefits of that medication. This information is given with the intention of persuading them to comply with treatment. The same might apply when a person refuses to go to occupational therapy, or to see the psychologist, or to answer the door to the CPN.

It is often assumed that if the person were really in possession of the full 'facts' then they would inevitably reach the same conclusion as the professional. This makes a nonsense of the idea of 'informed choice' as the only choice which is deemed to be 'informed' becomes that which the professional prescribes. The possibility is rarely entertained that the person may have reviewed the evidence and reached a different conclusion, or that they may have access to evidence (the expertise of personal experience) that is not available to the professional.

Participation and involvement is impossible if dissent is viewed as ignorance.

> You cannot agree with each other, so we don't know who to believe. (. . . we will therefore do what we think is best for you)

or

> You don't represent all service users. (. . . we will therefore do what the ones who agree with us say)

A diversity of beliefs, politics, interests, backgrounds and experiences exists among service users, just as it does among service professionals and the population as a whole. The diversity of professional perspectives is seen as one of the strengths of multidisciplinary working. However, a similar diversity among service users is often viewed as a problem, or used as a way of dismissing what is said (Crepaz-Keay, 1996) rather than seeing it as a rich pool of wisdom that can be tapped to ensure that the necessary range of services and approaches is available.

It is true that some service users – like women, lesbians, gay men, people from minority racial and ethnic groups, those whose problems make it less easy for them to express their opinions – find it less easy to get their views heard. This is a challenge in achieving genuine and comprehensive user involvement in services.

Participation and involvement is impossible if dissent is discounted as 'unrepresentative'.

> We haven't got the resources. (. . . therefore we have to carry on as we have been doing)

Providing the services requested by users is often seen as the 'icing on the cake': something to be done if there are resources left after 'core' services (as defined by professionals) have been provided.

Resource constraints are ever present within mental health services, but the allocation of scarce resources is not some 'given': it involves some hard political decisions. It would be possible to prioritise the wishes of service users and to *stop* doing something that professionals thought was important: close some acute beds and provide a non-hospital crisis house, or reduce the number of professional posts in order to provide a peer advocacy service, for example.

Participation and involvement are impossible if users' wishes are always seen as 'optional extras'.

As well as simple disbelief, there are several ways in which the views of those with mental health problems are routinely marginalised within services (Perkins, 1996). These include:

- *Humouring*. Listening politely to what a person says and taking no notice of it: 'Yes dear, how interesting'.
- *Limiting information*. Presenting the person with only partial information or giving information in an indigestible and incomprehensible manner.
- *Limiting choice*. As well as limiting information about the options available, this can include making one thing contingent on another. Choice is severely limited if, for example, a person may only live in a particular place if they take their medication, or have lunch at a day centre if they attend a group. A person's choice may also be constrained if support is withdrawn if they choose something of which the professional does not approve: 'You can do that if you want, but I won't help you if you do'. Clearly there are limits to the behaviours which a professional can support: killing oneself or robbing a bank would clearly fall outside this. But professionals attempts to control often denies people support in taking many ordinary risks – like trying to get a job or live independently. The concept of choice is only meaningful if the person has the right, and necessary support, to make choices that professionals may consider 'wrong'.
- *Verbal persuasion*. The power of articulate argument against requests or choices that a person has made is sometimes graced with the term 'counselling' but is frequently more akin to bullying. Luckstead and Coursey (1995) found that 58 per cent of service users reported having been pressured into taking some form of treatment or therapy against their better judgement, and that the most common type of force used was verbal persuasion.

Beyond Altruism: The Challenge For Professionals

Involving service users is not an act of altruism: a benevolent 'empowering' of the 'disempowered'. Users have expertise that most professionals lack (unless they have used mental health services themselves): what it is like to experience mental health problems, face the challenge of life with such difficulties, and be on the receiving end of services. This 'expertise of experience' is essential if we are to create accessible, acceptable and effective mental health services.

If the rhetoric of user involvement and participation is to become a reality, then mental health workers have to value and heed what the recipients of their services have to say at all levels: from individual care planning, through the operation of teams and services, to the strategic planning and service development. It is easy to involve someone when they agree with you. The real challenge involves changing the balance of power within mental health services and acceding to users wishes when they are at odds with professional judgements.

Moving away from a model where expert professionals tell patients what to do hits at the very heart of what has traditionally been regarded as 'professionalism'.

The ubiquitous assumption that 'the professional knows best' is probably the greatest impediment to effective user participation and joint working. Such assumptions are based on the belief that the professional has access to a specialised body of knowledge that is not accessible to, and cannot be understood by, non-professionals (Greenwood, 1957). If this is the case then 'involving service users' is reduced to persuading them that the professional knows what is best for them.

Such beliefs about the nature of professional expertise not only prevent professionals heeding what users have to say when it differs from their views, they also result in 'victim blaming' when what the professional has to offer is ineffective or rejected.

When professionals are faced with demands for assistance they feel inadequate to meet, or when their viewpoint or service offerings are rejected, they blame the person's 'lack of insight', 'poor motivation' or other character flaws, rather than seeing it as their own inability to understand or respond to the client's life experience. (Ridgeway, 1988, p. 4)

Increasing numbers of service users are recognising the limitations of professional expertise:

Ex-patients . . . are beginning to turn to each other rather than to mental health professionals for emotional and instrumental support. They are finding that people with experiential knowledge (i.e. having learned through personal experience) are more able to understand their needs than are professionals who have learned through education and training. Moreover, they are finding the support and help they can give each other to be as valuable – or sometimes more valuable – than the interventions of trained professionals. (Wilson Besio, 1987, p. 1)

Conclusion

The expertise of experience is essential to the development of effective mental health services, and this expertise cannot be tapped without effective user participation. No real involvement or partnership is possible without mutual respect and an acknowledgement of the expertise possessed by both parties. This can only become a reality if our view of professionalism changes.

It is not the case that professionals lack skills and expertise, rather that we do not have a monopoly on wisdom and we do not always know best. Perhaps the real challenge is moving towards a position where professionals put their expertise at the disposal of service users, rather than making decisions for them and doing unto them.

Further Reading

Campbell, P. (1996) 'The history of the user movement', in T. Heller, J. Reynolds, R. Gomm, R. Muston and S. Pattison (eds), *Mental Health Matters*, London, Macmillan.
Faulkner, A. and Layzell, S. (2000) *Strategies for Living: A Report of User-Led Research into People's Strategies for Living with Mental Distress*, London, The Mental Health Foundation.
Leader, A. and Crosby, K. (1998) *Power Tools. A Resource Pack for those Committed to the Development of Mental Health Advocacy into the Millennium*, Brighton, Pavilion Publishing.
Perkins, R.E., Buckfield, R. and Choy, D. (1997) 'Access to employment: A supported employment project to enable mental health service users to obtain jobs within mental health teams', *Journal of Mental Health*, 6, 307–18.

References

Avon Measure Working Group (1996) *The Avon Mental Health Measure. A User Centred Approach to Assessing Need*, London, MIND Publications.
Barker, I. and Peck, E. (1996) User empowerment – a decade of experience, *Mental Health review*, 1(4), 5–13.
Bingley, W. (1990) *An Introduction to Advocacy*, London, Good Practices in Mental Health Information Pack.
Bond, G.R., Drake, R.E. and Meuser, K.T. *et al.* (1997) 'An update on supported employment for people with severe mental illness', *Psychiatric Services*, 48, 335–46.

Bowl, R. (1996) 'Involving service users in mental health services: Social services departments and the NHS and Community Care Act 1990', *Journal of Mental Health*, 5, 287–303.

Campbell, P. (1996) The history of the user movement, in T. Heller, J. Reynolds, R. Gomm, R. Muston and S. Pattison (eds), *Mental Health Matters*, London, Macmillan.

Campbell, P. (1996b) 'What we want from crisis services', in J. Read and J. Reynolds (eds), *Speaking Our Minds*, Milton Keynes, Open University Press.

Campbell, P. (1996c) 'Challenging loss of power', in J. Read and J. Reynolds (eds), *Speaking Our Minds*, Milton Keynes, Open University Press.

Campbell, P. (1997) 'Citizen Smith', *Nursing Times*, 93, 31–2.

Chamberlin, J. (1997) *On Our Own*, New York, McGraw-Hill.

Conlan, E. (1996) 'Shaking hands with the devil', in J. Read and J. Reynolds (eds), *Speaking Our Minds*, Milton Keynes, Open University Press.

Conlan, E., Gell, C. and Graley, R. *et al.* (1994) *User group Advocacy: A Code of Practice*, London, Department of Health Mental Health Task Force.

Crepaz-Keay, D. (1996) 'Who do you represent?', in J. Read and J. Reynolds (eds), *Speaking Our Minds*, Milton Keynes, Open University Press.

David, A. (1990) 'Insight and psychosis', *British Journal of Psychiatry*, 156, 798–808.

Department of Health (1998) *Modernising Mental Health Services: Safe, Sound and Supportive*, London, The Stationery Office.

Department of Health (1999) *National Service Framework for Mental Health*, London, Department of Health.

Department of Health (2000) *Effective Care Co-ordination in Mental Health Services: Modernising the Care Programme Approach*, London, Department of Health.

East Yorkshire Monitoring Team (1997) *Monitoring Our Services Ourselves: User-led Monitoring of Mental Health Services*, Beverley, East Yorkshire Monitoring Team.

Faulkner, A. and Layzell, S. (2000) *Strategies for Living: A Report of User-Led Research into People's Strategies for Living with Mental Distress*, London, The Mental Health Foundation.

Greenwood, E. (1957) 'The Attributes of a Profession', *Social Work*, 2, 45–55.

Health Select Committee (1993) *Report of the Inquiry Into Mental Illness Services*, London, HMSO.

Leader, A. (1995) *Direct Power*, Brighton, Pavilion Publishing.

Leader, A. and Crosby, K. (1998) *Power Tools. A Resource Pack for those Committed to the Development of Mental Health Advocacy into the Millennium*, Brighton, Pavilion Publishing.

Leete, E. (1988) *The Role of The Consumer Movement and the Persons with Mental Illness*; Presentation at the 12th Mary Switzer Memorial Seminar in Rehabilitation, Washington, DC, 15–16 June.

Lewis, A. (1934) 'The Psychopathology of Insight', *British Journal of Medical Psychology*, 14, 332–48.

Lindow, V. (1994) *Purchasing Mental Health Services: Self-help Alternatives*, London, MIND Publications.

Lindow, V. (1996) 'What we want from community psychiatric nurses', in J. Read and J. Reynolds (eds), *Speaking Our Minds*, Milton Keynes, Open University Press.

Luckstead, A. and Coursey, R.D. (1995) 'Consumer perceptions of pressure and force in psychiatric treatment', *Hospital and Community Psychiatry*, 26, 146–52.

NHS Executive Mental Health Task Force (1994) *Building on Experience: A Training Pack for Mental Health Service Users Working as Trainers, Speakers and Workshop Facilitators*, London, NHSE.

National Schizophrenia Fellowship (in conjunction with Royal College of Psychiatrists Research Unit, Royal College of Nursing Research Institute and University of East Anglia Department of Social Work) (2000) *CUES – Service User Version*, London, National Schizophrenia Fellowship.

Onyett, S.R., Heppleston, T. and Bushnell, D. (1994) 'A national survey of community mental health teams', *Journal of Mental Health*, 3, 175–94.

Perkins, R.E. (1996) 'Seen but not heard: Can 'user involvement' become more than empty rhetoric?', *The Mental Health Review*, 1, 16–20.

Perkins, R.E., Buckfield, R. and Choy, D. (1997) 'Access to employment: A supported employment project to enable mental health service users to obtain jobs within mental health teams', *Journal of Mental Health*, 6, 307–18.

Perkins, R.E. and Fisher, N.R. (1996) Beyond mere existence: The auditing of care plans, *Journal of Mental Health*, 5, 275–86.

Perkins, R.E. and Repper, J.M. (1998) *Dilemmas in Community Mental Health Practice: Choice or Control*. Oxford, Radliffe Medical Press.

Perkins, R.E. (1998) 'An act to follow?', *A Life in the Day*, 2, 15–20.

Read, J. (1996) 'What We Want From Mental Health Services', in J. Read and J. Reynolds (eds), *Speaking Our Minds*, Milton Keynes, Open University Press.

Ridgeway, P. (1988) *The Voice of Consumers in Mental Health Systems: A Call for Change*, Burlington, VT, Center for Community Change Through Housing and Support.

Rinaldi, M. (2000) personal communication concerning a survey conducted by Merton Mind.

Rogers, A., Pilgrim, D. and Lacey, R. (1993) *Experiencing Psychiatry: Users' Views of Services*, Basingstoke, Macmillan.

Rose, D. (1996) *Living in the Community*, London, Sainsbury Centre for Mental Health.

Sainsbury Centre for Mental Health (1997) *Pulling Together: The Future Roles and Training of Mental Health Staff*, London: Sainsbury Centre for Mental Health.

Sang, B. and O'Brien, J. (1984) *Advocacy: The UK and American Experience*, London, King's Fund.

Sayce, L. (2000) *From Psychiatric Patient to Citizen: Overcoming Discrimination and Social Exclusion*, London, Macmillan.

Showalter, E. (1985) *The Female Malady: Women, Madness and English Culture 1830–1980*, London, Virago.

Tanzman, B. (1993) 'An overview of surveys of mental health consumers' preferences for housing and support services', *Hospital and Community Psychiatry*, 44, 5.

Torrey, E.F. (1986) 'Finally, a cure for homelessness: but it takes some strong medicine', *Washington Monthly*, 10, 95–7.

Wilson Besio, S. (1987) *The Role of Ex-Patients and Consumers in Human Resource Development for the 1990s*, Burlington, VT, Center for Community Change Through Housing and Support.

CHAPTER 18

Training and Clinical Supervision

TIM BRADSHAW

Introduction

It was not until the early 1990s that psychosocial intervention (PSI) training courses began to be developed which were accessible to mental health staff who worked in routine practice settings. These courses were welcomed by clinicians eager to increase their clinical skills and become more effective in their work with seriously mentally ill (SMI) people. In addition to this enthusiasm from the professions there were also calls from policy-makers to make this training in evidence based practice more widely available (Onyett, *et al*. 1995; Department of Health, 1994, 1996, 1999). In order to meet the demand for training many new PSI courses have been established around the UK with a total of 32 courses at diploma level or above being identified in a recent survey (Brooker and Evans, 1998).

Training is now more accessible than ever before, however, prospective students will be keen to ensure that the course they enroll with is going to develop their skills and make them more effective in their practice. This chapter is written with the needs of these prospective students in mind and aims to provide them with information that will assist them to make an informed decision about where to study. In order to achieve this aim a brief review of the history of PSI training in the UK will be provided together with evidence regarding the effectiveness of this training. This will be followed by an analysis of what the key ingredients of these successful courses are and a description of the approaches that have been developed for teaching and supervising trainees.

Background

A large number of randomised controlled trials have demonstrated the benefits of providing interventions to the families of patients (Chapter 11), and more recent studies have shown the benefits of individual psychological therapy to patients with this diagnosis (Chapters 7, 8, 9 and 10). Therapists who carried out clinical work in these carefully controlled research trials were given specific training in the use of psychosocial interventions and their work was closely supervised. Until recently similar training was not accessible to staff working in routine healthcare settings, consequently these types of interventions have not been widely available to patients and their families as part of their standard care.

The first report of a PSI training programme developed for staff working in a routine service setting was by Tarrier *et al.* (1988a). The training aimed to teach a group of social workers a cognitive behavioural approach to family intervention which had been developed and piloted with families in an earlier research study (Tarrier *et al.*, 1988b, 1989). Although this training programme was not formally evaluated, the authors suggest that written feedback from the trainees was positive and the trainees felt the families had benefited from receiving the intervention.

Further training programmes were organised in Manchester in the late 1980s, this time the target group for training were community psychiatric nurses (Brooker *et al.*, 1992, 1994). Within the context of a research study, Brooker and his colleagues ran two training courses for CPNs who were working in a range of NHS services in the north of England. Evaluation of the training showed that the patients of the trainees worked with using PSI had reductions in the severity of their symptoms and improvements in their social functioning compared to standard care. Also, the family members who cared for them showed reductions in minor psychiatric morbidity associated with the burden of caring, and increased satisfaction with the services that they received. The findings of these studies suggested that mental health staff working in routine NHS settings could achieve superior outcomes of care for patients who suffered from schizophrenia using PSI compared to standard care (Brooker *et al.*, 1992, 1994).

Around the same time as Brooker's study, another group of workers, led by psychiatrist Julian Leff at the Institute of Psychiatry in London, were also developing and evaluating PSI training programmes for nurses (Lam *et al.*, 1993; Gamble *et al.*, 1994). These courses were based on a model of family intervention that had been developed and successfully tested by Leff and colleagues in two randomised controlled trials (Leff *et al.*, 1982, 1985, 1989, 1990). The courses were evaluated by assessing the effects that the training had on the trainee's knowledge about schizophrenia and their attitudes towards sufferers and their families. The results showed that the trainees made significant gains in their knowledge and attitudes from the start of the training to the end of the course and that these gains were maintained after nine months, during which time the trainees had continued to receive supervision with their clinical work.

In 1991, workers from Manchester and London decided to collaborate to develop a two-centred training programme, which would build on their combined experience of providing training in this area. The programme, named the 'Thorn Initiative', aimed to train nurses and from 1994 other mental health professionals, to work more effectively with seriously mentally ill people and their families (Gamble, 1995). The training course was organised in three modules, case management, psychological management of psychotic symptoms and family intervention, and was evaluated in three ways. First, the impact of the trainees' interventions on the symptoms and social functioning of the patients that they worked with was assessed. Second, changes in the trainees' knowledge about SMI and their attitudes towards patients and their families were assessed, and third, changes in the trainees' clinical skills were evaluated. The results of the evaluation showed that the trainees knowledge, attitudes and clinical skills were all improved and that the patients that they worked with demonstrated better clinical and social outcomes than would normally be expected with routine NHS care (Lancashire *et al.*, 1997a, 1997b).

In summary, the literature suggests that mental health professionals who are suitably trained in the systematic application of PSI are more clinically effective in their work with people with SMI and their carers, than staff who are not trained in these approaches (Brooker *et al.*, 1992). In response to these findings many new PSI courses have been developed across the UK during the 1990s. However, as highlighted earlier, it is essential that along with the rapid growth of new courses, that the quality of the training is maintained. The next part of this chapter describes the elements of effective PSI courses that prospective students should look for when choosing where to undertake their studies.

Components of Effective Training Courses

Box 18.1. provides a summary of the elements that were common to the successful PSI training courses. The way in which these courses organised training and clinical supervision to facilitate optimum development of their student's clinical skills will now be discussed.

Characteristics of Trainers

It is important that trainers who are responsible for delivering PSI training are clinicians who are experienced in the field of SMI work. While a theoretical understanding of the principles of PSI can be gained by reading appropriate literature, knowledge of how the interventions are applied in practice can only be achieved through experience. Trainers should possess advanced levels of clinical skill in PSI and remain actively involved in clinical work. If the trainers do not possess these attributes then it is likely to reduce their ability to develop good levels of clinical skills in their students.

The course team should preferably be multidisciplinary in nature and have input from other stakeholders of mental health services, ideally this should include users of mental health services and those who care for them. This is important to ensure that the beliefs and philosophies of those involved in planning and delivering mental health services, are those shared by the team who plan and teach the training course. Additionally, as with clinical teams, having members of more than one discipline increases the range of skills and expertise available in the delivery of the programme.

Box 18.1   Elements of effective PSI training courses

1. Tutors are skilled and experienced clinicians who remain clinically active.
2. Trainees undertake clinical work with patients using PSI approaches while training.
3. Structured clinical supervision of the students work with patients is provided.
4. Clinical skills are assessed and feedback and coaching is provided.
5. The stress-vulnerability model of schizophrenia (see Chapter 1) underpins all interventions that are taught.
6. The course team is multidisciplinary in nature and includes input from service users and carers to both the planning and the delivery of the programme.
7. The issue of implementation of PSI in services is addressed.
8. Training is evidence based.
9. Content includes engaging service users, completing a comprehensive assessment of their needs and developing collaborative formulations for problem areas.
10. Number of hours is sufficient to address the aims of the curriculum.
11. Teaching and learning strategies include participatory exercises and particularly role-play.

Prospective students of PSI courses are advised to inquire about the backgrounds and experience of trainers who are involved in teaching the course. They should find out which disciplines they come from, what post-basic training they have undertaken, what experience they have of working with people suffering from SMI and whether they continue to be actively involved in clinical work.

Course Content

The amount of information provided to students on training courses should relate to the length of the course and the learning objectives that the course leaders aim to achieve. For instance it is unlikely that a two-day PSI workshop will lead to the development of a high level of clinical skill, however it could reasonably be expected to introduce those who attend to the principles of PSI and the models which underpin practice. Whereas more lengthy courses may aim to provide students with a broad knowledge base about PSI and develop their skills in each of the main areas of practice (see Box 18.2). Alternatively they may focus on the development of a high level of skill in a particular area

Box 18.2 Appropriate course content for comprehensive PSI training courses

Core course content

- The stress-vulnerability model
- Definitions of SMI
- Aetiological models of SMI
- Psychiatric symptoms and syndromes; diagnoses and their implications
- Engaging service users
- Use of standardised assessment tools when assessing the needs of people with SMI
- Risk assessment and management
- Neuroleptic medication and its effective management in the treatment of SMI
- Ethical aspects of practice

Services and the SMI

- Government policy and SMI
- Models of case management
- Assertive outreach
- Users views of services
- How to involve users in services
- Homelessness and SMI
- The criminal justice system and SMI
- Working effectively in multidisciplinary teams
- Multi-agency working
- Developing effective services for the SMI

Social interventions

- Social support networks in SMI
- Using assessment data in problem identification and care planning
- Effects of employment and other daytime activity on outcomes in SMI
- Creating accepting communities and preventing social exclusion

Psychological interventions

- Cognitive behavioural approaches to treating medication resistant symptoms
- Cognitive deficits in SMI
- Treating negative symptoms in SMI
- Prodromal signs monitoring and relapse prevention
- Intervention in early psychosis

(Continued)

(*Box 8.2   Continued*)

Family intervention

- The concept of expressed emotion in families and professionals who care for the SMI
- Families and SMI
- Families and the burden of caring
- Assessing the needs of families
- Giving information to the families of people with SMI
- Helping families to manage stress
- Goal setting with families
- Overcoming barriers to the implementation of PSI in services
- Keeping up the momentum and continuing to develop skills

of practice where the evidence base is thought to be most robust, for example family intervention. The author is not arguing here for the superiority of one course design over the other, however I am suggesting that prospective students should carefully examine the aims and objectives of the course and consider if they can be realistically achieved within the time that is available.

As a minimum the content of a PSI training course should provide trainees with information about the nature of schizophrenia and other psychotic disorders. It should also introduce trainees to information regarding factors that influence the onset, course and prognosis of SMI. Trainees should be made aware of the effects of stress on people suffering from SMI and consider how interventions aimed at reducing stress or enhancing abilities to manage stress may be beneficial to patients (see Chapter 1).

In addition to providing factual information, courses should encourage trainees to explore their own attitudes, values and behaviour towards the seriously mentally ill. This is of particular importance for clinicians working with patients who exhibit co-morbid states where personality disorders or substance abuse are present, in addition to the diagnosis of SMI (see Chapter 14). Courses should also contain an ethical component, which helps trainees to explore the issues related to working with this client group.

Methods of Teaching and Learning

Table 18.1 illustrates a variety of learning outcomes for PSI courses together with suitable approaches to teaching and learning that may be used to meet these outcomes. PSI courses should make use of traditional approaches to teaching and learning such as lectures and group exercises, however trainers

Table 18.1 Learning outcomes and related approaches to teaching and learning used on PSI courses

Learning outcome	Teaching and learning strategy
1. Acquisition of theoretical knowledge About SMI relevant to Practice with this client group	Lecture Discussion Use of case examples
2. Development of positive attitudes and an empathic understanding of the needs of people with SMI	Lecture Group discussion Role play Presentation by service users
3. Acquisition of skills in the appropriate and competent use of standardised assessments (e.g. symptoms, social functioning, medication side effects etc.) . . .	Lecture Role play Observation of an experienced interviewer Supervised clinical practice
4. Acquisition of clinical skills necessary for effective interventions with the SMI therapist and their families	Role play Observation of a skilled Supervised clinical practice
5. Ability to work as an effective member of a multidisciplinary team	Lecture Group exercises Seminar presentations

should also use more novel and innovative approaches to help facilitate the development of their trainees clinical skills.

In order to improve trainees clinical skills courses must incorporate experiential methods of teaching and learning such as role play exercises, where trainees have the opportunity to practice their skills while being coached by the course tutors. Again this places emphasis on the importance of the tutors themselves having a high level of clinical skill in order that they can be effective role models for trainees. However, clinical skills cannot be taught entirely in the classroom and in order to ensure that trainees can transfer these skills to their clinical practice, it is essential that they work with a small number of people with a diagnosis of SMI using PSI while they are training. Issues related to clinical supervision with this work is discussed later in this chapter. The trainees' clinical work should be assessed formally and they should be expected to reach a predetermined level of clinical competence in order to pass the course. Thus placing equal emphasis on the importance of clinical skills as well as academic abilities. Trainees who do not meet the level of skill required can be provided with extra support and supervision to help them to improve their skills.

For trainees who are learning new skills having to expose their practice to this level of scrutiny can be very stressful and initially many of them go through a stage of feeling de-skilled. However, it is the opinion of the author that working with patients and receiving supervision with this work while training is central to the process of developing of good clinical skills. Prospective students of PSI courses should inquire whether the course they are intending to train on requires them to work with patients while they are training and how the course will assess their development of skills.

Clinical Supervision

The PSI training courses reviewed earlier in this chapter all included clinical supervision as a key component in helping trainees to develop their clinical skills. It is important that potential students of PSI courses have some understanding of what to expect from clinical supervision sessions and how to get the most out of them.

Models of Clinical Supervision

Within the context of this chapter 'models of supervision' simply refers to the way in which clinical supervision is organised. Previous PSI courses have tended to provide weekly supervision to students at the course center in small groups of about five trainees to one supervisor. Supervisors are normally clinicians with advanced clinical skills and experience of working with seriously mentally ill people. While this model has been shown to be effective in terms of helping trainees to develop good clinical skills and carry out effective interventions with their patients it nevertheless has a number of limitations. First, supervision time needs to be divided between all group members and trainees only get limited time to present their patients. Second, supervisors often have limited opportunity to directly assess the trainee's clinical skills by listening to tape recordings of their work. Third, because the course tutors facilitate the sessions, trainees often experience difficulty in continuing to get supervision once they complete the training. It has been suggested that difficulty in accessing appropriate supervision may be associated with the poor implementation of PSI by trainees once they complete the training (Brennan and Gamble, 1997). An alternative model that has recently been piloted by the COPE Initiative at the University of Manchester has tried to overcome some of these difficulties, a description of the model of clinical supervision that has been developed will now be provided.

The COPE Initiative Model of Clinical Supervision

The COPE initiative is a major new PSI training programme in northwest England. The programme represents an evolution of the Thorn Diploma described earlier but with a particular focus on overcoming barriers to the implementation of PSI. COPE is developing a network of supervisors in services across the North-West to support trainees in continuing to use PSI once they complete training. The criterion for clinical supervisors is staff who have previously completed the Thorn Diploma or equivalent training. This is believed to be important in order to ensure that all supervisors have appropriate knowledge and skills in PSI. To ensure consistency in the way in which supervision is carried out all clinical supervisors receive training to prepare them for their role. The supervisors are introduced to the model of clinical supervision; they are trained to use a scale to assess trainee's skills (Haddock *et al.*, 2001) and to provide constructive feedback to trainees regarding their strengths and areas for development. The supervisors are also encouraged to explore and problem solve specific difficulties that can occur in supervision relationships.

Supervisors meet with the trainees every two weeks, normally there are two trainees to each supervisor. Sessions last 60–90 minutes and focus on the discussion of clinical issues, with trainees presenting details of the patients that they are working with followed by discussion and problem solving of any difficulties that they have encountered. Between sessions the supervisor listens to a tape of the trainee's clinical work and assesses their progress in the development of clinical skills, feedback on the tape is provided at the next session. The aim is for each trainee to get feedback on their clinical work at least once a month while they are training on the COPE course. Clinical supervisors and the course team meet monthly to review the progress of trainees and to identify any individuals who may need additional support. The advantages of this model are that trainees get more time to discuss their patients than in group supervision, they get regular feedback on their strengths and areas for development, the supervisor has the opportunity to continually monitor their progress and it is more likely that the trainee will be able to continue to get supervision once they complete the course. Initial evaluation of the model by Bradshaw (1999) has shown that it is effective in developing trainee's clinical skills.

Getting the Most out of Clinical Supervision

The aims of clinical supervision on PSI training courses are relatively straightforward and relate to the development of the clinical skill and competency of the trainee and ultimately their ability to provide effective help to their patients. Three issues have been listed below which relate to how trainees can get the most out of clinical supervision, each of these will be explored in more detail.

(1) The conditions that need to be present for the aims of supervision to be met.
(2) The responsibilities of the trainee.
(3) The responsibilities of the supervisor.

Conditions for Effective Supervision

In creating the conditions that are necessary for clinical supervision to be effectively conducted it is helpful if at the outset the trainee and their supervisor get together to discuss what the aims of the supervision are and how it is intended that these aims will be met. This information together with practical issues such as the frequency with which they will meet should be documented in the form of a supervision contract (Box 18.3). Such contracts can be helpful because they embrace the spirit of supervision as being a collaborative endeavour and they provide a clear baseline regarding what the relationship is about which can be reviewed at regular intervals to assess if supervision is meeting its stated aims.

There should be a commitment by both parties to make best use of the limited time available in supervision sessions. Sessions should have some structure and each meeting should start by setting an agenda of the main issues that need to be discussed, responsibility for managing time and keeping the session focused on the agreed agenda should be established. The respective responsibilities of the trainee and the supervisor to one another should be discussed and issues such as whose responsibility it is to make a new appointment if a session has to be cancelled should be agreed.

The content of clinical supervision should be agreed, when training in PSI this will normally focus on the trainee's clinical work with their patients. The

---

Box 18.3   Guidelines for developing a clinical supervision contract

1.	**Type of supervision**	How will supervision be carried out? What model of supervision will the group adopt? What will be the style of supervision? What is the purpose/aim of supervision?
2.	**Theoretical orientation**	Which theoretical model is it recognised that practitioners adopt in their clinical work?
3.	**Boundaries**	What will be the responsibilities of the supervisor and supervisee? What issues will be discussed?
4.	**Documentation**	How will records be maintained and by who?
5.	**Structure of session**	How will the session be organised and time managed?
6.	**Confidentiality**	How will issues relating to safe/professional practice be managed?
7.	**Evaluation**	When will supervision be evaluated and how will this be carried out?

aim of sessions should be to gain a better understanding of patients' problems, develop formulations to help conceptualise their current difficulties and identify suitable interventions that may help the trainee to work with their patients to overcome these difficulties. Sessions will often involve playing samples of audio-tapes to gain feedback on a particular intervention, role playing problem situations to help gain new insights into the patients current difficulties and exploring the application of interventions which may be helpful to the patient.

Responsibilities of Trainees in Supervision

In order to get the most out of supervision trainees need to be prepared to expose their practice to scrutiny by discussing their cases openly and honestly with their supervisor.

This can be anxiety provoking, particularly for experienced clinicians that are more accustomed to giving advice to others. However, if trainees are to get most out of supervision it is important that they are prepared to show the limitations of their knowledge of PSI by asking questions and openly discussing their feelings of being de-skilled when trying to learn and implement new approaches to intervention.

Trainees should prepare for supervision sessions by reviewing the cases that they are working with and considering what aspects of their patients' problems or their own practice they would like to explore with their supervisor. This preparation may include presenting an initial formulation of a patients problem which helps to explain its development and maintenance or playing a short section of audio tape in order to get feedback on the use of a particular skill or intervention. Trainees will get most out of supervision if for each item they include on the agenda they have a specific question to ask their supervisor, and co-trainee where appropriate, in relation to their clinical work that they wish advice or guidance with.

Trainees should take notes during supervision or even tape-record the sessions this will aid their recollection of the items that are discussed and help to ensure continuity in the themes that are discussed from one session to the next.

Responsibilities of the Supervisor

The supervisor has responsibility to ensure that the trainee is meeting the requirements of the training course in relation to the number of patients that they are working with and the nature of those patients' problems. They have responsibility to monitor the progress of the trainee's clinical work and to ensure that their interventions are appropriate for the needs of the patients that they work with. Feedback from supervisors should be provided in a sensitive and supportive way and it is important that supervisors recognise how stressful learning new approaches to clinical interventions can be. Equally important is that supervisors help trainees to set themselves specific, clearly defined and realistic targets in relation to particular aspects of their clinical work that they need to improve and that progress on these areas is regularly reviewed.

Example of Supervision in Practice

Brian had been qualified as a mental heath nurse for 12 years and had gained most of his experience working in acute in-patient settings. He was currently studying on a Diploma course in PSI and was receiving fortnightly clinical supervision from a graduate of the course who worked in his own service. During their first supervision session Brian and his supervisor drew up a contract for how supervision would be organised. They agreed that sessions would focus on the discussion of clinical issues and that at each meeting Brian would present a patient that he was working with and identify a problem that he wanted to discuss.

At the next session the agenda was set for Brian to present the case of a 22-year old man named Mark who was an in-patient following his third acute episode of psychotic illness. Brian had been working with Mark for several weeks, initially the work had concentrated on gaining his trust and assessing Mark's problems. Brian had just completed a KGV symptom assessment scale (Krawiecka *et al.*, 1977) with Mark, however he described feeling very uncomfortable with the interview and being concerned it had damaged his relationship with Mark. The main supervision question raised by Brian was to discuss issues related to the value of structured assessments such as the KGV.

Initially Brian's supervisor asked him to specify what concerns he had about the interview so that they could examine them more closely. Brian raised three specific concerns, first, that he had sounded hesitant and inarticulate when using the scale. Second, that the scale had not helped him to gain a better understanding of Marks problems and that he had only used it because of the requirements of the PSI training course. Third, that Mark had found the interview stressful and may have perceived the detailed questioning as intrusive. Having identified Brian's concerns the supervisor then suggested that they consider the validity of each in more detail. As an initial step it was decided that they would listen to the audio-tape of the session together and Brian would stop the tape and replay any examples of times when he had sounded hesitant and inarticulate. When Brian listened to the tape he found that although he had sounded a little anxious and had opened the session by almost apologising to Mark that he was 'going to ask him a lot of questions', he did not sound hesitant or inarticulate. In fact Brian was surprised by the clarity of the questions he had asked Mark. Brian's second area of concern was that the interview had not helped him to get a better understanding of Mark's problems. The supervisor encouraged Brian to describe everything that he had learned about Mark's symptoms from the assessment and which areas caused him most distress. Brian was able to comprehensively describe the exact nature of Mark's symptoms, their frequency, duration and severity and the degree of control Mark perceived he had over each one. Furthermore Brian had some additional information about why the symptoms were distressing and how they effected Mark's everyday life.

In concluding the supervision session Brian was asked to summarise what he thought had been most useful about the session and what he thought had been least useful. Brian said that he had enjoyed the session and now realised that although he had been anxious using the KGV assessment he had not come over as badly as he had originally thought, also he was surprised how much information he had gained using the scale. The thing he liked least about the session was having the supervisor listen to him on the tape and confessed that he had been anxious that the supervisor would criticise his skills. The supervisor thanked Brian for his honesty and asked if he still had any concerns remaining about using interviews such as the KGV symptom scale in the future. Brian replied that although he now recognised their usefulness he was still concerned about how Mark had experienced the interview. The supervisor asked if there was anyway Brian could evaluate this concern, Brian decided it would be useful to tell Mark of his concern and ask him whether he had found the interview stressful.

At the next supervision session the first agenda item set was to review Mark's feedback in relation to the KGV interview. Brian said that Mark had agreed that the interview had been stressful at times because he had found it hard to concentrate, however he also stated that it was the first time since he had been in hospital that anyone had shown real interest in finding out more about his problems and that he felt confident that Brian now understood him better and would be able to help him. Brian felt encouraged by Mark's comments and more confident about the usefulness of the interventions. His supervisor encouraged him to reflect on what had been the most useful aspect of the exercise from a learning perspective, after some discussion Brian concluded two main points. First, that just because doing something new feels uncomfortable it does not mean it is not useful or can not become easier with practice and, second, that in all aspects of clinical work it is worthwhile getting feedback from the patient on whether they are happy with the approaches that you are trying to use. Finally the supervisor added a note of caution that while the KGV had been shown to be a useful scale for assessing symptoms in Mark's case that there are some patients who may find the questioning intrusive and that the interviewer should be sensitive to this and be prepared to either use less structured means of assessment or simply concentrate on engagement in the early stages of working with the client.

Summary

The above example of clinical supervision has attempted to illustrate the model that we have been developing on our PSI training courses. The model focuses predominantly on the educational function of clinical supervision and on bridging the well documented gap between theory and practice. However, it also encompasses other functions of clinical supervision such as raising standards through the development of evidence based practice and supporting practitioners who are experiencing raised anxiety levels due to learning to use new clinical skills. While it is recognised that such a structured model of supervision would not be appropriate in every clinical environment it is suggested that this is a suitable model for practitioners who are learning to use evidence-based psychotherapeutic approaches to care.

Prospective students of PSI training courses should ask the course leaders about what arrangements are in place for clinical supervision. They should ask about the model of supervision that has been developed, what the criteria for supervisors is and how feedback and coaching regarding their clinical skills development will be provided.

Conclusion

PSI is a new and exciting development in the training of mental health workers who work with people who suffer from SMI. The concepts that are taught can normally be easily integrated into most professionals philosophical frameworks for conceptualising mental health and ill health. The interventions that are taught embrace the humanistic aspects of practice that are commonly introduced in the basic training of different mental health professionals. Additionally, they provide clinicians with a range of more structured interventions and approaches to therapy that research has demonstrated have the potential to reduce patients symptoms and improve their quality of life (Fadden, 1998; Haddock and Slade, 1996).

There is increasing evidence that this type of training is in demand from mental health professionals and in response to this demand many new training courses have been established. Practitioners who are fortunate enough to be able to attend a recognised PSI training programme will find it a rewarding and enriching experience and will enjoy increased job satisfaction by having more options to offer their patients. However, those eager to undertake training should consider the training that is on offer carefully and ask themselves whether it is really likely to lead to them developing enhanced clinical skill and becoming more effective in their interventions.

Further Reading

Haddock, G., Devane, S., Bradshaw, T., Tarrier, N., McGovern, J., Baguley, I. and Lancashire, S. (2001) An Investigation into the Psychometric Properties of the Cognitive Therapy Scale for Psychosis (CTS-Psy), *Behavioural and Cognitive Psychotherapy*, 29(2), 221–35.

Padesky, C. (1996) 'Developing Cognitive Therapist Competency: Teaching and Supervision Models, in P. Salkovskis (ed.), *Frontiers of Cognitive Therapy*, New York, Guildford Press.

References

Bradshaw, T. (1999) *An Investigation into the Effects of Structured Clinical Supervision on the Knowledge, Attitudes and Practice of Mental Health Nurses Undertaking Post Basic Training in Psychosocial Interventions*, unpublished MPhil thesis, University of Manchester.

Brennan, G. and Gamble, C. (1997) 'Schizophrenia family work and clinical practice', *Mental Health Nursing*, 17(4), 12–15.

Brooker, C. and Evans, J. (1998) *Charting the growth of psychosocial interventions training for mental health professionals in the United Kingdom*, The School of Nursing, Midwifery and Health Visiting. University of Manchester.

Brooker, C., Falloon, I., Butterworth. A., Goldberg, D., Graham-Hole, V. and Hillier, V. (1994) 'The Outcome of Training Community Psychiatric Nurses to Deliver Psychosocial Intervention', *British Journal of Psychiatry*, 165, 222–30.

Brooker, C., Tarrier, N., Barrowclough, C., Butterworth. A. and Goldberg, D. (1992) 'Training Community Psychiatric Nurses for Psychosocial Intervention: Report of a pilot study', *British Journal of Psychiatry*, 160, 836–44.

Department of Health (1994) *Working in Partnership: A collaborative approach to care*. Report of the Mental Health Nursing Review Team, London, HMSO.

Department of Health (1996) The Spectrum of Care: Local services for people with Mental Health Problems, London, HMSO.

Department of Health (1999) *The National Service Framework for Mental Health*, London, The Stationery office.

Fadden, G. (1998) 'Family Interventions', in C. Brooker and J. Repper (eds), *Serious Mental Health Problems in the Community: Policy, Practice and Research*, London, Bailliere Tindall.

Gamble, C. (1995) 'The Thorn Nurse Training Initiative', *Nursing Standard*, 9(15), 31–4.

Gamble, C., Midence, K. and Leff, J. (1994) 'The effects of family work training on mental health nurses' attitude to and knowledge of schizophrenia: a replication', *Journal of Advanced Nursing*, 19, 893–6.

Haddock, G., Devane, S., Bradshaw, T., Tarrier, N., McGovern, J., Baguley, I. and Lancashire, S. (2001) 'An Investigation into the Psychometric Properties of the Cognitive Therapy Scale for Psychosis (CTS-Psy)', *Behavioural and Cognitive Psychotherapy*, 29(2), 221–35.

Haddock, G. and Slade P.D. (1996) *Cognitive-Behavioural Interventions with Psychotic Disorders*, London, Routledge.

Lam, D.H., Kuipers, L. and Leff, J.P. (1993) 'Family work with patients suffering from schizophrenia: the impact of training on psychiatric nurses' attitude and knowledge', *Journal of Advanced Nursing*, 18(2), 233–7.

Lancashire, S., Haddock, G., Tarrier, N., Baguley, I., Butterworth, A., and Brooker, C. (1997a) 'Effects of training in psychosocial interventions for community psychiatric nurses in England', *Psychiatric Services*, 48(1), 39–42.

Lancashire, S., Haddock, G., Tarrier, N., Butterworth, A. and Baguley, I. (1997b) 'Training Community Psychiatric Nurses in Psychosocial Interventions in SMI: The Thorn Nurse Initiative', *The Clinician*, 12, 45–8.

Leff, J., Kuipers, L., Berkowitz, R., Eberlein-Vries, R. and Sturgeon, D. (1982) 'A controlled trial of social intervention in the families of schizophrenic patients', *British Journal of Psychiatry*, 141, 121–34.

Leff, J., Kuipers, L., Berkowitz, R. and Sturgeon, D. (1985) 'A controlled trial of social intervention in the families of schizophrenic patients: Two year follow-up', *British Journal of Psychiatry*, 146, 549–600.

Leff, J., Berkowitz, R., Shavit, N., Strachan, A., Glass, I. and Vaughn, C. (1989) 'A trial of family therapy v. a relatives group for schizophrenia', *British Journal of Psychiatry*, 154, 58–66.

Leff, J., Berkowitz, R., Shavit, N., Strachan, A., Glass, I. and Vaughn, C. (1990) 'A trial of family therapy v. a relatives group for schizophrenia: Two-year follow-up' *British Journal of Psychiatry*, 157, 571–7.

Krawiecka, M., Goldberg, D.P. and Vaughan, M. (1977) 'A standardised psychiatric assessment scale for rating chronic psychotic patients' *Acta Psychiatrica Scandinavica*, 55, 299–308.

Onyett, S., Pillinger, T. and Muijen, M. (1995) *Making Community Mental Health Teams Work*, London, The Sainsbury Centre.

Tarrier, N., Barrowclough, C. and D'Ambrosio, P. (1988a) 'A training programme in psychosocial intervention with families with a schizophrenia member', *Behavioural Psychotherapist*, 27, 2–4.

Tarrier, N., Barrowclough, C., Vaughn, C., Bamrah, J.S., Porceddu, K., Watts, S. and Freeman, H. (1988b) 'The community management of schizophrenia: A controlled trial of a behavioural intervention with families to reduce relapse', *British Journal of Psychiatry*, 153, 532–42.

Tarrier, N., Barrowclough, C., Vaughn, C., Bamrah, J.S., Porceddu, K., Watts, S. and Freeman, H. (1989) 'The community management of schizophrenia: A Two year follow-up of a behavioural intervention with families', *British Journal of Psychiatry*, 154, 625–8.

Conclusion

Over the past fifty years substantial developments have been made in the understanding and treatment of schizophrenia and other psychotic disorders. We have moved from a solely disease orientated biological model to a new conceptualisation known as stress-vulnerability which acknowledges the role of environmental and psychological factors in relation to the course and outcome of psychosis. This model has led to the development of a range of innovative evidence based psychosocial interventions all of which reinforce the need for professionals to form collaborative working alliances with service users and their families.

In the chapters of this book we have reviewed some of the most recent innovations in psychosocial interventions for people who suffer from psychosis. We have considered approaches for helping individuals to cope with the considerable demands of community living, for helping them to manage distressing symptoms, for working in partnership with friends and relatives and for improving the routine management of neuroleptic medication. Throughout the book the authors made reference to the research evidence that supports the effectiveness of these approaches.

Over the past decade there have been many references to the value of psychosocial interventions in government policy documents the most recent and most significant of these being the *National Service Framework for Mental Health*, published by the Department of Health in 1999. Groups representing service users have also been vociferous in their calls for alternative and complimentary treatments to medication.

However, despite the research evidence for the effectiveness of PSI, user groups expressions of approval for the interventions and government calls to implement these approaches with the SMI the evidence suggests that PSIs are only rarely practised in routine NHS settings. The reason for this slow transfer of the interventions from research to routine practice are at present unclear but the research that has been conducted suggests the explanation is likely to be complex and multifaceted. In concluding this final chapter we would like to express our sincere hope that this book may contribute to raising the profile of PSI and may result in an increase of the use of these valuable interventions by workers who practice in routine service settings.

Index

Abnormal Involuntary Movement Scale
    78
accessibility to services   48–9, 241
action plans on relapse prevention   74,
    133, 135–6
activity scheduling   90–2, 125–6
adherence   76–7, 79–80
advocacy   241–2
aetiological models   191
agranulocytosis (side-effect)   73
agricultural employment   162
akathisia (side-effect)   71
Alleged Lunatics' Friend Society   239,
    241
alogia   118, 121
altruism   247–8
Anderson, C.   168
anergia   118
anhedonia   118, 119, 121
anticholinergic medication   72, 74
antipsychotic drugs   30, 31, 68–81,
    102
anxiety   78, 84–100
assertive community treatment model
    56–7
assertive outreach   59–60
assessment   78, 102–15
    by case managers   60–1
    in cognitive behavioural therapy
        88–9
    in dual diagnosis   189, 195, 198
    of family   147–8, 149–50
    of insight   212
    of negative symptoms   119–21
    of patient   148–9
    of resources   120
    of risk   217
    scales of see scales of assessment

structured   228
    see also interviews
asylums see institutions
atypical neuroleptics   69
autonomic effects (side-effect)   72
autonomic hyperreactivity   13

Baker, Paul   19, 21, 22
Ball, R. et al.   223
Barker, I.   238
Barrett, Syd   20
Barrowclough, C.   145, 151, 154
Bartels, J. et al.   209
baseline score, relapse   134
Beck, A.   102
Beck, A.T.   84, 85
Beck, A.T. et al.   110
behaviour   85, 144, 208–9
    see also cognitive behavioural therapy
behavioural experiments   95–7, 111
Bentall, R.P.   15, 112
benztropine   74
bi-carmeral mind   18, 19
bi-directional model, in dual diagnosis
    191
biochemical disturbance   10
Birchwood, M. et al.   42, 131, 132,
    134
bisexuals   20
Blake, William   20
Bleuler, Eugene   6, 7
Bowl, R.   238
Boyle, Mary   7, 9
Brenner, M.H.   161
British County Asylums Act (1808)
    28
British Networks for Alternatives to
    Psychiatry   239

Brockington, I.F. *et al.* 9
brokerage model of service delivery 54, 55
Brooker, C. 252
Brown, G. 163
Bulwer-Lytton, Rosina 239

Calgery Depression Scale 78
Camberwell Family Interview 222
Campaign Against Psychiatric Oppression 239
campaign groups 239
Campbell, P. 40, 47
carbamazepine 74
care in the community 27, 31, 176–7, 184
care programme approach 54, 61
carers 11, 33, 133, 178, 240
Carey, John 19
case examples, illustrations and vignettes *see* case studies
case management 53–64
case manager roles 60–2, 68
case studies
   case management (Martin) 59
   clinical skills in dual diagnosis (Christine) 195–201
   communication training (Alan) 153–4
   community networking 179–80
   educational role (Alan) 150–1
   engagement in family intervention 146–7
   negative symptoms (Tom) 126–8
   neuroleptic drugs (Fred) 75–6
   organic training 231–2
   panic attacks (John) 97–9
   patient and family assessment (Alan) 149–50
   problem-solving (Alan) 153
   relapse 132
   relapse prevention (Sarah) 137–9, 140, 141
   risk (Bill) 214–16
   supervision in practice 262–3
CBT *see* cognitive behavioural therapy
Chadwick, P. *et al.* 42
Challis, D.J. 60
Chamberlin, J. 238, 240

checklist of potential service developments 34
chlorpromazine 70
choice 241, 245, 246
Churchill, Sir Winston 20
citizen advocacy 241
clinical case management model, of service delivery 55–6
clinical practice model 210
clinical psychologists 31
clinical skills, acquirement of 257, 258–63
clinical supervision, in training courses 258–63
closed questions 123–4
clozapine 70, 73
co-morbidity 190
co-therapists 145
cogentin 74
cognitive behavioural therapy 42–3, 84–7, 104–5, 210
   assessment 88–9
   interventions 41, 90, 106–14, 154–5
   in risk 210
   see also behaviour; therapies
cognitive triad 85
Coleman, Ron 22
collective ward stress 230
common factor models, in dual diagnosis 191
communication 105, 153–4
community care 27, 31, 176–7, 184
community, defined 177–8
Community Mental Health Centre Construction Act (1963; USA) 53
community networking 179–80, 184–5
community psychiatric nurses *see* nurses
community teams 56–7
compulsory treatment 11, 243
Congress of Mental Medicine (1885) 8
Conlan, Edna 240
consent 79, 80
contemporary policy development 27, 31–4
continuous low dosage strategy 74
conventional antipsychotics 69
COPE Initiative Model of Clinical Supervision 258–9

coping topics   14, 97, 107–8, 109, 144
Core Arts organisation   23
core beliefs, working with   113–14
core competencies of mental health
    workers   44
Corrigan, P.   230
cost of treatment   63, 69
counselling   39, 246
courses, training   252, 254–256
Coursey, R.D.   246
crime statistics   208, 209
critical incident replay   89
CUES (Carers' and Users' Expectation
    of Services)   240

danger level signs of relapse   135
dangerousness   205–7
Davies, B.P.   60
Davies, Hywel   10
decision-making   238
Deegan, P.   40
Delphi Opinion Survey   197
delusions   6, 108–12, 118, 209
dementia praecox   4, 5, 6
depression   78, 84–100
developing countries   162
development-acquisition model   57
diagnosis of schizophrenia   7, 8–9
diaries   89, 90, 93, 94, 112
    for relapse   136, 141
direct work with the client   61–2
disease model of schizophrenia   4
disengagement   154–5
disorganisation in negative symptoms
    118
distraction techniques   112
dopamine   69
dopamine receptors   69, 117–18
drapetomania   20
drug dosage, adjusting   77–8
Drury, V.   222
dual diagnosis
    aetiological models   191
    assessment   189, 195, 198
    definitions   190
    interventions   194–5
    treatment   192, 193–4
dysaesthesia aethiopica   20
Dysfunctional Attitude Scale   114

dysphoria (side-effect)   72, 135
dystonia (side-effect)   71

early psychotic experience   135
Early Signs Scale, for relapse   131, 132,
    135
early warning signs of relapse   79, 133,
    134–5, 214
education   124, 150–1, 211–14, 229
effective working relationships, principles
    of   45–8
electroconvulsive therapy   30
Ellis, A.   84
Emery, G.   84
emotional blunting   118, 119
employment   161–71, 242
    work models   167–9
empowerment/power   29–31, 240,
    243, 247
engagement   58–9, 87, 103, 114,
    182
    failure of   155
    in family intervention   146–7, 228
environmental protectors   14
environmental stressors   13, 168, 191
Epidemiologic Catchment Area Study
    (USA)   190
epilepsy   20
equal opportunities   242, 243
Escher, S.   10, 21
ESS *see* Early Signs Scale, for relapse
Estroff, S.   43
evaluation   62, 184–5, 240
Evans, J.   162
expressed emotion   144, 222–5
extra-pyramidal side-effects   69, 70,
    71–2

Fadden, G.   145, 225
Falloon, I.R.H. *et al.*   153, 155
families   11, 30, 143–56, 228
    and expressed emotion   224–5
    family intervention   30, 47, 143,
        146–7, 228
    and negative symptoms   117
    and PSI training programmes   252
    in risk   207–8, 216–17
Fisher, N.R.   238
Five Minute Speech Sample   223

five-factor model (Padesky and Greenberger) 135, 136
focusing therapy 112–13, 210
formulation 89–90, 106
Foucault, M. 28
Fowler, D. *et al.* 42, 114
Frame, Janet 20

Gandhi, Mahatma 20
General Medical Bill (1856) 30
genetic predisposition 12
Glasgow Media Group 206
goals 89, 124–6, 147, 152, 229
Goering, P.N. 41
good practice principles 77–80
government policies 167, 177, 185, 237, 267
Green, Peter 20
Greenberg, L. *et al.* 212
Greenberger, D. 135
Griffiths, R.D. 164
group psychosocial interventions 229
guided discovery 93, 97, 105, 108
guidelines, practice 103–6

Haddock, G. 112
Hage, Patsy 21, 22
hallucinations 6, 10, 70, 112–13, 118, 209
haloperidol 70
Hawton, K. *et al.* 88
Health of the Nation White Paper (1992) 31–32
hearing voices 10, 18–24, 111–12, 209
Hearing Voices Network 22, 242
heart disease 11
Helfgott, David 20
helping relationship 39–50
Herz, M. 131
Herz, M. *et al.* 132
high expressed emotion behaviour 144
Hogarty, G. *et al.* 48
Homer 19
homework 104, 107, 112, 126
homicide 22, 23, 205
homosexuals 20
Honig, A. 209
Hooper, R. 169

Hopkins, Sir Anthony 20
Hospital Anxiety and Depression Scale 78
hot and cold bath therapy 68
houses of correction *see* institutions
humouring 246
Huxley, P. 63

identification, in family intervention 146
in-patient environments 226–30
in-patient services, critique of 225–6
incompetence, user labels of 243–4
Individual Placement Support 166, 167
individual psychosocial interventions 229
informal assessment 78
information 150–1, 241, 245, 246
informed choice 245
informed consent 79, 80
insight 211–14, 244
institutionalisation 31, 121
institutions 221–33
    asylums 28–9, 30, 31, 53
    houses of correction 27
    long stay 176–7
    madhouses 28
    workhouses 28, 177
insulin-coma therapy 68
integrated treatment, in dual diagnosis 193–4
intensive case management model 57
interaction, style of 123–4
Interactive Staff Training Model 230
intermittent or targeted treatment 74
International Congress of Mental Science (1889) 8
international research 162–7
interpersonal skills 44–5, 228
interventions 209–211, 221–233
    cognitive behavioural therapy 41, 90, 106–114, 154–155
    dual diagnosis 194–5
    family intervention 30, 47, 143, 146–7, 228
interviews 107, 148, 195, 198, 201, 222
IPS *see* Individual Placement Support

Jaynes, J.   19, 21, 23
Johnson, B.   47
Joyce, G.C.   19
Jung, Carl Gustav   20
Juninger, J.   209

Kavanagh, D.   224
kemadrin   74
key area handbooks   32
key workers   53, 54
Kingdon, D.G.   10
Kraepelin, Emil   4, 5, 6, 7, 30
Kuipers, E.   223

labels of schizophrenia   3–4, 30
Langlands, Alan   238
Leader, Alan   239
Leff, Julian   252
lesbians   20
limbic system   69, 70
Lindqvist, P.   217
Link, B.   209
lithium   74
local advice services   178
local communities, working with
    180–1
long-term support   176–7
Luckstead, A.   246

McCandless-Glincher, L. *et al.*   131
McCann, G.   207
McCracken, S.   230
McGurrin, M.C.   162
madhouses *see* institutions
maintaining behaviours   85
management   29, 53–64, 147, 151–5,
    218
    of neuroleptic drugs   68–81
marginalisation of user views   246
Marshall, M.   64
measuring instruments for relapse   131
media   205, 206, 207, 225
medical power   29–31
medication   11, 14, 80–1
    anticholinergic   72, 74
    neuroleptic   30, 31, 68–81, 102
Melville, C.   131
Mental Health Act (1959)   31
Mental Health Foundation   24

mental health nurses *see* nurses
mental health professionals
    core competencies   44
    role   60–2, 68, 181–2, 195, 244
    training   253, 264
    and user involvement   247
mental health services   12, 23, 178,
    193, 241–3
Mental Health Task Force, Department
    of Health   239
mental health workers *see* mental health
    professionals
Mental Patients Union, UK   239
mesocortical pathways   69
mesolimbic pathways   69, 70
meta-analysis   62, 161
Milton, John   19
models   244
    aetiological   191
    of case management   55–8
    of clinical practice   210
    of clinical supervision   258
    disease model of schizophrenia   4
    five-factor model (Padesky and
        Greenberger)   135, 136
    social disability model   169
    stress-vulnerability models   5, 12–15,
        167–9, 210, 267
    transactional model of stress   151
monitoring systems   133, 136, 240
Moore, E.   223
Moore, E. *et al.*   222
moral management epoch   29
Morgan, S.   54
mortality rates   206
motivation   194–5, 201
Mueser, K. *et al.*   62, 131

Nash, John, Jr.   20
*National Service Framework for Mental
    Health*   32–4, 239, 267
negative automatic thought   85, 92–5,
    97
negative symptoms
    assessment of   119–21
    consequences of   121–2
    identifying   117–19
    misinterpretation of   121
    treatment for   122–6

neighbourhood networking   175–86
nervous system   69–70
neuroleptic malignant syndrome (side-effect)   72–3
neuroleptic medication   30, 31, 68–81, 102
neuroleptic-induced deficit syndrome (side-effect)   73, 121
neuroleptic-induced pseudo-parkinsonism   121
neurons   69
neurotransmitters   69, 70
'normal' population, schizophrenic symptoms in   9–10
normalising rationales   105
Nuechterlein, K.H.   14, 131
nurses   11, 31
    interpersonal skills   44–5, 228
    role in dual diagnosis   195
    training   61, 224–5, 252

occupation *see* employment
offending behaviour   208–9
Ogden, John   20
olanzapine   70
Onyett, S.   54
Onyett, S. *et al.*   238
open questions   123–4
opportunities, in neighbourhood networking   183–4
organic training   230–1

Padesky, C.A.   135
panic   87
parallel services   193
patient assessment   148–9
Peck, E.   238
peer advocacy   241, 242
Perkins, R.E.   238
Perry, A.   132
personal protectors   13–14
personal strengths model, of service delivery   57
personal therapy   48
pharmacokinetics   70
physical health checks   78–9
Pilgrim, D.   44, 47
Pinel, P.   28, 29
planning, by case managers   61

policy developments   27–34
    government policies   167, 177, 185, 237, 267
    political economy   29
politics and policies of schizophrenia   26–35
poly-pharmacy   73–4
Poor Law Commission   29
positive symptoms   117
post-traumatic stress disorder   11
poverty, economic   11, 32
poverty of speech   118
power/empowerment   29–31, 240, 243, 247
practice guidelines   103–6
pre-contemplative state, in dual diagnosis   195
Primary Care Groups   186
primary negative symptoms   118, 119
problem-solving   14, 147, 152–3, 210, 229
procyclidine   74
prodromal period   130, 131
professional advocacy   241
professional models   244
protocol, of family interventions   143, 145–6
pseudo-parkinsonism (side-effect)   71
PSI *see* psychosocial interventions
psychiatric nurses *see* nurses
psychiatry, history of   28, 29
psychodynamic psychotherapy   40
psychoeducation   211–14, 229
psychological treatment for anxiety and depression   84–100
psychomotor poverty   118
psychosocial interventions   41, 47, 80–1, 221–33, 251–3
    family   143, 144
    in in-patient environments   226–30
    and medication   80–1
psychosocial stressors   30, 168
psychotherapeutic approaches   39, 40
Psychotic Antecedent and Coping Interview   107

questions, open and closed   123–4

rating scales   78, 189
Read, J.   241

reality distortion   118
receptors   69, 117–18
record-keeping   78
rehabilitation   58, 164, 165
relapse   45, 74, 130, 136, 141
   case studies   132, 137–9, 140, 141
   danger level signs of   135
   early warning signs of   79, 133,
      134–5, 214
   percentages of   68, 102, 130, 131
   prevention action plans   74, 133,
      135–6
relapse prevention manual   136–7
relatives *see* families
Relatives Assessment Interview   148
Repper, J.   47, 162
Repper, J. *et al.*   45, 47
research   103, 143, 162–7, 240
residents' associations   178
resources   13, 120, 246
respect   243
review, by case managers   62
revolving chair therapy   68
Ridgeway, P.   243
risk   205–18
risperidone   70
Robinson, Crabb   20
Robinson, D. *et al.*   130
Rogers, A.   44, 47
Rogers, C. *et al.*   40
role awareness, mental health workers
      60–2, 68, 181–2, 195, 244
Romme, M.   10, 21, 22

safety behaviours   85
Sayce, L.   241
scales of assessment   78, 114, 119–20,
      148–9, 189
   Early Signs Scale   131, 132, 135
Scheid, T.L.   168
schema based interventions   113–14
Schingler, Aidan   22
schizophrenia concept
   contemporary view of   11–15
   diagnosis   7, 8–9
   disease model of   4
   and employment   161–71
   history of   5–8
   labels of   3–4, 30

politics and policies of   26–35
   treatments   84–100
Schneider, K.   7
Scull, A.   28
secondary negative symptoms   118
secondary persistent psychiatric illness
      model, in dual diagnosis   191
secondary substance misuse model, in
      dual diagnosis   191
Sedgewick, P.   29
self-advocacy   241, 242
self-help   242
self-injury   206
self-neglect   206
self-organisation   242
sequential service delivery, in dual
      diagnosis   193
serotonin   69, 70
service delivery   54–8, 193
service gap syndrome, in dual diagnosis
      190
service user movements   239
services
   accessibility to   48–9, 241
   checklist of potential developments
      34
   critique of in-patient   225–6
   local advice   178
   mental health   12, 23, 178, 193,
      241–3
   parallel   193
   providing integrated treatment
      193–4
   for substance misuse   193
sessions, structure of   104, 122–3, 147
sexual dysfunction   11
sexual side-effects   72
Shepherd, G. *et al.*   43
side-effects   11, 30, 69, 70–3, 121, 135
Skipworth, J.   217
Slade, P.D.   112
sleep deprivation   10
Smith, Mike   22
Snyder, K. *et al.*   223
social disability and access model of
      work   169
social exclusion   11, 185
Social Functioning Scale   120
social psychiatry movement   29

social stressors 30
Socratic dialogue 93, 97, 105, 108
Sound Minds organisation 23
staff 206, 222–5, 227, 230, 240
  see also nurses
stakeholders, input from 253
standardised assessment 78
stereotypes 22, 205, 206
Steuve, A. 209
Strauss, J.S. 43
stress 10, 11, 12, 168, 230
  management 147, 151–5
stress-vulnerability models 5, 12–15,
  167–9, 210, 267
stressors 13, 30, 168, 191
structured assessments 228
structured interviews 107
Stylianos, S.K. 41
Subotnik, K.L. 131
substance misuse 189–202
suicide 11, 23, 206
supervision contract 260, 262–3
supervisor responsibilities 261–2
support, effective 42–3
supported accommodation 177
supported employment 165, 166
Survivor's Poetry organisation 23
Swanson, J. 209
synaptic gap 69
syndrome, defined 5

talking therapy 40, 44, 102
tardive dyskinesia (side-effect) 31,
  71–2
targets for mental illness treatment
  31–2
Tarrier, N. 132, 145, 151, 154, 222,
  252
Tarrier, N. *et al.* 43, 252
task assignments 126
teaching methods *see* training
team working 56–7, 63–4
tenant organisations 178
theories, professional *see* models
therapies 48–9, 68, 112–13, 162, 210
  talking therapy 40, 44, 102
  see also cognitive behavioural therapy;
    treatment
Thorn Initiative 61, 252, 253

thought disorder 6, 113, 118, 209
thought transference 10
threat/control override symptoms 209
Tien, A.Y. 21
training 61, 227, 230, 240, 251–64
  in assessment procedure 78
  in communication skills 153–4
  nurses 61, 224–5, 252
  organic 230–1
  in risk management 218
  staff 227, 230, 240
transactional model of stress 151
treatment
  for anxiety and depression 84–100
  compulsory 11, 243
  costs 63, 69
  in dual diagnosis 192, 193–4
  ECT 30
  for negative symptoms 122–6
  strategies 73–5
  targets for 31–2
  voluntary 31
  see also cognitive behavioural therapy;
    therapies
Tuke, William 28, 29
Turkington, D. 4, 10

UK Advocacy Network 242
unemployment 168
United States 164
users 237, 241–5
  marginalisation of users' views 246
  user involvement 238–40, 247
  user needs 43–5

verbal persuasion 246
victim blaming 247
vocation *see* employment
voice hearing 10, 18–24, 111–12, 209
voluntary organisations 175, 193
voluntary treatment 31

Walsch, Neale Donald 22
Wannamaker, Zoë 20
ward culture 230
Warner, P. 161
Warner, R. 29
warning level signs of relapse *see* relapse
Watkins, John 22

weight gain   11, 72
Weldon, Georgina   239
Wessely, S.   208
Wilson, Brian   20
Wing, J.K.   163

work *see* employment
workhouses *see* institutions
working relationships, principles of
        45–8
World Health Organization   211